# DOCTORS, POLITICS AND SOCIETY: HISTORICAL ESSAYS

# THE WELLCOME INSTITUTE SERIES IN THE HISTORY OF MEDICINE

**Forthcoming Titles**

Doctors and Ethics: The Earlier Historical Setting of Professional Ethics
*Edited by Andrew Wear, Johanna Geyer Kordesch and Roger French*

The History of Health and the Modern State
*Edited by Dorothy Porter*

French Medical Culture in the Nineteenth Century
*Edited by A. La Berge and M. Feingold*

The History of Medical Education in Britain
*Edited by V. Nutton and Roy Porter*

Medicine in the Enlightenment
*Edited by Roy Porter*

Academic inquiries regarding the series should be addressed to the editors W. F. Bynum and Roy Porter at the Wellcome Institute for the History of Medicine, 183 Euston Road, London NW1 2BE, UK

# DOCTORS, POLITICS AND SOCIETY:
# HISTORICAL ESSAYS

*Edited by*
*Dorothy Porter and Roy Porter*

Rodopi

Amsterdam – Atlanta GA 1993

First published in 1993
by Editions Rodopi B. V., Amsterdam – Atlanta, G A 1993.



Design and Typesetting Christine Lavery, the Wellcome Trust
Printed and bound in the Netherlands by Editions Rodopi B. V.,
Amsterdam – Atlanta, G A 1993.



**British Library Cataloguing in Publication Data**
A catalogue record for this book is available from the British Library
ISBN 90-5183-510-8

**CIP-GEGEVENS KONINKLIJKE BIBLIOTHEEK, DEN HAAG**

Doctors

Doctors, politics and society : historical essays / ed. by
Dorothy Porter and Roy Porter. — Amsterdam - Atlanta, GA 1993 :
Rodopi. — Ill. — (Clio Medica 23 / The Wellcome Institute series
in the history of medicine)
Met index, lit. opg.
ISBN 90-5183-510-8 geb.
Trefw.: geneeskunde ; geschiedenis / gezondheidszorg ;
overheidsbeleid ; geschiedenis


Printed in The Netherlands

# Contents

# Acknowledgements

What could be more important nowadays than the politics of medicine? Yet, in the view of the contributors to this volume, the political involvements of doctors have never received from medical historians the attention they deserve. Consciously and unconsciously, political matters have been erased from the received histories of medicine, toned down or slanted. The aim of this volume is to put the politics back, where it belongs, in the history of medicine.

The volume has arisen out of a one-day symposium held at the Wellcome Institute for the History of Medicine in September 1991. Bernard Brais, Elizabeth Fee, Frank Honigsbaum, Dorothy Porter, Charles Webster and Paul Weindling gave papers at that conference, revised versions of which are published here. Our thanks to all of those. We have been further fortunate in securing papers for this volume from John Eyler, Anne Hardy, Edward T. Morman, Janet Semple, Susan Gross Solomon and Robert K. Webb. Our particular gratitude goes out to these authors for agreeing to board our ship, and proving such co-operative and punctual travellers.

We would also like to thank Frieda Houser of the Wellcome Institute for her invaluable administrative aid for the conference and the volume; Caroline Prentice for her superb research assistance; and Dr Kim Cross, Christine Lavery, and their colleagues, at the Wellcome Trust for the expertise and efficiency of their technical aid in preparing this work for the press.

As this book goes to press we have heard of the sad death of Janet Semple and would like to dedicate this book to her memory.

# Notes on Contributors

**Bernard Brais** acquired his medical and neurological training at McGill University in Montreal, Canada. From 1986 to 1988 he was a Hannah Institute for the History of Medicine postgraduate fellow at the Wellcome Institute. He completed an M.Phil. thesis at University College London on Jean-Martin Charcot and his neurological school. He is presently a postgraduate fellow in neurogenetics at McGill University.

**John M. Eyler** is a member of the Department of History of Medicine at the University of Minnesota. His interests include the history of public health, epidemiology, and health policy. He is the author of *Victorian Social Medicine: The Ideas and Methods of William Farr.* He has recently completed a book manuscript on the career of Sir Arthur Newsholme.

**Elizabeth Fee** is Professor of History and Health Policy at the Johns Hopkins University School of Hygiene and Public Health, and holds a joint appointment in the Institute of the History of Medicine at Johns Hopkins. She is the author of *Disease and Discovery* (Johns Hopkins University Press, 1987), and co-editor of *AIDS: The Burdens of History* (University of California Press, 1988), *The Baltimore Book: New Views of Local History* (Temple University Press, 1991), *A History of Education in Public Health* (Oxford University Press, 1991), and *AIDS: The Making of a Chronic Disease* (University of California Press, 1992). She is author of numerous articles on the history of medicine and public health and editor of the historical section of the *American Journal of Public Health.*

**Anne Hardy** read history at Oxford, where she obtained her doctorate in 1981. She subsequently held research fellowships at Nuffield College and the Wellcome Institute. She has published several articles on disease and public health in the eighteenth and nineteenth centuries, and is the author of *The Epidemic Streets: Infectious Disease and the Rise of Preventive Medicine in London 1855–1990* which will be published by Oxford University Press in 1993. She is currently a lecturer at the Wellcome Institute for the History of Medicine.

**Frank Honigsbaum** has written extensively on the history and operation of the National Health Service, including a definitive study of how the NHS was created. His most recent work deals with Oregon's controversial health rationing plan and its implications for Britain.

**Edward T. Morman** is Lecturer in the History of Science, Medicine, and Technology, and Curator of the Historical Collection of the Institute of the History of Medicine, at the Johns Hopkins University. He has published articles on the history of hospitals and of public health, and is currently developing undergraduate and medical school courses on race, science and medicine. He serves as bibliographer for the Sigerist Circle, and prepared the bibliography for *Women, Health and Medicine in America* (Garland, 1990).

**Janet Semple** studied History at Oxford University and subsequently worked at the London County Council, Nuffield College and the J. Walter Thompson Company. She has also taught, worked for publishers and marked examination papers. In 1984 she obtained a MSc in Government at the London School of Economics and went on to write a Ph.D. thesis on Jeremy Bentham's panopticon prison. This is being published by the Oxford University Press under the title of *Bentham's Prison.* She has also contributed articles to newspapers and journals. She now works at the Bentham Project at University College London.

**Susan Gross Solomon** is Professor of Political Science at the University of Toronto. She is the author of *The Soviet Agrarian Debate: Controversy in Social Science, 1923–1929* and co-editor of *The Social Context of Soviet Science and Health and Society in Revolutionary Russia.* She is currently writing a history of Soviet social hygiene in the inter war period, with special emphasis on Soviet-German medical relations.

**R. K. Webb** is Professor of History, Emeritus, at the University of Maryland, Baltimore County. He formerly served as professor of history at Columbia University from 1953 to 1970 and as editor of the *American Historical Review* from 1968 to 1975. He has held two Guggenheim fellowships, two major grants from the National Endowment for the Humanities, and a fellowship from the American Council of Learned Societies and has been a visiting fellow at the Victorian Studies Centre, University of Leicester; the Institute for Advanced Study; the Research School of Social Sciences at the Australian National University; the Center for the History of

Freedom at Washington University, St. Louis; and at St. Catherine's College, Oxford. His publications include *The British Working-Class Reader, 1790–1848: Literacy and Social Tension* (1955); *Harriet Martineau, a Radical Victorian* (1960); *Modern England from the Eighteenth Century to the Present* (1968, 1990); and (with Peter Gay) *Modern Europe* (1973). His current field of research is the history of English Unitarianism, on which he has published a number of articles and chapters.

**Charles Webster** has worked in Oxford since 1969. He is currently a fellow of All Souls College. His main activities relate to medicine and science in early modern Europe and health care and welfare in the twentieth century.

**Paul Weindling** is Senior Research Officer at the Wellcome Unit for the History of Medicine, University of Oxford. He is the author of *Health, Race and German Politics between National Unification and Nazism, 1870–1945* (Cambridge, 1989), and *Darwinism and Social Darwinism in Imperial Germany: the Contribution of the Cell Biologist Oscar Hertwig (1849–1922)* (Stuttgart, 1991). He co-edited *Information Sources for the History of Science and Medicine* (London: 1983), and is co-editor of *Social History of Medicine.*

# Introduction

That colossus amongst British reformers, Jeremy Bentham, argued that 'the art of legislation is but the art of healing practised upon a large scale'; his plans for building a better society involved the establishment of a ministry of health.[1] Bentham's perception of the parallel of medicine and politics, and his agenda for administrative action neatly encapsulate the concerns and scope of this volume. Covering the period from the French Revolutionary era to the present, and dealing with Germany, France, the USA and Soviet Russia as well as Britain, it comprises a series of essays that examine the interfaces between medicine and politics, focusing primarily upon the philosophies and plans of medical reformers themselves, sometimes wearing their medical, and sometimes their political, hats.

Analogies between the body natural and the body politic have been drawn since antiquity. People have spoken, for example, in interchangeable terms of the 'constitution', healthy or unhealthy, of individuals or states; or of the relations between the head and its members. Comparisons between the doctor and the statesman have likewise been commonplace, as part of the self-promotion of the professions but also within everyday parlance.[2] Top politicians have liked to represent themselves as physicians to society, expert and paternalist, diagnosing social disorders, setting the nation upon salubrious regimes or, occasionally, giving it a stiff dose of necessary medicine; 'it's not working if it's not hurting', became the inevitable catchphrase in the early 1990s of Conservative ministers glossing their attempts to deal with economic recession. And the politicians' pretensions have been the butt of satirists. Ever since Gillray, leading cartoonists have revelled in portraying society as a sick man being fought over by cantankerous and clumsy politicians in the guise of doctors, or rather as 'state quacks'.[3] And, employing similar metaphors, critics for their part were wont to claim the body politic was ailing, infected by the disease of monarchy or aristocracy, and bled white by their exorbitant taxes. Radicals have recommended salutary venesection or surgery, wielding the knife to rid the nation of a dropsical nobility or a cancerous king. Offering schemes for socio-economic revitalization, the *arbitristas* in seventeenth-century Spain liked to visualize themselves as physicians of the nation; but it was above all during the Enlightenment that intellectuals assumed that role. As Peter Gay has elegantly shown, the *philosophes* made particular play of acting the role of physician to the state.[4] The reasons are clear. Through Galileo and Newton, the techniques of natural science had acquired immense prestige as analytic tools. Thanks to the work of Vesalius and Harvey, anatomy was laying bare the hidden workings of the human body. At last, medicine itself might be seen as progressive, and perhaps doctors were beginning to rise in social esteem.[5] In those circumstances, there were evident attractions for reformers to present themselves as anatomists of state; such an image neatly squared with the self-presentation of the 'party of humanity' – they liked to see themselves as no mere superficial dabblers but as radical diagnosticians of a corrupted constitution. Through such moves, medicine would be incorporated, both figuratively and literally, into the 'social science' that it was the aspiration of the Enlightenment to forge. Here lies the context of Bentham's comparison between the healer's and the politician's art.

Within traditional macro/microcosm frameworks, it was easy, in a parallel way, for physicians to regard themselves as rulers of the body, charged with imposing regimen upon a patient. With great elaboration, medieval surgeons like Henri de Mondeville portrayed the body as a townscape, with its orifices likened to gates and portcullises and the head to a tower. In such a model, diseases became invading troops laying siege to the fortress, and the physician was the bodyguard or commander of the defensive forces.[6] Susan Sontag has implied that such military metaphors – which she distrusts as harmful – tainted medicine at the time of the advent of bacteriology ('germ warfare') and abdominal surgery in the second half of the nineteenth century; but the truth of the matter is that the vision of the body as a nation fought over by disease and the doctors has been current for centuries.[7] And especially after the invention of printing, it became common for doctors to write manuals offering the reading public at large medico-philosophical advice for enhanced personal and social well-being.[8]

From the eighteenth century, doctors and the state began to become involved in a growing dialogue that has progressed, without cease, to the present day, though at a different pace and in rather different directions in the various nations of Europe.[9] Mercantilist thinking encouraged the idea that the well-being of the people was the true object of royal policy.[10] The systematization and universalization of bureaucracy in German-speaking Europe as part of the programme known as cameralism led to huge chains of official appointments for medical men (chains that proved fetters as well as providing security). City governments and princely courts had their standing medical councils.[11] Within the newly-licensed, official medical bureaucracy, many medical decisions – for instance regarding smallpox inoculation – assumed a political dimension (did it have official public sanction?).[12] After 1700, medical professors at German-speaking universities were often summoned to give official counsel on administrative bodies, and they commonly served in a public capacity in courts of law.[13] The notion of 'medical police', formulated above all by Johann Peter Frank, united governments and doctors in the cause of producing an orderly, healthy, demographically sound society. There were comparable developments in France. Under Louis XVI, elite doctors belonging to the Société Royale de Médecine were granted official powers to control quackery and regulate medicines. The Revolution itself produced a host of schemes for putting medical training on a sounder public footing and for instituting public health schemes that in the event came to little, undermined by the politics of the Terror and the exigencies of war and public debt.[14]

But it was the nineteenth century that produced the most profound and lasting liaisons between medicine and the state. The root cause was massive social change. The demographic and industrial revolutions, rapid urbanization and all the health problems associated therewith experienced through much of Europe and on the eastern seaboard of the United States created situations in which mounting socio-political disorder and growing threats of disease were clearly interrelated.[15] As industrial 'shock towns' were assailed by filth diseases and waves of epidemics, most scandalously cholera, health reformers found it attractive to think of themselves as protectors and saviours of society. Towards the close of the eighteenth century, the agricultural writer, Arthur Young, deemed the greatest of all public benefactors he who made two ears of corn grow where there was but one before. If the pre-1800 hero was the agronome, the hero of industrial society, alongside engineers and entrepreneurs, might be the medical man: perhaps a Jenner, offering to deliver society from smallpox; perhaps a Snow, come to disconnect the Broad Street pump and end the scourge of cholera; or, later, a Pasteur (not himself medically trained) rescuing people from infectious diseases.

The Victorian era was an age prone to hero-worship,[16] but there were, of course, problems in this vision of doctor as hero. After all, the traditional pukka physician had served the elite and had never displayed notable social responsibility: elite London physicians fled the plague in 1665. But the emergent speciality of public health seemed fortunately to throw a bridge across the traditional gulf between clinical medicine (prizing its intimate, private patient/doctor relationship) and society at large.[17] However controversial, the public health profession could at least present itself as civicly responsible. In innumerable ways and with good reason, nineteenth-century society remained deeply suspicious about medics – remember George Bernard Shaw's characterization of the profession as a conspiracy against the laity; nevertheless, it became plausible for the first time for doctors to turn prophets. The utopias of earlier centuries had been the visions of divines, moralists and philosophers. Now, in works like Benjamin Ward Richardson's *Hygeia* (1876), medical men portrayed health and hygiene as the cornerstones of a New Society and the doctor as its priest.[18] It is perhaps no accident that in *Uncle Vanya* (1900) Chekhov, himself a physician, has another doctor, Astrov, serve as a mouthpiece for his anxieties for Russia's future.[19] Especially after 1850, mainstream social scientists, impressed by Comtean Positivism and Darwinian evolution, grounded their models of social statics and social dynamics on a biomedical basis. If society at large was a superorganism, politics might essentially be a matter of medical management.[20]

Such dreams and schemes began to seem capable of realization, as medical men and their supporters increasingly occupied positions of power and patronage. In Britain, after the extremely chequered career of Edwin Chadwick – not of course a medical man – Sir John Simon, chief medical adviser to the Privy Council, became a genuinely commanding health statesman;[21] in Third Republic France, as Jack Ellis has demonstrated, a remarkably large cohort of medical men won seats as deputies.[22] From the late nineteenth century, with Bismarck's social insurance schemes setting the pace, the state increasingly assumed a large measure of responsibility for health and medical care.[23]

This picture of a growing entente down the centuries between medicine and politics contains more than a grain of truth. But as told so far, it presents only half the story. For though, from the French Revolutionary era, with the development of professional reform and of rational administration, the worlds of medicine and politics were undoubtedly coming into closer alignment, the nature of the association was to remain deeply problematic and vigorously contested. How would medicine be politicized and politics medicalized? What mode of legitimization did medicine offer to politicians? What kind of power might physicians exercise over politicians? Would parliaments be able to suborn or seduce the doctors? Or would medicine possess an authority of its own, a scientific expertise above the party political fray? – or indeed, viewing this possibility in another light, would the *notion* that medicine possessed an intrinsic authority, an independent, scientific expertise, above the fray of party politics, itself serve as a convenient ideological prop for politicians or a way of passing the buck? In the endless horse-trading between practitioners and politicians, what were the swings and roundabouts, who had what to gain and what to lose?

Medical historians have obviously not been unaware of these issues. But there has been a tendency in traditional scholarship, especially in histories of public health, to simplify questions of medical politics, through the assumption that the growing rapport between medicine and the state visible during the nineteenth century was both desirable and foreordained, the ultimate outcome being state medicine, the creation of the welfare state and, in Britain, the National Health Service. Individuals and actions expediting those destinies thereby became 'progressive' and opposing forces 'reactionary'. Thus even in admirable works of scholarship like Samuel Finer's *The Life and Times of Sir Edwin Chadwick* (1952), it is taken for granted that national improvement hinged upon the uptake by the state of utilitarian sanitary reform and the public employment of sanitarians. Hence Chadwick's enemies were enemies of health and Chadwick's fall must have been retrograde.[24] As Elizabeth Fee and Edward Morman indicate in 'Doing History, Making Revolution: the Aspirations of Henry E. Sigerist and George Rosen', the socialist George Rosen's major contributions to the historiography of public health presupposed, in Whiggish and unproblematic ways, that the history of public health is self-evidently a story of the successive incorporation of doctors within the state.[25]

But reality was nothing like so simple. In recent years, historians of various hues – Marxist, feminist, libertarian, even professional doctors – have been questioning the teleological 'rightness' of the rapport between medicine and the state. Is such an entente incontrovertibly good for the state? for medicine? or indeed for the people? These traditional truths have been questioned. Michel Foucault notably threw a different light on the fusion of expertise and government, standardly approved in Fabian histories: rather than advancing democracy, welfare and social justice, the alliance of *savoir* and *pouvoir* could be seen as an intensification of a controlling rationality.[26] Feminists have construed such measures as the 1860s Contagious Diseases Acts in England, and legislation regulating contraception and abortion in Germany, not as ways of safeguarding the public health but as modes of controlling female bodies and sexuality.[27] These are matters pursued in detail in Susan Gross Solomon's contribution to this volume, 'The Demographic Argument in Soviet Debates over the Legalization of Abortion in the 1920s', which shows that in the intense policy debates over such questions in the early Soviet state the expressed wishes of women took a back seat, while economic needs took priority rationalized through certain ideologically tendentious notions of 'progressive' social policy.[28]

In *Dangerous Sexualities*, Frank Mort has advanced an astute analysis of the political ambiguities of applied medicine.[29] On the one hand, Mort reminds us that medically-sponsored health legislation was routinely professionally self-serving, flexing medical muscles and angling for reinforced prestige. Insofar as medical legislation brought 'progress', that was in large measure the progress of the vested interests of the medical establishment. On the other hand, Mort simultaneously stresses the degree to which, in England, multifarious countervailing political pressures limited the medical profession's capacity to achieve its own parliamentary goals or even clearly to agree upon them in the first place. The Contagious Diseases Acts were passed – but then repealed; compulsory smallpox vaccination was introduced, then watered down; eugenics legislation was stifled at birth.[30] Why? Such medicalizing goals were often unpopular – and, by the late nineteenth century, with the advent of mass democracy, politicians had to have an eye to the ratings. Ministers themselves frequently felt little respect for medical men, or at least, did not want to be seen as supping too often with an commonly unpopular profession. Moreover doctors themselves were often profoundly divided. It would be a mistake to picture the medical profession as a monolith, pressing surely and successfully for the incorporation of medicine within the state.[31] As the opposition of British doctors first to National Insurance (1911) and then to the National Health Service (1948) shows with crystal clarity, large segments of the medical profession feared being gobbled up by the state; their idea of medical politics, argues Charles Webster in his essay below on Lord Dawson, was the preservation of their autonomy. Often it was not doctors but reformers and politicians, including Jeremy Bentham and Edwin

Chadwick, who had the most grandiose plans for health within a future rational society – not least, plans for the reform of the medical profession.[32] In short, without descending into nominalism or throwing up our hands in analytic despair, it is important to recognize that as doctors and politicians became jointly involved in grappling with the problems, and deploying the resources of, the modern, corporate, bureaucratic state, that interplay spawned a never-ending proliferation of new tensions and conflict-points.[33]

Having sketched in the broad outlines and hinted at complexities, it is at this point that we reach the starting-point for the studies to follow, which concentrate, chiefly though not exclusively, upon individuals whose aim was to rivet knowledge and power, applying medical theory and practice to public affairs with a view to social improvement. Most of the essays focus upon medically qualified men, but not all: Jeremy Bentham was a social and legal reformer, Lyon Playfair primarily a chemist. All, however, in various ways occupied the public stage. Some did so with great eminence at the highest level: Christopher Addison became the first British Minister of Health and eventually a Viscount; Bertrand Dawson, the President of the Royal College of Physicians, was elevated to the House of Lords; Lyon Playfair was an MP, Bourneville a deputy in the French parliament; Arthur Newsholme rose to become Medical Officer to the Local Government Board. Others held medical or academic office, for example Henry Sigerist, who was director of the Institute of the History of Medicine at Johns Hopkins University, or John Ryle, who gave up the Regius Chair of Physic at Cambridge University to become the first Professor of Social Medicine at Oxford. Others, like Jeremy Bentham, or Thomas Southwood Smith, were most famous perhaps because of their tireless agitation, writings and force of personality.

Not surprisingly, these men (and it is notable that all were males) shared in large measure the missionary impulse. As many essays amply show, these campaigners frequently expressed deep discontents with the organization of medicine, past and present, and the derelictions of duty committed by a profession more interested, apparently, in doing well than making well. The health needs of the people, many claimed, had been neglected by profession and politicians alike. As Dorothy Porter shows in her 'John Ryle: Doctor of Revolution?', Ryle felt revulsion at the mercenariness of a profession addicted to lucrative private practice, and called for a new discipline of 'social medicine' that would compel medics to address the true health needs of the population.[34]

Several of the figures discussed in this book advanced radical critiques of the socio-political system at large. As Elizabeth Fee and Edward Mormon show, though an independently wealthy *haut bourgeois*, Henry Sigerist, one of the scholarly pioneers of the history of medicine, was a passionate Marxist, eager for capitalism's demise and seeing in the Soviet Union a better future, both social and medical.[35] Though Sigerist's friend, Ryle never joined the Communist party, but he equally identified the pre-war Soviet health system as the model for the future provision of services. In public and private, Ryle expressed his conviction that free-market capitalism was morally and medically bankrupt: health could not decently be reduced to a market-place commodity with a price-tag on it.[36]

Radicalism, however, takes many forms. Somewhat over a century earlier, Jeremy Bentham had looked to liberal individualism to reform the medical profession and revitalize the health of the community. As Janet Semple shows in her 'Bentham', the great utilitarian believed it was the state's duty to purge and reorganize the medical profession itself, eliminating its monopolistic traits, so that it could better serve the public interest and maximize the greatest happiness of the greatest number.[37] Bernard Brais's 'Désiré Magloire Bourneville and French Anticlericalism during the Third Republic' also focuses upon campaigns against entrenched vested interests, but in this case the campaigners were radical medical men. Charcot's *protégé* and henchman in Third Republic France, Bourneville contrasted medicine and the Catholic Church as the great progressive and reactionary forces in modern society. In matters regarding health, hospitals, education and medical research, insisted Bourneville and his comrades, the state should cease to heed the superstitious prejudices of the Church and instead implement the progressive policies indicated by medical science.[38]

But if a certain spirit of criticism and change unites many of the *dramatis personae* of this book, it is no less important to emphasize the vast divergences in their intellectual allegiances and programmes and in the strategies they adopted. As a counterweight to Bourneville's anti-clerical viewpoint, the role of religion in providing intellectual and ethical foundations for medical reformism must never be underestimated. In previously published work, John Pickstone has underlined the role of personal faith in girding into action that notable early-Victorian campaigner for education and public health. Kay-Shuttleworth was committed to the moral reform of the unwashed ragged classes as much as he was concerned to reduce their unnecessary premature mortality from epidemic disease. For Kay, public hygiene was an evangelical campaign which continued the late eighteenth-century humanistic mission of individual and social 'improvement'.[39] Parallels may be drawn with Robert Webb's account of Thomas Southwood Smith, 'Southwood Smith: The Intellectual Sources of Public Service'. Southwood Smith combined a passionate Unitarianism with a profound commitment to utilitarianism (a friend of Bentham, he delivered a celebrated funeral lecture over Bentham's corpse, in the midst of a raging thunderstorm).[40] Accepting much of Hartley's religious materialism and convinced of the uniformity and universality of natural law in Creation, Southwood Smith emphasized the ultimate unity of moral and medical imperatives, knowledge and action.[41] Revelation of deficiencies of health in the nation inevitably required their rectification. Southwood Smith emphasized the inner chain of relations between social conditions, disease and ill-health, and showed it to be a religious, moral and a medical duty – all were ultimately inseparable – for human faculties to be applied to bring about improvement, via literacy, education, and medical intervention. Indeed, it was not uncommon for *philosophe* doctors to adopt medical materialism as the basis – copper-bottomed and scientific, as they saw it – of a system of ethical values and action. The late eighteenth-century medical radical, Thomas Beddoes, believed that medicine itself – or at least the biomedical understanding of life – should be the cornerstone of ethics as a whole. Chemist, physiologist, and, perhaps, atheist, Beddoes was disposed, like his French contemporaries, the Idéologues, to adopt a materialist perspective upon the entire panorama of animated existence.[42] Beddoes ridiculed the attempts of Cartesian dualists to draw sharp divides between mind and brain, spirit and flesh – such socialists overlooked 'the inseparable connection between moral and medical topics'.[43] Drawing in part on his own clinical experience with psychosomatic complaints, Beddoes denied any rigid ontological differentiation between the physical and the moral, and insisted that all true ethical systems must be bodily-based. No code of living or even lifestyle could be *moral*, unless grounded upon, and conducive to, the permanent well-being of man as an organic being. Physiology was the foundation of all sound morals, for 'the science of human nature is altogether incapable of division into independent branches':[44]

> Every code of morals must ground its precepts on a comprehensive view of the laws that regulate feeling, and deliver the conditions of an offensive and defensive league, having for its object the well-

> being of individuals. Without accurate ideas therefore of the causes that affect the personal condition of mankind, how is it possible to conceive any progress in genuine morality? And will not every addition to this branch of knowledge necessarily tend to purify morals – that is, to introduce into the social compact covenants more beneficial to the parties? Without reference to the body, it is equally impossible to unfold the nature of the mind. Physiology therefore – or, more strictly, *biology* – by which I mean the doctrine of the living system in all its states, appears to be the foundation of ethics and pneumatology.

Thus there was an ethics of medicine; but, more importantly still, medicine itself must be the measure of valid ethics.

Positions such as Beddoes's, insisting that a true understanding of human moral and social destiny must derive from a grasp of man as a biomedical creature, became highly attractive to nineteenth-century medical reformers. As Brais shows, Bourneville and his colleagues espoused comparable views, partly under the influence of Comtean Positivism with its notion of a scientific morality revealed by the historical evolution of the human mind.[45] Rather as Southwood Smith used Necessarianism as a shibboleth, Bourneville and his fellow positivists depicted the progress of science both as a great objective fact about human development and also as a party badge, distinguishing the paladins of science from obscurantists and reactionaries. No accident that Bourneville edited a journal called *Le Progrès Médical*. Yet one man's medico-scientific 'progress' may look differently to others. In 'Heinrich Zeiss, Hygiene and the Holocaust', Paul Weindling examines the career of that early twentieth-century German bacteriologist, whose evolutionary, epidemiological, biological and anthropological views were at the cutting edge of contemporary medical research. The implications of Zeiss's life and work cannot but trouble us nowadays.

Alongside other vocal members of the German scientific community, Zeiss developed theories of racial hierarchy, health and destiny which purportedly demonstrated the superiority of so-called Aryan peoples and hence, through what he termed 'geomedicine', provided 'scientific' grounds for Teutonic hegemony. To Zeiss, such views doubtless appeared fully justified, scientifically speaking, but they conveniently squared with his personal prejudices and the ideological needs of an increasingly militant Reich in the interwar years, craving *Lebensraum*: he was an eager recruit to the Nazi party. As numerous historians have documented,[46] medical researchers and medical beliefs were deeply implicated in the extermination programmes of the Third Reich, not least through their eager development and deployment of eugenics and race hygiene.[47] Reinforcing his earlier publications, Weindling's paper contends that it would be a mistake to expect to find a small cadre of 'Nazi' medical men and scientists who 'abused' medico-scientific knowledge, as distinct from the great majority of sound and reputable experts. Rather the scientific community at large embraced certain core beliefs. Not least amongst them was the conviction that 'science' generated both factual knowledge and concomitant moral imperatives: evolution entailed ethics and biomedicine should be the well-spring of state policy.[48]

Yet, once again, we should not expect to find simplicity. For even amongst those who proposed science as the yardstick of policy, the question of what precisely constituted biomedically rational action was deeply contested. Should policy be entrusted to experts to enforce? Or, if the scientific was the natural, and evolution was nature's way, should not nature be left to take her course? Several essays in this volume address the conundrum of contrasting imperatives for action in medical politics, examining issues of welfare and wealth against the criterion of the constitutionality of the (more or less) democratic state.

Such issues arise, time and again, in the activities of one of the most prominent British medico-scientific lobbyists of the latter half of the nineteenth century, Lyon Playfair. In 'Lyon Playfair and the Idea of Progress: Science and Medicine in Victorian Parliamentary Politics', Anne Hardy examines the principles whereby as an MP and as a member of numerous medico-scientific boards and commissions Playfair attempted to lay down science policy. He deplored public ignorance of science and its ignominiously pitiful representation in British civic life. He ardently believed that medical and scientific knowledge should shape public policy, for example in matters of public health, and was profoundly committed to defending and strengthening professional power.[49] Yet, like so many Victorian medical and scientific activists, he was also a vehement believer in individualism, freedom and competition within the market economy, fearing that remnants of the old, aristocratic and nepotistic state would act as clogs on enterprise and investigation. Though pressing medicine's claims, he certainly had no dream of a socialist or centralizing alliance of medicine and science with the state, with a view to social reorganization. In certain medical and public health matters, Playfair pressed for extended legislation to protect the public; in other instances, and following John Stuart

Mill, Playfair believed the priority lay not in legislation but information. Unlike some contemporary medical men who were administering the public health system, he did not believe legislation could 'buck the market'. Sir John Simon held that if the state could not interfere in the iron law of wages, it could supplement working-class living standards by ensuring a supply of sanitary dwellings, unadulterated food and drugs, clean water and an urban infrastructure which would prevent the spread of epidemic infections. While Playfair did not share this vision of the public health mission, he did see the need politically to support the doctors who entered state service. He argued forcefully for the secure and full-time salaried appointment of qualified doctors as public health officers and promoted their political independence from the vested interests of their local government employers. While being wary of excessive state intervention, he was quite prepared to argue for strong health policing in some matters. Again, unlike Simon, Playfair fully endorsed the extension of the Contagious Diseases Acts universally to cover the civilian population. He did not believe that the health of prostitutes should be inspected only in garrison towns. He also saw the need for the state to play a role in the regulation of the professional and education standards of medical practice itself. In this he was a complete ally in Simon's campaign for a single portal of entry as the principal means of reforming medical education. But Playfair's ambiguity concerning state intervention was characteristic of nineteenth-century medical and scientific politics. The work of Christopher Hamlin on the politics of pure water reveals similar deep divisions amongst medical and scientific experts regarding the desirability of state intervention.[50]

The stance taken a generation later by Arthur Newsholme, the doyen of public health experts, marks a change. In 'The Sick Poor and the State: Newsholme on Poverty, Disease and Responsibility', John Eyler reveals Arthur Newsholme finding different answers to questions concerning the explanation of poor health and disease in industrial Britain. These issues had been to the fore since the debates surrounding the passing of the New Poor Law (1834). Edwin Chadwick had argued that disease created poverty, and so believed this provided a mandate for investing state funds in public health measures. By the close of the nineteenth century, supporters of 'degenerationist' theories and above all the eugenist lobby were newly arguing, on the contrary, that sickly people were the product of unhealthy bioplasm inherited from their biologically inferior forebears. Money spent on public health and social improvement measures was largely money wasted – it could even be counter-productive; the root of the problem lay in the lumpen proletarian residuum itself and its wretched genetic inheritance. Entering this long-running debate as a spokesman for the public health profession, Newsholme fiercely contested the eugenist claim to biologically-based destitution. He insisted that poverty was the prime cause of disease, and that public health must operate from a 'social standpoint'. Eyler depicts Newsholme seeking greatly to expand the authority of preventive medicine to design and implement measures of social reform. Newsholme found a place to express his views amongst his Fabian socialist friends such as the Webbs, but he held back from independent parliamentary socialism. He urged the Webbs to support the creation of a state-unified health service run by public health officers employed by a central government department. He still believed, however, that environmental and social improvement should ultimately focus upon improving the moral character of the indigent. Once again, medical, moral and ideological strands were interwoven.[51]

But Newsholme set a standard for others to follow. John Ryle saw Newsholme as a direct predecessor in the development of social medicine and relied heavily upon Newsholme's study of Soviet health care for modelling his own ideas. In Ryle the medicine of the social, however, had much more powerful links with socialist politics. Ryle made a connection between the politics of epistemology and the politics of economic and social reform. Holism was a philosophy to be lived as well as a theory of knowledge. For Ryle this translated into a mission to re-invigorate medicine and reform society at the same time. In the late 1930s Ryle reflected the spirit of a generation of intellectuals who believed 'science was social relations'. In particular, as J. D. Bernal expressed it, science and communism were one of the same flesh. As Dorothy Porter shows below, for Ryle, changing the disciplines of medicine was a means to changing society as a whole, not only through the social relations of health but by recasting the moral imperative of progress itself.

Ryle's view was powerfully influenced by his admiration for the reconstruction of medicine and health care in the post-revolutionary Soviet Union. Here, Susan Solomon shows how doctors finally got a stake in the operations of the state. They invented a new 'political medicine' called social hygiene, dedicated to improving the people's health rather than simply eliminating disease. The new socio-political medicine, wedded to the ideals of the revolution, finally allowed doctors to become state technocrats and enabled them to take their place in the new 'progressive era' of the rationally ordered society. The question of abortion permitted the medical profession to move into a field of expertise which went beyond the issues arising out of the termination of individual pregnancies and assumed a wider field of competence in demographic and social questions. It is interesting, as Solomon notes, that major sectors of the profession attempted to steer clear of these wider responsibilities and to restrict themselves to narrower 'medical' matters.

Two other essays forming a neat pairing in this volume, however, warn against any simple view of the elective affinities between medicine and the state, Frank Honigsbaum's 'Christopher Addison: A Realist in Pursuit of Dreams',[52] and Charles Webster's 'The Metamorphosis of Dawson of Penn'.[53] Addison and Dawson were contemporaries; Addison became the first Minister of Health (1919), and Dawson rose to become President of the Royal College of Physicians. They formed, in a sense, the two senior statesmen for medicine in Britain. Yet they appear to have had surprisingly little contact with each other's ideas. Honigsbaum remarks that at no point in his work at the Ministry of Reconstruction during the last years of the First World War did Addison (himself a former medical practitioner and professor of anatomy) consult Dawson or the College of Physicians. Addison ultimately employed Dawson on his new Medical Council at the Ministry of Health to pursue the planning of a comprehensive health service. But Addison failed to anticipate that Dawson's preoccupation with resisting a salaried service would thwart his dream of a state-funded system. Addison was wedded to the nationalization of health care, and became more radical with the years. Once a Liberal politician, he eventually joined the Labour Party in its struggle to establish a welfare state. But Addison's urgency and haste often meant that he overlooked the important conflicts and alliances endemic in getting his ambitious schemes implemented. And, despite his long political experience, he still fell foul of personal naïvety. His career almost collapsed at one point as the result of Lloyd George's disloyalty. Most importantly, Addison failed to use his influence to win the medical profession to his cause. Perhaps Addison's failures resulted from the fact that relations between political representatives and the medical profession were haphazard, and their priorities poorly aligned.

Webster shows, for his part, that despite a high posthumous reputation for his medical planning report of 1920, Bertrand Dawson was and became an ever-stronger enemy of a state medical service. Dawson believed that whole-time salaried employment of doctors would produce a state service that was a soulless machine, and he lived bitterly to regret his initial flirtation with medical collectivism. He considered that his early advocacy of collective planning had played into the hands of socialists and Bolsheviks. Having originated the idea of 'health centres', Dawson emphasized that such collectivism in medicine could only function on condition that the traditional liberties of the medical profession were preserved. Most important of all, the stimulus induced by free-market rivalry was sacrosanct. The interplay of doctors and politics thus reflects the internal politics of the medical profession and of political caucuses as much as it shows responsiveness to national need or any supposed overarching emplacement of the bureaucratic state.

This book thus poses important questions about the role of medicine in the modern political order. In what ways have doctors mounted a medical critique of the evils of emergent industrial and urban society? How have they envisaged medicine putting them right? What role have they staked out for medical men, and the medical profession as a whole, in forging a healthier, more efficient, just and rational society? What do such plans say about the political objectives – and also the real political power – of physicians? In what ways has the political establishment itself responded to, and accommodated, the plans for medico-political change advanced by leading medical spokesmen? All these questions pertaining to health politics are obviously still crucially unresolved in the late twentieth century.

The book also poses the question of the development of the doctor as social actor. This idea crystallized with the Enlightenment, in the visions and writings of activists like Thomas Beddoes, Erasmus Darwin and Cabanis.[54] They held out a dream in which the physician could become the legislator of the new moral world. The doctor's duty was to instruct the people in the lessons of living, because without understanding these, how could they possibly make the wider choices of life? A vision was being offered of the doctor as intellectual guru, rather as Coleridge thought of the new intelligentsia, the clerisy, called to serve as moral leaders of the future. No servile tradesman, no sycophantic courtier, no technocratic fixer, the new social doctor would be the humanist physician become priest and preceptor to humanity. Herein was formulated a new, upstanding vocational vision for medicine as a modern profession, a new breed of intellectuals committed to truth and progress, to enquiry and experiment, that could sway the destiny of nations. Doctors would be able to pursue national improvement. They would succour the people. They would, as Virchow put it, serve as the natural attorneys of the poor.[55]

Yet there was a profound tension in this vision. If, as political and social animals, reformist doctors tended to be libertarian, egalitarian, and of democratic leanings, how were these goals to be squared with the models and metaphors that medicine presupposed? For the fundamental relations of clinical medicine surely hinge upon hierarchies of expert authority (active physician, passive patient) based not, of course, as then, on wealth, rank, patronage or pull, but on science and skill. Two incommensurable images thus clashed in reformists' projections of a good society. On the one hand, a heartfelt *liberté* and *égalité*. On the other hand, the protocols of the technocrat.[56]

In this tension lies, of course, the essence, and the contradictions, of so many reforming movements, radical and socialist, ever since, not least those to which medical practitioners have subscribed; simultaneously espousing some sort of liberationist faith in the people, but also a more *dirigiste* notion that the people had to be saved from their own follies, and guided to a better future by enlightened sanitarians, utilitarians, social engineers, social scientists, St Simonians, Comtian positivists, Fabians, the Party, or whoever, in the name of public health, progress and order, the greatest happiness of the greatest number, national efficiency, the public good or the dictatorship of the proletariat.[57]

The doctors' dilemmas register the ambiguities of the Enlightenment towards the masses – epitomized in Voltaire's supposed anxiety that, were the servants ever freed from their false consciousness, one would have to count the spoons.[58] Classically, the tension implicit between '*for* the people' and '*by* the people' was to be resolved through the medium of education: the wise pedagogue would help the people effect the transition from being passive and grateful recipients of good to becoming agencies of good in themselves. It is no accident that so many medical reformers, from Beddoes through Southwood Smith, were zealots for education.

The issues were never clearly resolved. In Britain, the kind of alliance that might have been forged between political and medical radicals did not cohere. Medics wrung their concessions out of the early Victorian state but then retreated into professional conservatism. The politics of medical change became atomized. As Adrian Desmond has recently shown, reformist currents within the profession were concerned mainly with occupational change (the career open to talent), without strong commitments to radical social change.[59] By the close of the nineteenth century, the English medical profession had grown entrenched and sleek, having carved out for itself new professional restrictive practices that masqueraded as ethics and seemed to elevate it above the vulgarities of trade and the ignominy of subservience. In Third Republic France, physicians achieved a sizeable representation in Parliament, but used their muscle-power to protect privileged interests.[60] Over the last century, it has mainly been in the Third World that the alliance between doctors, radicals and revolutionaries has come to the fore, notably in our own day in Salvadore Allende and Che Guevara. What the future holds remains unclear.

## Notes

1. Jeremy Bentham, quoted in Mary Mack, *Jeremy Bentham: An Odyssey of Ideas*, 1748–92 (London: Heinemann, 1962), 264. Bentham continues: 'it is the common endeavour of both to relieve men from the miseries of life. But the physician relieves them one by one: the legislator by millions at a time'. He also states that 'Medicine, commonly so called ... has for its basis the observations of the axioms of pathology, commonly so called. Morals is the medicine of the soul. The science of legislation is the practical part of this medicine ... God forbid that any disease in the constitution of a state should be without its remedy': John Bowring, *The Works of Jeremy Bentham,* 11 vols (Edinburgh: Simpkin, Marshall and Co., 1843), 1, 304–5, 367. See also Benjamin Spector, 'Jeremy Bentham, his Influence upon Medical Thought and Legislation', *Bulletin of the History of Medicine*, xxxvii (1963), 25–42. For discussion, see, in this volume, Janet Semple 'Bentham's Utilitarianism and the Provision of Medical Care'.
2. For the body politic and the image of macrocosm and microcosm, see E. M. Tillyard, *The Elizabethan World Picture* (London: Chatto and Windus, 1943); L. Barkan, *Nature's Work of Art: the Human Body as Image of the World* (New Haven, Conn.: Yale University Press, 1975); J. B. Bamborough, *The Little World of Man* (London: Longman, Green, 1952); H. Baker, *The Dignity of Man: Studies in the Persistence of an Idea* (Cambridge, Mass.: Harvard University Press, 1947); Miri Rubin, *Corpus Christi. The Eucharist in Late Medieval Culture* (Cambridge: Cambridge University Press, 1991); Ernst H. Kantorowicz, *The King's Two Bodies: A Study in Medieval Political Theology* (Princeton, N.J.: Princeton University Press, 1957). William Harvey likened the heart to the king: Christopher Hill, 'William Harvey and the Idea of Monarchy', *Past and Present,* xxvii (1964), 54–72, reprinted in Charles Webster (ed.), *The Intellectual Revolution of the Seventeenth Century* (London: Routledge & Kegan Paul, 1974), 160–81.
3. See Kate Arnold-Forster and Nigel Tallis (comps), *The Bruising Apothecary: Images of Pharmacy and Medicine in Caricature* (London: Pharmaceutical Press, 1989); Ronald Paulson, *Representations of*

*Revolution, 1789–1820* (New Haven, Conn.: Yale University Press, 1983); Herbert M. Atherton, *Political Prints in the Age of Hogarth* (Oxford: Clarendon Press, 1974); M. Dorothy George, *English Political Caricature 1793–1832* (Oxford: Clarendon Press, 1959). For instance, a Cruikshank cartoon called *Doctor Sangrado Releeving John Bull of the Yellow Fever* shows Pitt (Sangrado) taking the Briton's guineas (p. 14). Charles Fox was often portrayed as a Bedlamite lunatic. The name Buonaparte ('Boney Part') lent itself to anatomical caricature.

4. P. Gay, 'The Enlightenment as Medicine and as Cure', in W. H. Barber (ed.), *The Age of the Enlightenment. Studies Presented to Theodore Besterman* (Edinburgh: St Andrews University Publications, 1967), 375–86; *idem, The Enlightenment,* 2 vols (New York: Knopf, 1967–9); for discussion, see Roy Porter, 'Was There a Medical Enlightenment in Eighteenth Century England?', *British Journal for Eighteenth Century Studies,* v (1982), 46–63; *idem, The Enlightenment* (London: Macmillan, 1990).
5. For a conspectus, see Roy Porter, 'Medical Science and Human Science in the Enlightenment', in Christopher Fox, Roy Porter and Robert Wokler (eds), *Inventing the Human Sciences* (San Francisco: University of California Press, 1993).
6. Marie-Christine Pouchelle, *Corps et Chirurgie à l'Apogée du Moyen-Age* (Paris: Flammarion, 1983; English trans., Cambridge: Polity Press, 1990).
7. Susan Sontag, *Illness as Metaphor* (New York: Farrar, Straus & Giroux, 1978; London: Allen Lane, 1979); *idem, AIDS as Metaphor* (Harmondsworth: Allen Lane, 1989).
8. Paul Slack, 'Mirrors of Health and Treasures of Poor Men: Uses of the Vernacular Medical Literature of Tudor England', in C. Webster (ed.), *Health, Medicine and Mortality in the Sixteenth Century* (Cambridge: Cambridge University Press, 1979), 237–74; Roy Porter (ed.), *The Popularization of Medicine, 1650–1850* (London: Routledge, 1992).
9. C. M. Cipolla, *Cristofano and the Plague: A Study in the History of Public Health in the Age of Galileo* (Berkeley: University of California Press; London: Collins, 1973); *idem, Public Health and the Medical Profession in the Renaissance* (Cambridge: Cambridge University Press, 1976); *idem, Miasmas and Disease. Public Health and the Environment in the Pre-Industrial Age* (New Haven and London: Yale University Press, 1992); A. W. Russell (ed.), *The Town and State Physician in Europe from the Middle Ages to the Enlightenment* (Wolfenbüttel: Herzog August Bibliotek, 1981).
10. Jonathan Barry and Colin Jones (eds), *Medicine and Charity Before the Welfare State* (London: Routledge, 1991).
11. C. F. Mullett, 'A Century of English Quarantine (1709–1825)', *Bulletin of the History of Medicine,* xxiii (1949), 527–45; Paul Slack, *The Impact of Plague in Tudor and Stuart England* (London:

Routledge & Kegan Paul, 1985). Slack emphasizes that the difficulties caused by plague were primarily seen as problems of public order requiring 'policing' methods.

12. A good introduction is offered by George Rosen, *From Medical Police to Social Medicine* (New York: Science History Publications, 1974). See also Mary E. Lindemann, 'Producing Policed Man: Poor Relief, Population Policies, and Medical Care in Hamburg, 1750–1806' (Ph.D. dissertation, University of Cincinnati, 1980); *idem*, 'Aufklärung and the Health of the People: Volksschriften and Medical Advice in Braunschweig-Wolfenbüttel, 1756–1802', in Rudolf Vierhaus (ed.), *Kultur und Gesellschaft in Nordwestdeutschland zur Zeit der Aufklärung* (Zurich: 1978). See also Andreas-Holger Maehle, 'Conflicting Attitudes Towards Inoculation in the Enlightenment', in Roy Porter (ed.), *Medicine and the Enlightenment* (Amsterdam: Rodopi, 1993); and Mary Lindemann, 'The Enlightenment Encountered: Medical Practice and Enlightenment in Northern Germany, 1750–1820', in the same book.
13. Johanna Geyer-Kordesch, 'German Medical Education in the Eighteenth Century: The Prussian Context and its Influence', in W. F. Bynum and R. Porter (eds), *William Hunter and The Eighteenth-Century Medical World* (Cambridge: Cambridge University Press, 1985), 177–206.
14. Matthew Ramsey, *Professional and Popular Medicine in France, 1770–1830* (New York: Cambridge University Press, 1988); *idem*, 'The Repression of Unauthorized Medical Practice', *Eighteenth Century Life*, vii (1982), 118–35; *idem*, 'The Politics of Professional Monopoly in Nineteenth-Century Medicine: The French Model and its Rivals', in G. L. Geison (ed.), *Professions and the French State, 1700–1900* (Philadelphia: University of Pennsylvania Press, 1984), 225–305; *idem*, 'Property Rights and the Right to Health: The Regulation of Secret Remedies in France, 1789–1815', in W. F. Bynum and R. Porter (eds), *Medical Fringe and Medical Orthodoxy, 1750–1850* (London: Croom Helm, 1987), 79–105; *idem*, 'Public Health in France', in Dorothy Porter (ed.), *The History of Health and the Modern State* (Philadelphia: University of Pennsylvania Press, 1993); William Coleman, *Death is a Social Disease. Public Health and Political Economy in Early Industrial France* (Madison, Wis.: University of Wisconsin Press, 1982). For schemes for medical reform in the Revolutionary era, see George Rosen, 'Political Order and Human Health in Jeffersonian Thought', *Bulletin of the History of Medicine*, xxvi (1952), 32–44; Dora Weiner, 'Le droit de l'homme à la santé: une belle idée devant l'Assemblée constituante: 1790–1791', *Clio Medica*, v (1970), 208–23; *idem*, 'Public Health Under Napoleon: the Conseil de Salubrité de Paris, 1802–1815', *Clio Medica*, ix (1974), 271–84; L. J. Jordanova, 'Guarding the Body Politic: Volney's Catechism of 1793', in Francis Barker *et al.* (eds), *1789: Reading Writing Revolution. Proceedings of the Essex Conference*

*on the Sociology of Literature, July 1981* (Colchester: University of Essex, 1982), 12–21; Dora Weiner, *Citizen Patient* (Baltimore: Johns Hopkins University Press, forthcoming); David Vess, *Medical Revolution in France, 1789–1796* (Gainesville: University Presses of Florida, 1975).

15. See for example F. B. Smith, *The People's Health, 1830–1910* (London: Croom Helm, 1979); Anthony S. Wohl, *Endangered Lives: Public Health in Victorian Britain* (London: Dent; Cambridge, Mass: Harvard University Press, 1983); and, for a wider and suggestive survey, R. J. Evans, 'Epidemics and Revolutions: Cholera in Nineteenth-Century Europe', *Past and Present*, cxx (1988), 123–219.
16. See Waiter Houghton, *The Victorian Frame of Mind* (New Haven: Yale University Press, 1957).
17. For recent surveys of public health see Dorothy Porter, 'Public Health', in W. F. Bynum and Roy Porter (eds), *The Companion Encyclopaedia of the History of Medicine* (London: Routledge, 1993); *idem*, 'Introduction', in *idem*, (ed.), *The History of Public Health and the Modern State* (Amsterdam: Rodopi, 1993); John Duffy, *The Sanitarians: A History of American Public Health* (Urbana and Chicago: University of Illinois Press, 1990); Jane Lewis, *What Price Community Medicine?* (Brighton: Harvester, 1986); *idem*, 'The Public's Health: Philosophy and Practice in Britain in the Twentieth Century', in Elizabeth Fee and Roy Acheson (eds), *A History of Education in Public Health. Health that Mocks the Doctors' Rules* (Oxford: Clarendon Press, 1991), 195–229; Fitzhugh Mullan, *Plagues and Politics: The Story of the United States Public Health Service* (New York: Basic Books, 1989); see also Sir Arthur Salusbury MacNalty, *The History of State Medicine in England* (London: The Royal Institute of Public Health and Hygiene, 1948); George Rosen, *A History of Public Health* (New York: M.D. Publications, 1958); Jeanne L. Brand, *Doctors and the State: The British Medical Profession and Government Action in Public Health, 1870–1912* (Baltimore: Johns Hopkins University Press, 1965); C. F. Brockington, *Public Health in the Nineteenth Century* (Edinburgh & London: E. & S. Livingstone, 1956); *idem, A Short History of Public Health* (London: J. & A. Churchill, 1966); W. M. Frazer, *A History of English Public Health, 1834–1939* (London: Ballière, Tindall & Cox, 1950). For Pasteur as hero, see Bruno Latour, *The Pasteurization of France* (Cambridge, Mass.: Harvard University Press, 1988).
18. For visionary works, see Benjamin Ward Richardson, *Hygeia, a City of Health* (London: Macmillan, 1876). See also H. W. Rumsey, *Essays on State Medicine* (London: Churchill, 1856).
19. On Chekhov and the doctors see William B. Ober, 'Chekhov among the Doctors: The Doctor's Dilemma', *Bulletin of the New York Academy of Medicine*, xlix (1973), 62–76; Rose Melzer, 'Chekhov's Doctors', *Adler Museum Bulletin*, vii (1981), 15–19.

20. See John Simon, *English Sanitary Institutions* (London: Churchill, 1890); for background ideas in social science, see S. Collini, D. Winch and J. Burrow, *That Noble Science of Politics: A Century of Intellectual History* (Cambridge: Cambridge University Press, 1984); Stefan Collini, *Public Moralists: Political Thought and Intellectual Life in Britain, 1850–1930* (Oxford: Oxford University Press, 1991).
21. R. Lambert, *Sir John Simon 1816–1904 and English Social Administration* (London: MacGibbon & Kee, 1963).
22. Jack D. Ellis, *The Physician-Legislators of France. Medicine and Politics in the Early Third Republic, 1870–1914* (Cambridge: Cambridge University Press, 1990).
23. For the lead-up to the National Health Service, see Derek Fraser, *The Evolution of the British Welfare State: The History of Social Policy Since the Industrial Revolution* (London: Macmillan, 1973); F. Honigsbaum, *Health, Happiness and Security. The Creation of the National Health Service* (London: Routledge, 1989); J. Pater, *The Making of the National Health Service* (London: Kings Fund, 1981); Charles Webster, *Problems of Health Care: The National Health Service Before 1957* (London: HMSO, 1988).
24. S. E. Finer, *The Life and Times of Sir Edwin Chadwick* (London: Methuen, 1952).
25. See George Rosen, 'What is Social Medicine? A Genetic Analysis of the Concept', *Bulletin of the History of Medicine*, xxi (1947), 674–733; *idem*, 'Toward a Historical Sociology of Medicinc. The Endeavor of Henry E. Sigerist', *Bulletin of the History of Medicine*, xxxii (1958), 500–16; *idem*, 'Critical Levels in Historical Process: A Theoretical Exploration Dedicated to Henry Ernest Sigerist', *Journal of the History of Medicine and Allied Sciences*, xiii (1958), 179–85; *idem*, 'Social Science and Health in the United States in the Twentieth Century', *Clio Medica*, xi (1976), 245–68; *idem*, *A History of Public Health* (New York: M.D. Publications, 1958); see also E. Morman, 'Scholarship as Advocacy: George Rosen as Historian and Public Health Educator', in *Abstracts of American Association for the History of Medicine 65th Annual Meeting, Seattle, Washington* (Seattle: AAHM, 1992), 1 (paper delivered at the 65th Annual Meeting of the Association, 30th April– 3rd May 1992); Dorothy Porter and Roy Porter, 'What Was Social Medicine? An Historiographical Essay', *Journal of Historical Sociology*, i (1988), 90–106. Sigerist wrote in 1946: 'nobody will deny that the physician is playing an increasingly important part in society': H. E. Sigerist, 'The Place of the Physician in Modern Society', *Proceedings of the American Philosophical Society*, xc (1946), 275–9.

    There is now a fine historiography on the growth of welfare states and their attendant politics. See amongst others E. P. Hennock, *British Social Reform and German Precedents. The Case of Social Insurance 1880–1914* (Oxford: Clarendon Press, 1987); J. R. Hay, *The Origins of the Liberal Welfare Reforms 1906–1914* (London:

Macmillan, 1975), Wolfgang J. Mommsen (ed.), *The Emergence of the Welfare State in Britain and Germany, 1850–1950* (London: Croom Helm, 1981); Pat Thane, *The Foundations of the Welfare State* (London: Longman, 1982); Douglas E. Ashford, *The Emergence of Welfare States* (Oxford: Blackwell, 1986); Douglas E. Ashford and E. W. Kelley (eds), *Nationalising Social Security in Europe and America* (Greenwich, Conn.: JAI, 1986).

For discussion of Whig history, see Herbert Butterfield, *The Whig Interpretation of History* (London: Bell, 1931); A. R. Hall, 'On Whiggism', *History of Science,* xxi (1983), 45–59.

26. Michel Foucault, *Discipline and Punish: The Birth of the Prison* (London: Harmondsworth, 1979); for discussion see Scott Lash, 'Genealogy and the Body: Foucault/Deleuze/Nietzsche', in Mike Featherstone, Mike Hepworth and Bryan S. Turner (eds), *The Body. Social Process and Cultural Theory* (London: Sage, 1991), 256–80; B. S. Turner, 'The Practices of Rationality: Michel Foucault, Medical History and Sociological Theory', in R. Fardon (ed.), *Power and Knowledge: Anthropological and Sociological Approaches* (Edinburgh: Scottish Academic Press, 1985), 193–213; and *idem, Medical Power and Social Knowledge* (Beverly Hills, Calif.: Sage, 1987); David Armstrong, *The Political Anatomy of the Body* (Cambridge: Cambridge University Press, 1983). For feminist critiques, see Barbara Ehrenreich and Deirdre English, *Complaints and Disorders: The Sexual Politics of Sickness* (New York: Old Westbury, 1974). For libertarian critiques, see Thomas S. Szasz, *The Manufacture of Madness* (New York: Dell, 1970; London: Paladin, 1972); *idem, The Myth of Mental Illness: Foundations of a Theory of Personal Conduct* (London: Granada, 1972; revised edn, New York: Harper and Row, 1974); I. Illich, *Limits to Medicine: The Expropriation of Health* (Harmondsworth: Penguin, 1977). For critiques from within medicine, see T. McKeown, *The Role of Medicine: Dream, Mirage or Nemesis* (London: Nuffield Provincial Trust, 1976); *idem, The Rise of Modern Population* (London: Edward Arnold, 1976).
27. Judith R. Walkowitz, *Prostitution and Victorian Society: Women, Class, and the State* (Cambridge: Cambridge University Press, 1980); Paul McHugh, *Prostitution and Victorian Social Reform* (London: Croom Helm, 1980); Cornelie Usborne, *The Politics of the Body in Weimar Germany. Women's Reproductive Rights and Duties* (London: Macmillan, 1992).
28. For further writings on Soviet health policy and its backgrounds, see Susan Gross Solomon, 'The Expert and the State in Russian Public Health: Continuities and Changes Across the Revolutionary Divide', in Dorothy Porter (ed.), *The History of Health and the Modern State* (Amsterdam: Rodopi, 1993); John F. Hutchinson, *Politics and Public Health in Revolutionary Russia, 1890–1918* (Baltimore: Johns Hopkins University Press, 1990); Alec Nove, 'Is

There a Ruling Class in the USSR?', in Anthony Giddens and David Held (eds), *Classes, Power and Conflict. Classical and Contemporary Debates* (London: Macmillan, 1992), 588–604; Murray Yanowitch, 'Work, Hierarchy and Management "Participation" in the Soviet Union', in *ibid.*, 605–28; Elizabeth Garnsey, 'Competing Interests and the Soviet Occupational System', in *ibid.*, 629–42.

29. Frank Mort, *Dangerous Sexualities: Medico-Moral Politics in England Since 1830* (London and New York: Routledge & Kegan Paul, 1987).
30. For opposition to compulsory vaccination, see Dorothy Porter and Roy Porter, 'The Politics of Prevention: Anti-Vaccinationism and Public Health in Nineteenth-Century England', *Medical History*, xxxii (1988), 231–52.
31. Medical professionalization needs more investigation. See, for instance, Dorothy Porter, 'Stratification and its Discontents: Professionalisation and the English Public Health Service, 1848–1914', in E. Fee and Roy Acheson (eds), *Health that Mocks The Doctors' Rules. A History of Education in Public Health* (Oxford: Oxford University Press, 1991), 83–113; Elizabeth Fee and Dorothy Porter, 'Public Health, Preventive Medicine and Professionalisation in England and America, 1848–1914', in A. Wear (ed.), *The History of Medicine in Society* (Cambridge: Cambridge University Press, 1992), 249–75; on the role of the medical profession as the new public health 'priests' of society see D. Porter, 'How Soon is Now? Public Health and the *BMJ*', *B.M.J.* ccci (1990), 738–40; John V. Pickstone, 'The Professionalization of Medicine in England and Europe: The State, the Market and Industrial Society', *Japanese Journal of Medical History*, xxv (1979), 1–31. More broadly, see H. J. Perkin, *The Origins of Modern English Society 1780–1880* (London: Routledge, 1969); *idem, The Rise of Professional Society. England Since 1880* (London: Routledge, 1989); and for America, see Paul Starr, *The Social Transformation of American Medicine* (New York: Basic Books, 1982). For more theoretical discussion see Terence J. Johnson, *Professions and Power* (London: Macmillan, 1972); W. J. Reader, *Professional Men: The Rise of the Professional Classes in Nineteenth-Century England* (London: Weidenfeld & Nicolson, 1966); E. Freidson, 'The Theory of Professions: State of the Art', in R. Dingwall and P. Lewis (eds), *The Sociology of the Professions* (London: Macmillan, 1983), 19–37; D. Rueschemeyer, 'Professional Autonomy and the Social Control of Expertise', in R. Dingwall and P. Lewis (eds), *The Sociology of the Professions* (London: Macmillan, 1983), 38–58; Guy Benveniste, *The Politics of Expertise* (London: Croom Helm, 1973); for discussion specifically of professionalization and medicine see E. Hughes, 'The Making of the Physician', *Human Organization*, xiv (1956), 22–5; N. Parry and J. Parry, *The Rise of the Medical Profession: A Study of Collective Social Mobility* (London: Croom Helm, 1976); R. K. Merton, *Some*

Merton, *Some Thoughts on the Professions in American Society* (Providence: Brown University Papers, 37, 1960); *idem*, 'Some Preliminaries to a Sociology of Medical Education', in R. K. Merton, G. Reader and P. L. Kendall (eds), *The Student Physician* (Cambridge, Mass.: Harvard University Press, 1957), 3–79; Barbara Rosenkrantz, 'The Search for Professional Order in Nineteenth Century American Medicine', in J. Leavitt and R. Numbers (eds), *Sickness and Health in America. Readings in the History of Medicine and Public Health* (Madison, Wis.: University of Wisconsin Press, 1985), 219–32; Ivan Waddington, *The Medical Profession in the Industrial Revolution* (Dublin: Gill and Macmillan, 1984), 53–95; Irvine Loudon, *Medical Care and the General Practitioner 1750–1850* (Oxford: Clarendon Press, 1986); Rosemary Stevens, *Medical Practice in Modern England. The Impact of Specialisation and State Medicine* (New Haven: Yale University Press, 1966); George Rosen, *The Structure of American Medical Practice 1875–1941* (Philadelphia: University of Pennsylvania Press, 1983), 38–108; Frank D. Campion, *The AMA and U.S. Health Policy Since 1940* (Chicago: Chicago Review Press for the AMA, 1984); M. Jeanne Peterson, *The Medical Profession in Mid-Victorian London* (Berkeley: University of California Press, 1978), 244–82.

32. For the wider question of the role of Benthamite Utilitarianism in bringing about the 'nineteenth-century revolution in government', see Oliver MacDonagh, 'The Nineteenth Century Revolution in Government: A Reappraisal', *Historical Journal*, i (1958), 52–67; G. Kitson Clark, 'Statesmen in Disguise: Reflections on the History of the Neutrality of the Civil Service', *Historical Journal*, ii (1959), 19–39; J. Bartlett Brebner, 'Laissez-faire and State Intervention in Nineteenth-Century Britain', *Journal of Economic History*, viii (1948), Supp., 59–73; Henry Parris, 'The Nineteenth-Century Revolution in Government: A Reappraisal Reappraised', *Historical Journal*, iii (1960), 17–37; Robert M. Gutchen, 'Local Improvements and Centralization in Nineteenth Century England', *Historical Journal*, iv (1961), 85–96; Jennifer Hart, 'Nineteenth Century Social Reform: A Tory Interpretation of History', *Past and Present*, xxxi (July 1965), 39–61; L. J. Hume, 'Jeremy Bentham and the Nineteenth Century Revolution in Government', *Historical Journal*, x (1967), 361–75; William C. Lubenow, *The Politics of Government Growth: Early Victorian Attitudes Toward State Intervention 1833–1848* (Newton Abbot: David and Charles, 1971); S. E. Finer, 'The Transmission of Benthamite Ideas 1820–50', in Gillian Sutherland (ed.), *Studies in the Growth of Nineteenth Century Government* (London: Routledge & Kegan Paul, 1972), 11–32; David Roberts, 'Jeremy Bentham and the Victorian Administrative State', *Victorian Studies*, ii (1959), 193–210; *idem*, *Paternalism in Early Victorian England* (New Brunswick, N.J.: Rutgers University Press, 1979).

33. For an understanding of modern political regimes emphasizing their pluralistic nature, see A. Giddens, *The Constitution of Society: Outline of a Theory of Structuration* (Cambridge: Polity, 1984); Michael Mann, *The Sources of Social Power. A History of Power from the beginning to A.D. 1760*, 3 vols (Cambridge: Cambridge University Press, 1986); Anthony Giddens and David Held (eds), *Classes, Power and Conflict. Classical and Contemporary Debates* (London: Macmillan, 1992); *idem, Central Problems in Social Theory* (London: Macmillan, 1979); *idem, The Constitution of Society* (Cambridge: Polity Press, 1984); *idem, Profiles and Critiques in Social Theory* (Berkeley: University of California Press, 1982); John Holloway and Sol Piccotto (eds), *State and Capital: A Marxist Debate* (London: Edward Arnold, 1978); David Held, *States and Societies* (London: Basil Blackwell, 1990); Simon Clarke (ed.), *The State Debate* (London: Macmillan, 1991); T. Skocpol, *States and Social Revolutions: A Comparative Analysis of France, Russia and China* (Cambridge: Cambridge University Press, 1979); J. Hall, *Powers and Liberties* (New York: Oxford University Press, 1985); M. Zeitlin (ed.), *Political Power and Social Theory* (Greenwich, Conn.: JAI Press, 1980), vol. 1; C. Tilly (ed.), *The Formation of National States in Western Europe* (Princeton, N.J.: Princeton University Press, 1975); P. Anderson, *Lineages of the Absolute State* (London: New Left Books, 1974).
34. See Dorothy Porter, 'Changing Disciplines: John Ryle and the Making of Social Medicine in Twentieth Century Britain', *History of Science*, xxx (1992), 119–47.
35. It would be fascinating to have a full-length study of Western medical men who either visited the Soviet Union or learned about it at second hand and then wrote paeans of praise to the new communist medical system. For intellectuals and fellow travellers in the inter-war years see G. Werskey, *The Visible College* (London: Allen Lane, 1978); David Caute, *The Fellow Travellers: A Postscript to the Enlightenment* (New York: Macmillan, 1973). See Henry Sigerist, *Medicine and Health in the Soviet Union* (New York: Citadel Press, 1947).
36. See Dorothy Porter, 'John Ryle: Doctor of Revolution?', in this volume. See also J. A. Ryle, *Changing Disciplines* (London: Oxford University Press, 1948).
37. On Bentham see also Mary Mack, *Jeremy Bentham: An Odyssey of Ideas, 1748–1792* (London: Heinemann, 1962); J. Dinwiddy, *Bentham* (Oxford: Oxford University Press, 1989); Ross Harrison, *Bentham* (London: Routledge & Kegan Paul, 1983).
38. See also Jack D. Ellis, *The Physician-Legislators of France. Medicine and Politics in the Early Third Republic, 1870–1914* (Cambridge: Cambridge University Press, 1990); Jan Goldstein, *Console and Classify: The French Psychiatric Profession in the Nineteenth Century* (Cambridge: Cambridge University Press, 1987).
39. See also J. V. Pickstone, 'Ferriar's Fever to Kay's Cholera: Disease

and Social Structure in Cottonopolis', *History of Science*, xxii (1984), 401–19. For early nineteenth-century religion, see F. K. Brown, *Fathers of the Victorians: The Age of Wilberforce* (Cambridge: Cambridge University Press, 1961). For an American parallel, see Charles Rosenberg and Carol Smith-Rosenberg, 'Pietism and the Origins of the American Public Health Movement', *Journal of the History of Medicine and Allied Sciences*, xxiii (1968), 6–34.

40. Ruth Richardson and Brian Hurwitz, 'Jeremy Bentham's Self Image: An Exemplary Bequest for Dissection', *B.M.J.* ccvc (1987), 195–8.
41. See for Hartley and Priestley, Elie Halévy, *The Growth of Philosophic Radicalism*, 2 vols (London: Faber and Faber, 1928).
42. On the Idéologues, see M. Staum, *Cabanis. Enlightenment and Medical Philosophy in the French Revolution* (Princeton, N. J.: Princeton University Press, 1980); S. Moravia, 'The Enlightenment and the Sciences of Man', *History of Science*, xviii (1980), 247–58; on Beddoes, see Roy Porter, *Doctor of Society: Thomas Beddoes and the Sick Trade in Late Enlightenment England* (London: Routledge, 1991).
43. Thomas Beddoes, *Hygëia: or Essays Moral and Medical, on the Causes Affecting the Personal State of our Middling and Affluent Classes*, 3 vols (Bristol: J. Mills, 1802), vol. 1, essay iii 83.
44. T. Beddoes, *Contributions to Physical and Medical Knowledge, Principally from the West of England* (London: T. Longman and O. Rees, 1799), 3, 4.
45. For a luminous discussion of the power of late nineteenth-century positivism and scientism, see Nancy Leys Stepan, *'The Hour of Eugenics', Race, Gender and Nation in Latin America* (Ithaca: Cornell University Press, 1991).
46. Benno Müller-Hill, *Murderous Science: Elimination by Scientific Selection of Jews, Gypsies and Others, Germany 1933–1945*, trans. by George R. Fraser (Oxford: Oxford University Press, 1988); Robert N. Proctor, *Racial Hygiene: Medicine Under the Nazis* (Cambridge, Mass. and London: Harvard University Press, 1988); Geoffrey Cocks, *Psychotherapy in the Third Reich: the Göring Institute* (New York: Oxford University Press, 1985); D. Gasman, *The Scientific Origins of National Socialism: Social Darwinism in Ernst Haeckel and the German Monist League* (London: Macdonald, 1971); Nancy Stepan, *The Idea of Race in Science* (Hamden, Conn.: Archon Books, 1982).
47. Daniel Kevles, *In the Name of Eugenics: Genetics and the Uses of Human Heredity* (New York: Knopf, 1985).
48. For introductions to scientistic sociology, see Robert C. Bannister, *Sociology and Scientism. The American Quest for Objectivity 1880–1940* (Chapel Hill: University of North Carolina Press, 1987); Lester R. Kurtz, *Evaluating Chicago Sociology* (Chicago: University of Chicago Press, 1984); J. David Lewis and Richard L. Smith, *American Sociology and Pragmatism. Mead, Chicago Sociology and Symbolic Interaction* (Chicago: University of Chicago Press, 1978); Julius Weinberg, *Edward Alsworth Ross and the Sociology of*

*Progressivism* (Madison: University of Wisconsin Press, 1972); Dennis Smith, *The Chicago School. A Liberal Critique of Capitalism* (London: Macmillan, 1988). For a Marxist variant on these ideas see J. D. Bernal, *The Social Function of Science* (London: Routledge, 1940; first edition London, 1939), 353–6. For discussion of the political-epistemology of Bernal's book, see Mikulás Teich, 'Reflecting on the Golden Jubilee of Bernal's *Social Function of Science*', *History of Science*, xxviii (1990), 411–18. For Bernal himself see Maurice Goldsmith, *Sage. A Life of J. D. Bernal* (London: Hutchinson, 1980).

Also consult Weindling's other writings: *Health, Race and German Politics Between National Unification and Nazism 1870–1945* (Cambridge and New York: Cambridge University Press, 1989); *idem*, 'Public Health in Germany', in Dorothy Porter (ed.), *The History of Health and the Modern State* (Amsterdam: Rodopi); *idem*, 'The Modernization of Charity', in Jonathan Barry and Colin Jones (eds), *Medicine and Charity Before the Welfare State* (London: Routledge, 1991), 190–206; *idem* 'The Medical Profession, Social Welfare, and the Birth Rate in Germany, 1914–18', in J. Winter and R. Wall (eds), *The Upheaval of War: Family, Work and Welfare in Europe 1914–1918* (Cambridge: Cambridge University Press, 1988), 417–37.

49. Playfair defended scientific vivisection, for example. See Nicolaas A. Rupke (ed.), *Vivisection in Historical Context* (London: Croom Helm, 1987); Richard D. French, *Antivivisection and Medical Science in Victorian Society* (Princeton: Princeton University Press, 1975).
50. Christopher Hamlin, *A Science of Impurity: Water Analysis and the Manufacture of Expertise in Nineteenth Century Britain* (Berkeley: University of California Press, 1990); see also his 'State Medicine in Britain', in Dorothy Porter (ed.), *The History of Health and the Modern State* (Amsterdam: Rodopi, 1993). On public health, liberty and government intervention, see Roy Porter and Dorothy Porter, 'The Enforcement of Health: the British Debate', in E. Fee and D. Fox (eds), *AIDS: The Burdens of History* (Berkeley: University of California Press, 1988), 97–120.
51. See also J. M. Eyler, 'Mortality Statistics and Victorian Health Policy: Program and Criticism', *Bulletin of the History of Medicine*, l (1976), 335–55; for Newsholme's own views, see A. Newsholme, *Evolution of Preventive Medicine* (Baltimore: Williams and Wilkins, 1927); *idem*, *The Prevention of Tuberculosis* (New York: E. P. Dutton & Co, 1908). On the opposition of public health to eugenism, see Dorothy Porter, '"Enemies of the Race": Biologism, Environmentalism and the Public Health in Edwardian England', *Victorian Studies*, xxxiv (1991), 159–78. On eugenics, see Geoffrey R. Searle, *Eugenics and Politics in Britain 1900–1914* (Leyden: Noordhoff, 1976); C. Webster (ed.),

*Biology, Medicine and Society 1840–1940* (Cambridge: Cambridge University Press, 1981); Donald MacKenzie, *Statistics in Britain, 1865–1930* (Edinburgh: Edinburgh University Press, 1981); Greta Jones, *Social Darwinism and English Thought: the Interaction between Biological and Social Theory* (Brighton: Harvester Press, 1980); *idem, Social Hygiene in Britain* (London: Croom Helm, 1986); Linda Clark, *Social Darwinism in France* (Alabama: University of Alabama Press, 1984); D. Gasman, *The Scientific Origins of National Socialism: Social Darwinism in Ernst Haeckel and the German Monist League* (London: Macdonald, 1971); S. Trombley, *The Right to Reproduce: A History of Coercive Sterilization* (London: Weidenfeld and Nicolson, 1988); Mark Haller, *Eugenics: Hereditarian Attitudes in American Thought* (New Brunswick, N. J.: Rutgers University Press, 1984); Robert Bannister, *Social Darwinism: Science and Myth in Anglo-American Thought* (Philadelphia: Temple University Press, 1979); A. Farrell, *The Origins and Growth of the English Eugenics Movement, 1865–1925* (Ann Arbor: University Microfilms, 1970); Paul Weindling, 'The Medical Profession, Social Welfare, and the Birth Rate in Germany, 1914– 18', in J. Winter and R. Wall (eds), *The Upheaval of War: Family, Work and Welfare in Europe 1914–1918* (Cambridge: Cambridge University Press, 1988), 417–37; Robert Proctor, *Racial Hygiene: Medicine Under the Nazis* (Cambridge, Mass.: Harvard University Press, 1989); Sheila F. Weiss, *Race Hygiene and the Rational Management of National Efficiency: Wilhelm Schallmayer and the Origins of German Eugenics, 1890–1920* (Ann Arbor: University Microfilms, 1983); Pauline M. H. Mazumdar, 'Eugenicists and the Residuum: the Problem of the Urban Poor', *Bulletin of the History of Medicine*, liv (1980), 204–15; *idem, Eugenics, Human Genetics and Human Failings. The Eugenics Society, its Sources and its Critics in Britain* (London: Routledge, 1992); Nancy Stepan, *The Idea of Race in Science* (Hamden, Conn.: Archon Books, 1982).

52. For Addison, see also Kenneth and Jane Morgan, *Portrait of a Progressive: the Political Career of Christopher, Viscount Addison* (Oxford: Clarendon Press, 1980).
53. For Dawson, see also Francis Watson, *Dawson of Penn* (London: Chatto and Windus, 1950).
54. Roy Porter, *Doctor of Society: Thomas Beddoes and the Sick Trade in Late Enlightenment England* (London: Routledge, 1991), Conclusion.
55. On Virchow, see Karl Figlio and Paul Weindling, 'Was Social Medicine Revolutionary? Rudolf Virchow and the Revolutions of 1848', *Bulletin of the Society for the Social History of Medicine*, xxxiv (1984), 10–18. See also Ellis, *The Physician-Legislators of France*; E. H. Ackerknecht, *Rudolf Virchow: Doctor, Statesman, Anthropologist* (Madison: University of Wisconsin Press, 1953), 105–18; David Pridan, 'Rudolf Virchow and Social Medicine in Historical Perspective', *Medical History*, ix (1964), 274–8.

56. On experts, see J. A. Passmore, *The Perfectibility of Man* (London: Duckworth, 1970); W. H. G. Armytage, *The Rise of the Technocrats; A Social History* (London: Routledge & Kegan Paul, 1965).
57. For medicine, the St Simonians and the politics of medical expertise in France see Frank Manuel, *The Prophets of Paris* (Cambridge, Mass.: Harvard University Press, 1962); K. Baker, 'The Early History of the Term "Social Science"', *Annals of Science*, xx (1964), 211–26; *idem, Condorcet: From Natural Philosophy to Social Mathematics* (Chicago: Chicago University Press, 1975); J. V. Pickstone, 'Bureaucracy, Liberalism and the Body in Post-Revolutionary France: Bichat's Physiology and the Paris School of Medicine', *History of Science*, xix (1981), 115–42; Dorinda Outram, 'Science and Political Ideology, 1790–1848', in R. C. Olby, G. N. Cantor, J. R. R. Christie, and M. J. S. Hodge (eds), *Companion to the History of Modern Science* (London: Routledge, 1990), 1008–23; Theodore M. Porter, 'Natural Science and Social Theory', in R. C. Olby, G. N. Cantor, J. R. R. Christie, and M. J. S. Hodge (eds), *Companion to the History of Modern Science* (London: Routledge, 1990), 1024–43; B. Haines, 'The Inter-relations between Social, Biological and Medical Thought, 1750–1850: Saint-Simon and Comte', *The British Journal for the History of Science*, xi (1978), 19–35.
58. H. C. Payne, *The Philosophes and the People* (New Haven: Yale University Press, 1976).
59. Adrian Desmond, *The Politics of Evolution. Morphology, Medicine and Reform in Radical London* (Chicago: University of Chicago Press, 1990).
60. Ellis, *The Physician-Legislators of France.*

# 1

## Bentham's Utilitarianism and the Provision of Medical Care

*Janet Semple*

Among the makers of the modern world Jeremy Bentham shares with Lenin the dubious distinction of remaining unburied; their corpses are displayed to the public gaze. There is a move to bury Lenin, but Bentham sits as yet unthreatened, dressed in his velvet jacket, grey trousers and large hat. Unlike Lenin, he chose to be there, believing that his body, his auto-icon, would be a sacred image of a new rationality and an inspiration to future generations of utilitarian philosophers. Few of the small numbers who visit Bentham at University College London are likely to know more about him than that he preached the doctrine of 'the greatest happiness of the greatest number'. This may seem an anodyne idea but it has destroyed empires. For Bentham attempted to teach the world that only representative democracy, freedom of information and free debate could stop rulers oppressing, despoiling and degrading their subjects; ideas that now appear to be triumphantly vindicated. He may be spared the final indignity of a decent burial. His philosophy must not be buried whereas Leninism would be better interred with Lenin.

Bentham's corpse has a special relevance for doctors, it should be a sacred relic of the medical world, a visible sacrifice marking a significant advance in the practice of surgery. The Anatomy Act of 1832 which ensured an adequate supply of bodies for dissection was the work of Bentham and Benthamites. Thereafter paupers from the workhouses whose relations could not afford funeral expenses could be handed over to the anatomists. Before then, dissection had been a cruel extension of punishment reserved for murderers; it now became, as Ruth Richardson in her masterly and moving study maintains, a punishment for the 'unpardonable offence' of poverty.[1]

As with many other aspects of his thought, Bentham's legacy in the field of medical research is ambiguous. Dissection with its associations of prurient curiosity, necrophilia and the complete destruction of the body offended against the customs, sentiments, superstitions and taboos of all classes of society. It even seemed to destroy the hope of life eternal. Every week in the General Confession of the Church of England, congregations reasserted their belief in 'The Resurrection of the body, And the life everlasting'. The Anatomy Act inevitably caused anguish, anxiety and fear among the poor. Bentham certainly agreed with the idea of using the bodies of the poor to supply the anatomy schools; he suggested that hospital patients might, by the act of applying for treatment, be deemed to have given consent to dissection. Bentham may have lacked an imaginative sympathy for the prejudices of the poor but he did have some regard for their sensibilities. He drew a crucial distinction between a post-mortem to discover the cause of death and dissection which anatomised the body. In a draft bill, he proposed that bodies claimed by relations should not be used except in cases with 'extraordinary symptoms' when a post-mortem to ascertain the cause of death could be performed; dissection was confined to unclaimed patients. He deferred to religious sentiments by suggesting that the remains should be afforded a Christian burial – at the expense of the anatomists. Also in contrast to the secrecy that later veiled the administration of the Anatomy Act, the names of the dissected were to be published in the newspapers.[2]

And at least Bentham did have the courage of his convictions and faced himself the physical humiliation of a public dissection. As a young man of 21 he had left his body to his friend, Dr George Fordyce, for medical research and with all the bombast of youth asserted that 'this my Will and special request I make not out of affectation of singularity, but to the intent and with the desire that Mankind may reap some small benefit in and by my decease, having hitherto had small opportunities to contribute thereto while living'.[3] As an old man he added to this simple request; with the feeble facetiousness of extreme age he postulated a 'farther use of the Dead to the Living' in the mass creation of auto-icons: 'If a country gentleman had rows of trees leading to his dwelling, the Auto-Icons of his family might alternate with the trees. Copal varnish would protect the face from the effects of rain.... There might be whole-length Auto-Icons and Auto-Icons of the head alone. In one case many generations might be deposited on a few shelves in a moderate sized cupboard.' For himself he decreed that his skeleton should be macerated, articulated in a sitting position dressed in his clothes and displayed in a box – where he remains to this day. 'Commemoration Clubs there will be, over which the names they bear will preside bodily in the Auto-Icon form ... Whom shall the Bentham Club have for its Chairman? Whom but Bentham himself? On him will all eyes be turned, – to him will all speeches be addressed.'[4]

This bizarre disposal of his remains may have had a reason beyond a pathetic striving for a shadow of immortality; it may have been designed to save him from the recycling, infinite segmentation and disappearance into the medical charnel-houses of the nineteenth-century hospitals. But nevertheless in his willingness to submit his body to the anatomists Bentham was unique among his contemporaries. None of his friends followed his example. Benthamites used his philosophy and his prestige to advocate the dissection of the pauper, but were unable to overcome their sentimental repugnance to the dissection of their own bodies. Bentham alone set an example hoping to encourage a wider public to overcome superstitious fears, an end not achieved until the twentieth century. In this, as in many other matters, Bentham was ahead of his time. His frail little corpse laid on the dissection table has the stark majesty of a Roman hero. Dead, he was a warrior in the cause of rationality, medical advance and human happiness. As his friend and doctor Thomas Southwood Smith said over his body:

> He had a great regard for the science of medicine ... . He knew that the basis of medicine is anatomy, and that the only means of acquiring a knowledge of anatomy is through dissection. He had an utter contempt of the prejudices which withhold the means of pursuing dissection. He was satisfied that there is but one way of putting those prejudices down: and that is, that those who are above them should prove it by giving their own bodies for dissection.[5]

In his contribution to this volume Professor Webb has unravelled the complex influences, religious as well as secular, Unitarian as well as utilitarian, in Smith's inspiration for his life of public service. Bentham's inspiration was more simple. It was drawn from the French Enlightenment and rational secular utilitarianism. His philosophy was based on the seemingly straightforward dictum that 'the greatest happiness of the greatest number' could provide the standard of right and wrong and on the seemingly simple view of human psychology and ethics that: 'Nature has placed mankind under the governance of two sovereign masters, *pain* and *pleasure.* It is for them alone to point out what we ought to do, as well as to determine what we shall do.'[6] This paper will discuss Bentham's utilitarianism as it provided a guide for administrative action; it will not attempt to deal with the complex philosophical problems posed by his theories or the difficulties that arise in deriving personal ethics from utilitarian premises. Bentham's political philosophy, rooted in happiness, has paradoxically become associated with gloomy cheese-paring rigidity. It is perhaps necessary that Bentham should be more clearly distinguished from Benthamites. Bentham argued that the only proper end of government is the greatest happiness of the greatest number of people, or as he preferred to call it later in life, 'the greatest happiness principle'. As a theory of government it has been attacked from two different fronts; firstly that it has led to arrogant insensitive reforms, killing initiative, spontaneity and true happiness; and conversely, that Bentham was a foolish optimist who blithely disregarded the realities of human suffering of which he was himself ignorant. John Stuart Mill with all the passion of the convert denounced Bentham on both counts: 'If he thought at all of any of the deeper feelings of human nature, it was but as idiosyncrasies of taste' and Mill belittled the philosophy as well as the personality of his erstwhile mentor: 'He had neither internal experience nor external.... He never knew prosperity and adversity, passion nor satiety ... he lived from childhood to the age of eighty-five in boyish health. He knew no dejection, no heaviness of heart. He never felt life a sore and weary burthen. He was boy to the last.'[7]

Mill and those who have accepted his valuation show a remarkable lack of sympathy for a reticent man who made no parade of his misfortunes. He had been a delicate child and in the first 12 years of his life he saw five little brothers and sisters and finally his mother die. In middle age he lost a young nephew, in old age a much-loved brother. Bentham's desire to better the lot of humanity was founded on a knowledge of pain. His use of language is partly to blame for these misapprehensions. 'Happiness' has a frivolous ring to it, but when Bentham analyses its components they seem sensible and sober enough. 'Subsistence, abundance, security, equality - to these heads may be reduced the fruits of good government.'[8] Without the means of subsistence, food and shelter to sustain life, no human existence is possible. Abundance, anything over and above, will provide the comforts and amenities of life. The more evenly these good things are spread among the population, the greater will be the sum of happiness. But absolute equality cannot be a proper object of endeavour for natural inequality of talents will make it unstable and bring it into conflict with security. Security is the overriding aim, a security that in Bentham's terms includes the basic liberties of the subject – security against injuries to person, property, reputation or condition in life, security against all oppressions from government, community or neighbours. Security alone is concerned with the future for it enables people to look forward in the knowledge that their lives and property will not be wantonly or capriciously destroyed. On this security of expectation Bentham's philosophy of government rests.

The utilitarian principle that governments should strive after the welfare of their subjects may seem boringly obvious today. But to treat it as a dull truism shows dangerous complacency. Bentham has been the victim of his own success. The widespread triumph of utilitarianism in the nineteenth century has made it seem the ideology of a new established order, but this obscures its essential nature; it remains revolutionary, even subversive. As Stendhal wrote in his description of the reaction after 1815, 'The words *liberty, justice,* and *happiness of the greatest number* are criminal; they give men's minds a habit of discussion.'[9] This habit of discussion is the very essence of Bentham's theory of government. Underlying it is a harsh belief that the interests of rulers are and always will be in diametrical opposition to the interests of their subjects. Whatever the rhetoric, divine sanction, natural law, the general will, or, in our day, the destiny of the nation or the rights of the workers, rulers will end up oppressing and exploiting their subjects. Ruling elites will automatically close ranks to protect their own, cover up mistakes, spend taxpayers money on schemes for their own benefit; and all will protect and extend their powers and privileges. Bentham was not so blind as to deny the existence of altruism, or self-sacrifice or of a selfless benevolence that could inspire a life dedicated to the public good. But such heroics were the exception and any system of administration that relied on them was built on sand. 'It is', he wrote, 'to the general tenor of human conduct, and not to any extraordinary deviations from it, on pain of being ineffectual all such arrangements must be adopted.'[10] During the last years of his life, Bentham came to the realization that the only way to avoid the evils inherent in government was to set up a representative democracy; for only in a democracy can subjects supervise, control and overthrow their rulers. It is the only form of government that will consistently aim at the greatest happiness because the people are themselves sovereign. The interest of every individual has a value equal to any other – each one counts for one and no one for more than one; and each man is the best judge of his own interests. But

Bentham also realized that democratic institutions alone cannot ensure the continuance of good government, they can too easily be subverted by the natural alliance of sinister interest, of corrupt representatives and corrupt governors. This harsh realism is in sharp contrast to the sentimentality of much democratic theory. In his *Constitutional Code* [11] he devised an elaborate system of election and supervision that would ensure that the interests of the rulers became identical with their duty to rule in the interests of their subjects. Public opinion played a crucial role in achieving this junction of interest and duty. Freedom of the press, freedom of discussion, constant debate and the widest dissemination of information would create a workable democracy; government would be open, responsible and responsive to the wishes and needs of the people. Officials' hold on power would be precarious, dependent not only on the acquiescence but on the active support of the people. Policy was subject to constant question and debate. An intellectual ferment sustained and perpetuated Bentham's state. Southwood Smith related Bentham's utilitarianism to his decision to submit his body to dissection. 'By this act, he carries by his own personal example, ... the greatest practical principle for the development and application of which he has raised to himself an immortal name'; that is the principle that the only right and proper end of a community is the 'maximum of the aggregate of happiness'.[12]

The dissection is only the final episode in a long story. As a young man Bentham came to London to embark on a legal career, but recoiling from the corruption of self-seeking lawyers, he refused to practise. An allowance from his father gave him a modicum of financial independence and he embarked on a life devoted to thinking, writing and the reform of the law. Despite the revelation that he possessed 'a genius for legislation' he took a keen interest in other subjects, in particular science, displaying the insatiable curiosity that is the hallmark of genius. Dr A. Dube's challenging new interpretation of Bentham's ethical theory emphasizes the centrality of his application of scientific methods to the study of man and society. He maintains that in Bentham's theory, acquisitiveness inspires men to work and so to the achievement of greater happiness, and is the driving force towards a better society. But Dube does not examine the sources from which these methods derived.[13] Bentham was painfully aware of the inadequacy of the education he had received at Westminster School and Oxford; he had learnt nothing but Greek and Roman myths and theology which he denounced as 'that scourge and reproach to human kind'.

With arrogant snobbery Oxford University had positively discouraged the study of chemistry, 'as a science useless if not pernicious, and which considering what it was and by whom taught could be fit only to make a man an atheist or fit him for an apothecary'. In a sad litany of his ignorance at Oxford, he later confessed: 'I knew nothing of anatomy ... I knew nothing of the manner in which man is preserved from the several calamities by which his health may be affected ... I learnt nothing of the air I breathed in ... I knew not what the sea contained'.[14] In the London of the 1770s he was able to remedy these deficiencies, becoming something of a polymath. Much effort has been expended on uncovering the roots of Bentham's philosophy in Hobbes, Helvétius, or Beccaria, but little on the influence of the scientists, Hunter, Bergman, Fordyce and Priestley, with whom he consorted and corresponded. He became a close friend of one of the most eminent physicians and chemists of the day, Dr George Fordyce, and attended his lectures 'on the practise of Physic'. He reconciled this with his other studies, for the extra work involved 'took me up but an hour before breakfast, which scarce ever is my time for writing'.[15] Fordyce introduced him to an exclusive club of scientific men where he rubbed shoulders with the great John Hunter himself. Bentham also studied chemistry under Fordyce and himself dabbled in experiments in botany and in the composition of gases and metals. He wrote to Joseph Priestley describing an improved 'Apparatus for generating airs'.[16] Priestley was 'exceedingly obliged' but although he had no objection to the apparatus he feared that 'it must be rather troublesome in practice'. But Priestley had a real respect for Bentham's efforts and ability. 'I have no doubt', he wrote on another occasion, 'but that if you were to go to work in good earnest you would do something considerable ... I shall be very glad to hear from you when you begin to do any thing.'[17] Bentham also assisted in the English translation of Torben Bergman's essay *On the Usefulness of Chemistry*. For most people this would be a taxing intellectual exercise, but with arrogant condescension, Bentham described himself as 'a man whose principal pursuits lie in a widely different line, and who was tempted to step aside for a few moments into this distant and more amusing field in quest of a relaxation that might sweeten the toil of a severer study'.[18]

Bentham never applied himself seriously to scientific experiment and the 'severer study' of law and punishment came to monopolize his attention. He first addressed the question of medical care when he debated the appointment of doctors for his panopticon prison;

he suggested that this might be a suitable post for a ship's surgeon. Bentham put much faith in his measures of preventive medicine, a rigid regime, hard work, warmth, cleanliness, exercise, light, air, an adequate but plain diet, regular sleep and an abstinence from alcohol. These he believed would prevent sickness in the prison and would therefore leave the doctor ample time to indulge a taste for chemical experiment. When, in 1797, he extended his panopticon principles to provision for the poor, he advocated a similar regime for paupers and his ambitions had expanded; he aspired now to preside over a great research establishment. Bentham's proposals were published in the *Annals of Agriculture* and for several years he hoped that the government would adopt them. To the end of his life he nursed a bitter disappointment that they had been ignored by the political establishment. Bentham's system of poor law provision was based on a network of 250 industry houses spaced around the country, no more than 10 3/8 miles apart. But the pauper population was predominantly in the arable areas of the south and east of England and a rational system would have concentrated relief there. Bentham had allowed his passion for symmetry to override considerations of common sense and geography. Each industry house would initially have contained 2000 people, but within 21 years this would have risen to 5000. So Bentham was envisaging a pauper community of a million – a staggeringly large proportion of a population of around nine million. All those needing relief would have to enter the house and they would be able to leave only when they had worked sufficiently to pay the cost of their provision. All the maimed, the sick, the able-bodied, the old, the children would be gathered in, some categories, such as beggars and prostitutes, by force. One of the least attractive aspects of Bentham's scheme is his detailed analysis of how every scrap of work could be extracted and every ability exploited.[19]

Bentham at first envisaged that these industry houses would be administered by government, but on further consideration, he realized that they would be more economically and efficiently managed by a joint stock company analogous to the East India Company; it was to be called the National Charity Company. Profit would provide the motive for good frugal management; public inspection and careful bookkeeping would ensure that the inmates were decently and humanely treated. This proposal to reform the poor law was far more than a practical scheme to manage workhouses. Bentham invested in it his hopes for the future of mankind, it would be a vast social experiment, a 'crucible of men', an ideal society highly regimented but safe, secure and dynamic; a society organized for the creation of wealth and the improvement of living standards. A component of this utopia was a national scheme for medical care which would have met the needs of the whole of the labouring population.

The treatment of the indigent is one of the most contentious areas in the application of utilitarian ideas. Some of the most repulsive and punitive aspects of the new poor law have been credited to Benthamites. Edwin Chadwick, the architect of the Amendment Act of 1834 and one of the commissioners entrusted with its administration, was a follower and friend of Bentham and his mentor's influence can be clearly seen in some of the provisions of the Act. It is not possible within the confines of this paper to deal adequately in any way with this complex and controversial question; but it might be instructive to distinguish Bentham more carefully from his followers. His ideas were nurtured in the soil of enlightened optimism and in a perhaps naïve belief in the rationality of man. He also made the assumption, derived from Adam Smith, that wealth could be indefinitely increased. In contrast, his followers were greatly influenced by the dismal science of later economists and above all by Malthusian theory. They inclined to see the growing population of the poor as a threat to living standards. To a writer in *The Edinburgh Review* in 1820, it seemed self-evident that 'the present redundant population of the country has been entirely produced by the Poor-Laws'. Relief must be abolished, albeit gradually; it had been madness to create this surplus population, but it would be cold-blooded cruelty to get rid of them by other than gentle means.[20] In contrast, Bentham saw population as a source of greater wealth and the engine of a dynamic economy. It is not possible to re-assess here Bentham's contribution to the poor law debate, but one general point can be made. The grinding exploitation of labour in which he delighted was to be employed not just to generate profits for a successful joint stock company, but also to create an alternative society in which the lot of the poor would be steadily ameliorated. The influence of scientific methods, the careful collection of facts, experiment, deduction and publication of results came to form the framework of his utilitarian theory of administration.

Bentham emphasized the crucial distinction between the poor, whom he defined as all those who needed to work for their subsistence, and the indigent, those who needed relief. And he was clear that the interests of each individual, poor or indigent, must be safeguarded. 'But what is possible to government,' he wrote, 'and what it is the duty of government to do is to abstain from doing any thing that shall put the poor man as such in a worse condition than the rich in any respect: whether in respect of his property, his liberty, his reputation, his life or his domestic or political rights. In all these respects the duty of government has been violated by the laws in being.' Wages were the very foundation of security and subsistence: 'The wages of the poor are the patrimony, the only property of the poor ... A country is rich or poor according to the condition of the majority of its inhabitants and the great, the vast majority of the inhabitants of every country is constituted by the poor.'[21] Relief of indigence was a necessity and must not be left to the caprice of private charity; it was a fundamental duty of government to ensure the subsistence and security of all members of the community. But it must never be forgotten that the indigent were maintained at the expense of the poor – work must therefore be a condition of receiving relief – and the condition of life of the pauper should not be superior to that of the labouring classes. Bentham did not argue that it should deliberately be made less attractive; the enforcement of less eligibility derived from Chadwick rather than Bentham. Bentham was temperamentally benevolent and preferred to dwell on the myriad advantages that his schemes would bring to the people: cheap travel, security for savings, assured employment, annuities and, above all, medical care.

Bentham had divided the country into areas centred on each industry house; the house would function as a dispensary and indeed might replace the county hospital. Within these areas, a medical curator and his apprentice doctors, sub-curators, would practise. The medical curator, possibly a former ship's surgeon, would be paid a salary, the sub-curators would give their services free. The doctors would be expected to minister to the needs not only of the paupers within the house but of the independent poor outside. Bentham believed that doctors should tender for the salaried positions, the man willing to do it for the least amount of money being the most acceptable. 'Where a man, of undisputed fitness, accepts a duty with *small pay,* or what is still better no pay at all, it is ... not only so much the better in point of *economy,* but the better for the *service.* From his taking the situation *with* a salary, all you can know is, that he likes the *salary;* from his taking the situation *without* salary, what you are *sure of* is that he likes the *service.*'[22] It is possible that in this suggestion is the origin of the system of tendering that contributed to the degradation and servile dependence of the Union doctors in the nineteenth century.[23] But

Bentham was acutely aware that the interest of doctors must be protected and be made to coincide with their duty. They would not be allowed to charge for their services to the poor nor make money by selling drugs. But there would be advantages in the service. The drugs dispensed would be the property of the government, 'brought under proper *professional* inspection, upon the largest and most economical scale, at the most advantageous market'. The quantity of the dosage and the quality of all drugs would be approved by a committee of the College of Physicians who would produce public reports of their efficacy.

Bentham carefully analysed the motives that would inspire the doctors: they would have the opportunity to practise; they would become known among the better-off labourers and the 'Friendly Society men'; they would have access to the superior drugs approved by the College of Physicians; and above all, they would gain in reputation, emulating the achievements of their fellows. Bentham does, however, rely partly on the altruism of the medical profession, but it is an altruism based on self-interest: 'backwardness in point of attendance, whether any thing be or be not to be got by it, is a failing neither frequent in the practice, nor natural to the situation, of this most beneficient and respectable of all temporal professions for tho' the *pocket* should fail to be enriched by visits to the poor, the stock of *experience,* of *skill* and thence of *reputation* can never miss of its increase. Accordingly, gratuitous assistance is as notoriously *abundant* in the medical profession, as in *others* it is rare.'[24] With midwives the junction of interest and duty was to be more directly enforced: 'the pay of the midwife ... might be made more or less dependent on *success. Half* the fee might be deducted, in the case of death, of either the *mother or child,* within the *month:* the *half,* or the whole of the *remainder,* in the case of the death of *both* within that period.'[25]

When it came to the question of the collection of information and statistics Bentham allowed full rein to his inventive genius. The industry houses were to be centres of a range of medical experiments based on the careful collection of information. A record would be kept of each case, details of the patient, the date when the illness began, its duration, nature and symptoms, the number of visits paid by the doctor, the regime suggested, the drugs prescribed, the subsequent symptoms and the outcome of the illness. Comprehensive morbidity and mortality statistics covering the whole of the labouring classes were to be collected and published. Correlations between health and weather, health and diet, health and abstinence from alcohol, health and occupation, health and locality were to be made. Such statistics would have laid the foundations of a comprehensive epidemiology. Normal health as well as disease was to be studied. The stages of child development were to be monitored. Bentham, a childless bachelor, nevertheless provided a list of the steps which if recorded would have created a framework for paediatrics. Each child was to have a progress book – a 'Calendar of Hebe' – in which would be recorded their age, and when certain developments took place, among them awareness of light, smiling, recognizing persons, appearance of first tooth, attempt to imitate sounds, standing supported, walking alone.[26] The validity of this plan has recently been recognized: 'The list shows Bentham's prescience in conceptualising the data that would need to be collected before we could properly understand the temporal steps in a child's development'.[27] Strength should be tested at regular intervals and the results correlated with diet; the medical effects of age of marriage and child bearing should be monitored. The industry houses would be centres of medical education. In 1797, Bentham did not discuss the controversial question of the dissection of human remains, but he suggested that the medical curators should give public lectures on veterinary medicine and that all domestic animals found dead should be conveyed to the house where the cause of death would be ascertained.[28]

The industry houses were to be instruments of scientific advance in all fields. Bentham enthusiastically extolled his vision in words that encapsulate his reliance on scientific methods and his passion for scientific discovery.

> Observation and experiment compose the basis of all knowledge. The basis, in proportion as it spreads in extent, swells in solidity and value. Hitherto the stock of relative *data,* or known facts, the materials of which this basis is composed, has been in almost every line ... scanty, accidental, irregular, incomplete, both as to time, and place, – the scattered fruit of the uncombined exertions of unconnected individuals. The institution of the proposed Company would afford the first opportunity ever presented to mankind, of enriching the treasury of useful knowledge by contributions furnished on a national scale, and on a regular and all-embracing plan; and would thus form an epoch.... The sciences which now await this epoch, for a degree of improvement altogether unattainable by any other means, would thus be raised to a pitch of certainty, to which neither example, nor, till now, so much as conception, has perhaps ever reached. The advancement of knowledge is performed ... as new lights are added to the old stock;

> in the way of dissemination, in proportion as the multitude of individuals, to whom any part of the existing stock of lights has been communicated, is increased.[29]

Bentham planned the publication of digests of medical statistics which would form the basis of informed discussion and the furtherance of knowledge. Each industry house would keep a medical register, returns from which would be sent to the College of Physicians in London. Abstracts of these would form a complete body of medical transactions in relation to the poor: 'An accumulating body of medical information, authentic and universal, would thus be annually poured into the treasury of useful knowledge. It is by such means, and such alone, that the progress of improvement, in this most important walk of science can be made to receive its utmost degree of acceleration.' These medical transactions would become required reading for all doctors and Bentham suggested that 'The obligation of *buying* it, might be made a condition of the *permission to practice* in the profession, in any of its branches'.[30] In these ideas on the collection and dissemination of medical information and statistics Bentham was well ahead of his time. It was not until 1911 with Lloyd George's Health Insurance Act that doctors were required to make any such returns – and in the event they were too random and disorganized to be of any use. It is only now with the use of computer technology that any semblance of reality can be given to Bentham's dream.[31]

The organization of medical care within the framework of the industry houses is a forerunner of Bentham's mature constitutional theory. He applied to government the scientific methods learnt in the lecture rooms of London doctors in the 1770s. He came to see the legislator's role as that of a physician ministering to the body politic; a society could sicken as could a man and might be healed by the methods derived from medical practice. He wrote: 'Arithmetic and medicine – these are the branches of art and science to which, in so far as the maximum of happiness is the object of his endeavours, the legislator must look for his means of operation: – the pains or losses of pleasure produced by a maleficent act correspond to the symptoms produced by a disease. Experience, observation, and experiment – these are the foundations of all well-grounded medical practice: experience, observation, and experiment – such are the foundations of all well-grounded legislative practice.'[32] When Bentham applied this analogy to penal law he drew conclusions that have profound implications for the infliction of punishment. Crimes were the disorders of society and so:

> Occupied on the penal branch of law, the legislator is its medical practitioner – its surgeon. In a surgical operation the cure is the benefit: the pain of the patient the burthen. The operations of the surgeon have for their object, the rendering the cure as prompt and as complete as possible, at the expense of as little pain as possible. The surgeon, when he cuts into the bladder of the patient for the extraction of a stone – does he say, the patient *deserves* to be so cut? Not he indeed: by no surgeon was any such absurdity ever uttered. The possessor of political power ... has, at all times, in all places, uttered it without a blush. Why? Because ... the magistrate – the legislator – such is man's nature – have been tyrants: tyrants having each of them, for the object of his acts as such – not the greatest happiness of the greatest number, but his own single greatest happiness.[33]

The Constitutional Code mirrors the panopticon industry houses; each relies on the collection, analysis, dissemination and free discussion of knowledge. What is lacking in Bentham's poor law proposals is the element of democracy; that came later. Bentham often failed in imaginative sympathy for the poor and displayed an almost callous disregard for their dignity. In the National Charity Company he created a machine for the regimentation and exploitation of labour down to the most minute detail. It was based on the utilization of every scrap of productive power from the old, the infirm, the disabled and little children. The Anatomy Act exemplifies the same unattractive side of utilitarian reform, riding roughshod over customary death rituals and beliefs, causing untold mental agony and adding to the corroding fear of poverty that haunted the English working class into the twentieth century. But there is another side to the argument: an essential ingredient of Benthamite security is that the law and its administration should be certain and uniform, it should exclude, as far as possible, the workings of chance and caprice – in Benthamite language, contingency must be minimized. These principles can be clearly seen in the security and certainty of the industry houses. The Anatomy Act also aimed to increase security by ending the chaotic chance of grave robbery which had left vulnerable all mourners and all those facing death. The Act backfired, creating uncertainty, fear and anguish. But perhaps one of the major reasons for this is that it was not subjected to public scrutiny. The passage of the Act was marked by a clever manipulation of parliamentary processes, it slipped through without adequate debate or consideration of alternative provisions. Its administration was shrouded in secrecy; the medical profession and the politicians colluded in deliberately stifling public debate until the twentieth century. This would have been anathema to Bentham. His theory of government depended on freedom of information and discussion, or as he put it, 'the uncorrupted, free and ever open Public Opinion Tribunal'; anyone endeavouring to suppress this freedom is 'an enemy to all happiness, to all virtue, to all mankind'.[34] And it should not be forgotten that Bentham's utilitarianism would have required universal manhood suffrage in the 1830s. The only limitation he suggested was a simple literacy test – and he believed that reading and writing could be easily mastered. He envisaged a democracy enlightened by education and debate. The franchise advocated by Bentham was not achieved until 1918. One might speculate that legislation such as the Anatomy Act and the Poor Law Amendment Act that criminalized poverty and degraded the poor would not have survived in Bentham's democracy. When the political parties had to win the votes of the working class the interests and sensibilities of the poor became a matter of consideration. The voice of the poor would have had to be heard in Bentham's land. But history and medicine took a different road; there is a paradox as yet unresolved between the intellectual arrogance of the utilitarians and their insistence on free debate. Bentham still sits, an ambiguous icon of his principles and of medical experiment: the legacy of both is still in dispute.

## Notes

1. R. Richardson, *Death, Dissection and the Destitute* (London: Routledge & Kegan Paul, 1987), 270–81. I am deeply indebted to this remarkable book for my treatment of the Anatomy Act throughout this paper.
2. R. Richardson, 'Bentham and "Bodies for Dissection"', *The Bentham Newsletter*, x (1986), 24.
3. *The Correspondence of Jeremy Bentham* (*C W*), ed. T. S. L. Sprigge (London: The Athlone Press, 1968), i 136.
4. J. Bentham, *Auto-Icon; or Farther Uses of the Dead to the Living* (not published), 3, 5.
5. T. Southwood Smith, *A Lecture Delivered over the Remains of Jeremy Bentham, Esq., in the Webb Street School of Anatomy and Medicine, on the 9th June 1832* (London, 1832), 62–3.
6. J. Bentham, *An Introduction to the Principles of Morals and Legislation* in *Utilitarianism*, M. Warnock (ed.), (London: Fontana Press, 1990), 33. Bentham's emphasis.
7. J. S. Mill, 'Bentham', in *Utilitarianism*, M. Warnock, (ed.),101, 96–7.
8. UC (Bentham Mss. at University College London), clxii 137.

9. *Le Chartreuse de Parme,* cited in F. B. Artz, *Reaction and Revolution 1815–1852* (New York and London: Harper, 1963), 4. Stendhal's emphasis.
10. UC, clxxii 228.
11. *Constitutional Code, Volume I* (*The Collected Works of Jeremy Bentham*), F. Rosen and J. H. Burns (ed), (Oxford: Clarendon Press, 1983).
12. Southwood Smith, *op. cit.*, 4, 7.
13. A. Dube, *The Theme of Acquisitiveness in Bentham's Political Thought* (New York, London: Garland Publishing Inc., 1991).
14. UC, clvi 2–7.
15. *Correspondence* (*CW*), i 240.
16. *Ibid.*, 210–16.
17. *Ibid.*, 225, 265.
18. UC, clvi 2–3.
19. *'Tracts on Poor Laws and Pauper Management'*, in *The Works of Jeremy Bentham*, J. Bowring (ed.), (11 vols., Edinburgh: William Tait, 1838–43), viii 358–433. See C. F. Bahmueller, *The National Charity Company. Jeremy Bentham's Silent Revolution* (Berkeley, Los Angeles, London: University of California Press, 1981) for a full if somewhat polemical account.
20. *The Edinburgh Review* or Critical Journal, 1820, xxxiii 95.
21. UC, cli 7b, 20.
22. UC, cliii 50. Bentham's emphasis.
23. This question is fully discussed in I. Loudon, *Medical Care and the General Practitioner 1750–1850* (Oxford: Clarendon Press 1986), 244–5.
24. UC, clii 46–7. Bentham's emphasis.
25. *Ibid.*, 53. Bentham's emphasis.
26. Bowring, viii 426.
27. *Paediatrics* (1981), 68, 447.
28. Bowring, viii 428.
29. *Ibid.*, 424–5.
30. UC, cliii 48 Bentham's emphasis.
31. I am indebted to Dr Ian Tait for this information.
32. Bowring, iii 224.
33. Bowring, ix 23. Bentham's emphasis.
34. *First Principles Preparatory to Constitutional Code* (*CW*), P. Schofield (ed.), (Oxford: Clarendon Press, 1989), 292.

# 2

## Southwood Smith: The Intellectual Sources of Public Service

*R. K. Webb*

In the study of the political or public career of a doctor – or of any professional – several possible strategies present themselves. First, most obvious and most important, is simply to set down in appropriate detail what happened, as that can be extracted from the documentary record. Then one might turn to the political or administrative dynamics underlying the public work: to understand them requires a deeper reading of the record informed by familiarity with the context in which the career was played out. There is, however, a range of antecedent questions that are more difficult to answer: what motives lay behind the choice of career and shaped its particular development? how were the mind and personality of the subject formed and adapted to a public role? how did the ideas of one person relate to those of contemporaries?

In the past century or so it has been fairly easy to cope convincingly with such questions. The self-revelation of autobiographies and diaries, which public figures provide in abundance these days, must always remain suspect, and the voluminous written record is often formal and evasive, with individuality sunk in committees or lost in the transience of telephone conversations. But the institutional matrices out of which public figures have emerged since the latter years of the nineteenth century – schools, universities and other academic bodies, government, the media, even the churches – are relatively homogeneous and well-understood sources of influences easy to identify and trace. And knowledge of these sources supplements a wealth of accessible information about family, education, evaluations of performance, economic status, medical history, and the like.

When Southwood Smith emerged as one of the founders of the

public-health movement in Britain in the second quarter of the nineteenth century, the context that we now take for granted as available (with due caution) for biographical extrapolation was far more complex and obscure. Local communities were more varied and more formative than they have been in the nationalized culture of the past hundred years; education was fragmented and much of it done entirely apart from any institutional structure; religion was central to a degree now unimaginable; and much information that is now commonplace has been lost or was never set down where a historian could find it. In this confusion, there is great temptation to rely on conventional or gross historical categories, to generalize from obvious associations, and to foreshorten through the application of unthinking prejudice – to equate, for example, self-education with poor education, religious nonconformity with narrowness, and a provincial background with provinciality.

Although much in Smith's life remains inaccessible, there is a remarkable range of published and unpublished work which, when properly set into its institutional and intellectual context, can illumine a career of the first importance in the history of medical administration and of the public service generally. This essay will, then, say less about what Smith did than about why and how he did it, less about the immensity of his accomplishment than about how that accomplishment fits into a larger personal and philosophical unity.

A suggestive way into this inquiry is offered by a debate that thirty years ago moderately exercised historians of Victorian Britain. It was concerned with the 'nineteenth-century revolution in government' – the extension of state intervention to new areas of concern and the transformation of the organs of the state and of their way of doing business – and, specifically, with the role of Jeremy Bentham and his followers in forcing and shaping this fundamental change.[1] As the debate unfolded, Dr George Kitson Clark intervened to point out that, while the present-day ideal of a professional, non-political, and anonymous civil service can be traced back at least to the 1830s, it was not realized until the late nineteenth century.[2] Many of the key figures in the Victorian revolution in government were well-known, controversial, and even notorious figures – among them Edwin Chadwick, Rowland Hill, J. R. Porter, and James Kay-Shuttleworth. Precluded for social reasons from serving as ministers, these 'statesmen in disguise' were not brought in at an early age to be formed in the service, but were appointed (under the often unjustly reviled system of patronage) in their thirties or even forties because their established reputations as 'veteran publicists and controversialists' or their advocacy of certain programmes qualified them as experts who could take on urgent tasks in a government otherwise quite unprepared to do so.

In the course of his argument, Dr Kitson Clark suggested that the country was fortunate at that juncture to have 'an unusually large number of people whose habits of mind fitted them for this task, men who could be trusted to apply to any problem careful systematic observation and self-confident and rigorous argument working from relatively simple and superficial first principles and not confused by too profound or intrusive a philosophy'. Among them, he said, would certainly have to be numbered the followers of Jeremy Bentham, 'but to call all such men Benthamites is certainly to narrow too much to one group a much more generalized contemporary cast of mind'. To make his point, he instanced (among others) those whose medical training had taught them the importance of systematic observation.

The career of Southwood Smith is remarkably pertinent to Kitson Clark's argument, for Smith was both a physician and an intimate of Jeremy Bentham's in the last decade of the philosopher's life. But Smith was also a Unitarian, at a time when that denomination in England was powerfully influenced by a philosophical and theological system called 'necessarianism'. Unitarians were few in number in English society, but important out of all proportion to their numbers, for most of the nineteenth century; committed necessarians were relatively few within the denomination but, again, important out of all proportion to their numbers, though for somewhat less of the century. One segment of that 'generalized contemporary cast of mind', Unitarians, and necessarians, also remind us of the striking intellectual pluralism of late eighteenth- and early nineteenth-century English society, in which men and women formed in many different but related ways came together in a common enterprise, without losing the identity, style, and confidence rooted distinctively in their varied origins.[3]

Harold Laski once said that Smith's public-health work had no more to do with his Unitarianism than Lord Halifax's desire for an accommodation with the Nazis had to do with his being a Trinitarian Anglican.[4] But to refute Laski in this particular case and to understand why Unitarianism helps so much in explaining Smith, it is necessary first to trace the main outlines of a religion whose tenets and force are now little appreciated.

English Unitarianism emerged as a distinct denomination in the last years of the eighteenth and the early years of the nineteenth century. Its principal base lay in English Presbyterianism, once the largest of the denominations that made up Old Dissent but which had been much reduced in numbers through defections (largely to the Congregationalists) brought about by the clash of a rising Evangelicalism with the heterodox ideas increasingly evident among younger ministers and prominent laymen. The Unitarians could also count some important recruits from the Church of England and from the orthodox Dissenters; the little remnant of the General Baptists that had survived an Evangelical schism in 1770 gradually became more closely allied to the Unitarians, while early in the nineteenth century a few congregations in Lancashire came over from the Methodists.

As a theology, however, Unitarianism long antedated the new denomination: it was one response to the impulse to rational religion broadly evident in both Church and Dissent in the eighteenth century. A significant number of healthy-minded individuals (as William James would have called them) were convinced that nature reflected the design and beneficence (and proved the existence) of God, but, unlike the Deists, they insisted on the continuing relevance and authority of Revelation and on the centrality of the life, death, and resurrection of Jesus Christ. The application of reason to religion inevitably came up against the central Christian dogma of the Trinity. As early as the 1630s, some English rationalists were well acquainted with the writings of the Continental followers of the Italian heresiarchs, Lelio and Fausto Sozzini, who had questioned the divinity of Christ, while others were pushed to similar conclusions by study of the Bible. For much of the Restoration period, the Church was embroiled in Socinian controversy, and by the second decade of the eighteenth century, anti-Trinitarianism had begun to have an impact in the ranks of Dissent, at first in the qualified form of Arianism, which maintained Christ's divinity but saw Him as subordinate to God the Father.

Despite this drift, orthodox and heterodox Dissent maintained an uneasy accommodation until mid-century when a powerful Evangelicalism commanding the allegiance of the majority came into inevitable conflict with the growing conviction among the latitudinarian few that Jesus was purely human – a doctrine that escaped what Unitarians were coming to see as the moral difficulties of a substitutionary Atonement and that also offered a powerful inducement to emulation. Gradually thereafter, Arianism was eclipsed by Unitarianism, as Socinianism was rechristened to avoid the overtones of abuse that clung to the older term.

What set early nineteenth-century English Unitarianism apart from Unitarian movements in other countries was the powerful influence of Joseph Priestley. Priestley is best known today as the discoverer of oxygen and as one of the founders of modern chemistry, a claim to fame almost matched by his celebrated political radicalism. In the past quarter-century, however, historians of science and of political thought have begun to recognize how deeply both enterprises were rooted in his religion. Raised as an orthodox Calvinist, Priestley quickly became an Arian after entering Daventry Academy in 1752 and then, having himself been an innovative teacher at Warrington Academy in the 1760s, he turned Unitarian in 1768 as a result of reading the just-published *Letter on the Logos,* written nearly 40 years earlier by the great Dissenting scholar Nathaniel Lardner. Much earlier, while a student at Daventry, Priestley had been persuaded by the conclusions in David Hartley's *Observations on Man,* which had appeared in 1749. The notion of a psychology dependent on the polarities of pleasure and pain and on the instrumentality of association of ideas drew on earlier writers, but Hartley, taking up a suggestion of Sir Isaac Newton, offered a novel explanation of the working of association of ideas through vibrations in nerves and brain in response to impressions on the senses. He placed his elaborated psychology in a grand religious framework that set him apart from his contemporary David Hume, whose psychology was moving in a parallel direction: compared with Dr Hartley as a reasoner, Priestley was to write, 'I consider Mr. Hume as not even a child'.[5]

Hartley made Priestley a determinist, or, as he called it, a necessarian.[6] Because men act in obedience to motives, Hartley and Priestley maintained that it was impossible for anyone to act differently while the state of the mind – its motives, the complex ideas formed by association from sense impressions – remained unaltered. All such actions to the end of time were present to God's foreknowledge, but Priestley insisted that he was no fatalist, that in acting a necessarian might feel as free as anyone; what he did deny was 'metaphysical liberty', the notion that one could choose to act differently without a prior change in the state of mind and so of motives.

Two related considerations were of particular significance for the future. One was an all-encompassing view of Providence. Evil, in this view, is part of a divine plan that we, with our limited capacities, cannot comprehend – that was a theological commonplace, as hundreds of funeral sermons attest. But the beneficent and all-seeing God of Hartley and Priestley, working not directly but through human agency, had provided a way to remedy and ultimately to eliminate evil. We suffer through ignorance of divine laws; our knowledge of those laws is steadily expanding, in the realm of morals as well as of nature. In consequence and in time, through education of one sort or another, all men could thus be made aware of their best interests and so brought to happiness, and the benevolent man or woman had an obligation to help on this great providential scheme. The second consideration, then, is a cosmic optimism that carried with it specific means of bringing about that consummation through the study of natural and moral philosophy, through education, and through the right ordering of institutions.

Priestley's materialism, also drawn from Hartley and confirmed by his own researches and those of other scientists of his time, posed a serious problem for some of his Unitarian followers, especially in the Victorian period, though Priestley had never insisted on its acceptance. The difficulty was that if mind was a function of the body, which was dissolved at death, belief in the resurrection of the dead through some unimaginable mechanism could (like the authentic miracles) rest only on biblical authority, a frail reed as biblical criticism (at which the Priestleyans were themselves pioneers) moved relentlessly forward. But a future life was essential to the necessarian scheme, for there happiness would be attained if it was not on earth; and by the end of his life, Priestley had become a convinced believer in universal restoration, the certainty that all men would be saved and the ultimate rejection of his ancestral Calvinism. In this view, life on earth is probative and educational, sin is remediable error, and the possibility of perfection, even on earth, was reinforced by the example of a fully human Jesus, who owed His perfection not to His divinity but to His having learned it.

Priestley was nearly half a century in arriving at the full development of his theology. That his younger followers could telescope that long evolution into a brief span of time was owing in part to the remarkable series of polemics that Priestley published in the decade and a half after his conversion to Unitarianism. Priestleyanism swept through the Dissenting academies in the 1780s, pushing Arians into Unitarianism and carrying some from the orthodox end of the spectrum swiftly to the opposite extreme. This theological radicalism was closely associated with political radicalism, given impetus by the American Revolution, by the political events of the 1780s, and, above all, by the French Revolution: it was a sermon preached in 1789 by Priestley's Arian friend Richard Price that triggered Burke's *Reflections* a year later.

The reaction was terrible – the riots in Birmingham in 1791, of which the prominent Unitarian community there was the principal target; Priestley's losses in those riots and his ultimate emigration to America (emulated in expectation or reality by many others); the transportation of the Rev. Thomas Fyshe Palmer to Botany Bay; the suspicion visited on Unitarians everywhere and the further decline of their congregations and their reputation. Most historians of religion have eagerly pointed to that falling-off, but the little band of survivors themselves thought by the second decade of the new century that the tide had turned and that in time they would sweep all before them.[7]

Although there were grounds for that confidence in the circumstances of the immediate postwar world, not least the legalization of anti-Trinitarian religion in 1813, the reality turned out to be quite different. With the capture of most of Dissent and much of the Church by Evangelicalism, the Unitarians were almost alone in maintaining the cause of liberal religion in the first three-quarters of the nineteenth century. They had a panoply of means to propagandize their views, both theological and philosophical, to confirm their members in their faith and to carry their message to the non-Unitarian world. Sermons, lectures, and discussion groups in congregations were reinforced by reading and conversation in families and in those circles of like-minded people that formed such a striking feature of provincial society: we have much evidence in letters and diaries to support this reinforcing role.[8] Denominational journals and newspapers, of internal importance but also recognized outside, were seconded by the extensive part played by Unitarians in the burgeoning general periodical and newspaper press of the period.[9] They tended to educate their children, girls as well as boys, in generally excellent schools, and these schools sometimes attracted pupils from outside the Unitarian fold. Manchester College, now at Oxford and the sole Unitarian remnant of the Dissenting academies, had a most distinguished career in the nineteenth century, educating lay as well as divinity students as late as the 1850s, while the University of London founded in the 1820s (that is, University College London) and the new provincial universities later in the century bore a notable Unitarian impress – hardly surprising in view of the key role played by education in the Unitarian scheme of things and of the importance of Unitarians in the political and intellectual culture of provincial towns.

To be sure, the Unitarians lost the Dissenting leadership they had inherited from their Presbyterian forebears to a newly aggressive and vengeful orthodoxy among Congregationalists and Baptists; they saw some of their number drift away to free thought or to the Church, though they continued to appeal to newly liberated minds in need of shelter against the winds of doctrine. By no means were all Unitarians theologically or philosophically literate, but the general outlines of this dogmatic faith were widely accepted; moreover, there was a definable and distinctive Unitarian culture which, particularly in the Priestleyan phase of the first half of the century, gave committed believers the means of testing and interpreting their experience, of ordering their priorities, of perceiving a way to analyse and resolve problems. That culture also reinforced the obligations Unitarianism imposed to follow its dictates in religious and secular society.

Thomas Southwood Smith was born at Martock, near Yeovil in Somerset, on 21 December, 1788. His parents, William Smith and Catherine Southwood, were strict Baptists, and the boy was early destined for the ministry.[10] In 1802 at the age of 14, he entered the Baptist Academy in Bristol (now Bristol Baptist College) on a generous scholarship that reflected the impression he made on the academy's leaders. But doubts set in, and Smith left the institution, by that action cutting himself off forever from his family. In 1808, he married Anne Read, the daughter of a Bristol manufacturer and a supporter of the Academy; the couple had two daughters, Caroline and Emily, who fell to their father's sole charge on the death of Anne, from fever, in 1812.

Although little information is now available about the course of Smith's life down to 1812, a few important contextual points must be made. One, rightly emphasized by Dr Poynter, is that the Baptist Academy, though strictly Calvinist in its theology, shared in the assumption characteristic of eighteenth-century religion that the study of natural philosophy and the study of religion were mutually reinforcing; accordingly, the Academy had a commendable array of scientific apparatus, though scientific instruction in Smith's time was only uncertainly part of the curriculum.[11]

A second point is the existence of an impressive range of material and psychological support within an enlightened provincial town and the Unitarian community in particular. Smith's parents knew the Unitarian minister at Crewkerne, William Blake, who was one of the boy's supporters in his application to the Academy – a salutary reminder that sectarian boundaries were sometimes more easily bridged then than later.[12] Through Blake the young Smith was also put into touch with an imposing network of leaders of both the medical profession and Rational Dissent. Blake's brother Malachi was a prominent physician in Taunton, and when Smith entered on his spiritual crisis, William Blake sent him for advice to John Prior Estlin, the Priestleyan minister of Lewin's Mead Chapel in Bristol, one of the most distinguished Unitarian congregations in the country. Estlin's son, John Bishop Estlin, was a celebrated eye surgeon in Bristol who was in turn closely connected with the famous Bristol physician Thomas Beddoes, who died in 1808. Perhaps more important than anyone was Benjamin Spencer, a Bristol surgeon who had himself left the Baptists many years earlier to become Unitarian and to pursue the study of medicine at Edinburgh.[13] When his wife's death brought a new crisis in Smith's life, it was his Bristol friends who arranged support from the Unitarian Fund for his studies at Edinburgh, where he went in 1812.

In Edinburgh, Smith pursued the study of medicine and the propagandizing of Unitarianism with equal success. He received his MD in 1816, and meanwhile had taken over the pulpit of the Edinburgh congregation, the ancestor of the present St Mark's Church in Castle Terrace, which can trace its remote ancestry to the 1630s but whose formal, if unsteady history since 1776 had been primarily as an offshoot of the English Universalist movement. Smith was also active in organizing the Scottish Unitarian Association, to proselytize for Unitarianism throughout the northern kingdom.[14]

Smith was remarkably well placed to inspire the Edinburgh congregation to new life. As a refugee from the rigours of Calvinism, he, like other Baptist recruits to Unitarianism at the same period,[15] was especially attracted by the doctrine of universal restoration, which, as we have seen, was the last element that Priestley added to his theological amalgam. But Smith was also a learned and cultivated man, far more able to appeal to the educated audience that Edinburgh offered than some of his humbler predecessors.[16]

In 1816, Smith published his Latin thesis for the doctorate, *De morbis mente laesa*, which proclaims his obligations both personal and intellectual.[17] Smith began this little work by expounding the Hartleian understanding of the working of the human mind and of the principle of association and then turned to the effects of disease in disrupting the associative process; he is mostly concerned with mania, marked by perturbation of the order and series of ideas, disruption of the connection of ideas to sensation, and the overthrow of judgement by interfering with the limitations on vividness and retention characteristic of the healthy mind. The discussion is limited, tentative and, in part, speculative – inescapably so, given the dearth of knowledge and, indeed, the impossibility of gaining much knowledge through direct observation. But there is nothing tentative about Smith's acceptance of associationist psychology or the dependence of the mind on the body; in this he was primarily obligated to the *Elements of the Philosophy of the Mind* by Thomas Belsham, the most important textbook of Hartleian psychology for that generation.[18] Belsham is the first name among the four men to whom the book is dedicated – the others are Benjamin Spencer, William Blake of Crewkerne, and John Evans, General Baptist minister at Worship Street, London. But for all the personal obligation Smith felt to the latter three, Belsham is the most important intellectual influence. Described by Smith in the dedication as Hartley's disciple and Priestley's friend, Belsham had undergone a notorious conversion to Unitarianism from orthodoxy in 1789, when he resigned as the head of Daventry Academy. He was appointed principal of the new Hackney College, which became a hotbed of radicalism in the 1790s and was finally closed by the trustees in 1796. He succeeded Priestley as minister at the Gravel Pit, Hackney, and later moved to the premier London congregation, Essex Street, founded by the former Anglican Theophilus Lindsey in 1774. Until his death in 1829, Belsham was the pre-eminent Unitarian theologian and the principal transmitter of the ideas of Hartley and Priestley to the next generation.

The debt to Belsham is equally evident in a much more important work that Smith published in the same year, *Illustrations of the Divine Government, tending to Show that Everything is under the Direction of Infinite Wisdom and Goodness and will Terminate in the Production of Universal Purity and Happiness*, a major contribution to Unitarian theology that grew out of lectures Smith began to deliver to his Edinburgh congregation in 1813. The book begins with a forthright statement of the argument from design, the laws of association, philosophical necessity, and the explanation of evil; the latter half of the book is given over to arguments for universal restoration. A hostile notice sent Smith to read Jonathan Edwards (much as Priestley had been sent to Edwards by Augustus Toplady), where he found his views on Providence reinforced, but whose dogmatic Calvinism also drove him to defend universal restoration with renewed vigour in the third edition of 1822, which was considerably expanded to deal with what Smith called 'the evils of the social state', including a long discussion of the Malthusian principle. To the young Harriet Martineau, then putting herself through a rigorous course of self-instruction in philosophy and theology, the book was a major factor in making her a confirmed necessarian.[19]

In 1816, Smith returned to Yeovil to combine the careers of minister and physician, a not uncommon linkage in the period.[20] In 1818, he remarried, his new wife the daughter of John Christie, a prominent London merchant active in denominational affairs.[21] In 1820, apparently owing to his wife's wish to be in London, the couple removed to the metropolis. The next year Smith qualified as a licentiate of the Royal College of Physicians, developed a private practice, and in time became consulting physician to the London Fever Hospital, the Eastern Dispensary, and the Jews' Hospital in Whitechapel.

His natural milieu was the tightly knit Unitarian society of Hackney and London, but before long he compromised himself with at least some of this group. His second marriage was not happy, and in the mid-1820s the couple separated, Mrs Smith going abroad with the son that had been born to them; the daughters from the earlier marriage remained with their father. After a time in bachelor quarters, Smith went to live with Margaret Gillies and her sister Mary, in Hampstead. Margaret Gillies was a painter of considerable talent who executed the woodcuts that had such a powerful effect on public opinion when they appeared as illustrations in the famous 1842 report on the labour of women and children in the mines. In 1844, Smith and Margaret Gillies set up a separate house in Highgate.[22]

This unusual arrangement did not go unnoticed. The Unitarian barrister and diarist Henry Crabb Robinson, who had been impressed on meeting Smith at John Christie's house in 1823, later declared him to be one of the most disagreeable men he knew. Joseph Hunter, the famous antiquary, minister at Bath when Smith was at Yeovil, and later deputy keeper of the public records, listed him as one of those radicals – along with Hazlitt, Godwin, and W. J. Fox – whose personal lives were impure. But Smith was not entirely cut off from Unitarian society, and he remained close to W. J. Fox, who had abandoned his wife to live with the composer Eliza Flower. This 'free-thinking, high-living clique' disturbed James Martineau, when his sister, through Fox, became a frequent visitor in the early 1830s. Apparently Harriet herself was sufficiently distressed by the rumours to wish, on finally meeting Smith at W. J. Fox's house, that she could only hear his 'tremendously interesting' conversation (through her new ear trumpet) without having to see his face, with its 'utterly vile' expression, which made him impossible to trust. Yet four years later, just before her temporary break with W. J. Fox over his domestic arrangements, she had chosen Smith as her doctor (she intended, like Bentham, to leave him her body for dissection) on the advice of a friend of Fox's who considered Smith 'the most wrongfully injured of men'.[23]

Whatever his standing with the London Unitarians, Smith entered a new and certainly overlapping circle when he met Jeremy Bentham in 1821. He was, apparently, one of the 'low radicals' who so distressed the Mills and the Austins whose influence on the old man had waned.[24] He regularly contributed to the *Westminster Review*, and, when Bentham died in 1832, there occurred the famous occasion at the Webb Street School of Anatomy when Southwood Smith lectured over the body, while a thunderstorm raged outside. Two days later, Richard Grainger, the distinguished anatomist and proprietor of the school, dissected the body. Smith later assembled the bones into a skeleton and preserved the head by putting it under an air pump over sulphuric acid to draw out the fluids, thus rendering it 'as hard as the skulls of the New Zealanders'; because all expression was gone from the face, he commissioned a wax image from portraits. The skeleton was then placed in a suit of Bentham's clothes, suitably stuffed, and the effigy was placed in a mahogany case with glass doors. This auto-icon – as Benthamite jargon had it (Carlyle called it 'that aboamenable Kipper') – was kept in Smith's consulting rooms in Finsbury and in 1850 was given to University College London, where it can be seen on application to the porter.[25]

After Bentham's death, Smith appears to offer a prime example of the celebrated Benthamite capacity at permeation.[26] In 1833, he served on the commission on the employment of children, inaugurating more than twenty years of official (and sometimes uneasy) collaboration with Edwin Chadwick. Chadwick chose Smith, along with James Kay-Shuttleworth and Neil Arnott, to write the path-breaking reports on the sanitary condition of London at the end of the thirties. Smith served on the commission on employment of women and children in mines, which reported in 1842, and in 1848 he was made a commissioner under the new Public Health Act, whereupon he gave up the private practice that he had maintained throughout his London career. When Chadwick fell from power in 1854 – a victim of anti-centralizing fervour and also of his own overreaching – Smith fell with him, but, because none of his government work prior to his service at the Board of Health had been paid, he was denied a pension until shortly before his death in 1861.[27]

But let us look further at the association with Bentham, taking advantage of Smith's published works and of some valuable manuscript sermons preserved in Dr Williams's Library.[28] Written partially in a now obsolete shorthand – Smith was not adept at it and used the notations largely for connectives and simple words, thus making the manuscripts relatively easy to decipher – these sermons are dated as to composition and as to the successive occasions on which they were delivered, down to his entry into government service in 1833.

Until 1821, Bentham had been only one name, and not the most frequently referred to, in Smith's usual Unitarian pantheon: Newton, Washington, Laplace, Hartley, Howard, Franklin, Fox, Clarkson, Romilly, Paley, Lardner, Lindsey, Price, and Priestley. Once in the establishment at Queen Square Place, however, Smith quickly acknowledged Bentham's centrality. His oration in Webb Street showed how fully he had mastered Bentham's writings, but what is remarkable is how little this new and close collaboration seems to have diverted a train of thought and activity begun long before. A casual glance at sermons written after 1821 will turn up phrases or even passages with a distinctly Benthamite ring. But references to pleasure and pain occur in the first edition of *Divine Government*, as they do in Hartley: they were part of the vocabulary of eighteenth-century psychology to which both Bentham and the Unitarians were heirs. When the tell-tale phrase 'the springs of action' occurs in a sermon written in 1825, that, too, is echoing Hartley and, in the sermon, is buried deep in an account of the associationist origins of benevolence.

Or consider this passage from 1826:

> Why is crime an evil, but because it produces suffering? And why is punishment a good, but because it diminishes crime? Without a tendency to that result, its infliction is altogether unjustifiable. One man robs another. You imprison the robber. That imprisonment is an evil. It is so much suffering. But if its effect be to prevent his robbing any more; or if, failing in that, the example operate as a check or warning to others, and deter them from committing depredations, there is good produced which overbalances the evil he endures in his punishment. Its infliction is therefore benevolent, but if it could infallibly be foreseen there would be no such consequence; if there would never be one robber the less, then that punishment would only be so much gratuitous and useless suffering. Its infliction would be mere malignity: the production of pain for its own sake. The production of evil can only be justified for the prevention of greater evil.

But this extended (and much the longest) echo of Bentham serves only as a corroborative rhetorical flourish, an illustration (such as all ministers use from reading or from fashionable current discussion), to give point to an argument. What Smith is really doing is offering an analogy for the remedial character of divine punishment visited on erring men, and the passage thus becomes a clinching argument for final restoration.

Much of the collaboration in the Bentham circle, which became particularly close after Smith's marriage broke up, has similar roots. The *Westminster Review* was as much a Unitarian as a Benthamite periodical, and Smith's first article in it in 1824 – on Bentham's *Chrestomathia*, his plan for a day school on the monitorial principle – merely expanded on his already strong interest in education, so central to a necessarian. In an article he had contributed to the *Monthly Repository* in 1822, and which had originated as a paper given to the Non-Con Club, a group of Unitarian radicals organized by Robert Aspland, Smith had already dealt with another monitorial plan 'for acquiring and communicating an accurate Knowledge of the Scriptures without Expense', in which a teacher would teach four boys for three years, those four boys another four, and so on until all the world (though he admitted that the strict mathematical increase was problematical) had been given the essential knowledge and had been brought by associationist principles to stand on the side of freedom in institutions, humanity in legislation, and purity in religion. Smith knew the scheme at first hand, for it was the plan of the institution founded in Bristol in 1817 by his old friend Benjamin Spencer.[29]

Again, Smith wrote much in the 1820s on legal topics. In 1824, he published Edward Livingston's project for reforming the Louisiana criminal code, at the suggestion and expense of John Abel Smith, just out of Cambridge and a member of the great banking family headed by Lord Carrington. It was apparently only through his Unitarian friend John Bowring that Bentham learned in 1830 about Smith's part in this publication, with the result that Smith was asked to write an article for the *Jurist* on Livingston's expanded penal code and procedural code, though in the event the article (if written) was never published.[30] This interest in penology and law, while no doubt powerfully reinforced by his growing acquaintance with Bentham's works and projects, descends directly from the necessarian emphasis on the corrective nature of punishment. Does God punish vindictively or on the principle of utility? Smith asked in one of his sermons. On utility, of course: so man's punishments must be useful and beneficial to the whole.

> Well were it if human governments could be taught that the respect which best secures obedience is produced by mildness and liberty, not by inflexibility, severity, and terror. The principle on which the divine

> ruler ensures moral obedience is applicable to political obedience also, and its adaptation elevates the good government of opinion above the brute force of tyranny.

The date is 1818. The debt is surely greater to Howard, Paley, the Whig reformers, and Romilly than to Bentham, and above all to the Unitarians, who drew their principles from a time when Bentham's works were little known and were preaching law reform for 20 years before Southwood Smith preached on it. When in 1829 he wrote an article on the application of Unitarian principles to the reformation of criminals, he still saw those principles not only as tests of the validity of penal practice, but as instruments of it.[31]

As Smith's career developed, however, other consequences of necessarian thought proved more important with respect to public service. In the *Illustrations* he had outlined a three-fold strategy by which those who had escaped from ignorance, vice, and misery could bring society through improvement to possible perfection: (1) the generalization of purely disinterested benevolence, or, at worst, realizing that an enlightened self-love must promote the welfare of others; (2) filling all the offices of state with men of this persuasion; and (3) educating the poor to be responsive to ideas, to knowledge of their own callings and of the simple laws of nature, and the fundamental principles and duties of government and Christianity. Southwood Smith himself did much philanthropic work, risking his life more than once by going into the appalling slums of London to treat and to observe. But he was able to carry out the injunctions of that three-fold strategy on a broader stage through intelligent administration and education. Though many of the details of his public work must have come from Bentham or from the men around him, he did not need Bentham for the basic model: that was provided by what in the *Illustrations* he repeatedly called (again following Hartley) 'the divine administration'.[32] God's simple, ingenious system was implemented through other beings, obedient to government by fixed and invariable laws. Sensation, as we have seen, gives rise to volition, and a particular volition leads certainly to a particular action. To understand perfectly the constitution of the animal and material worlds would give sovereign control over both, and so with man:

> The bodily frame and the natural temper of an individual may seem...ill adapted to execute the work which the Deity has determined to perform by him: yet no force is employed to induce him to do it. He is not compelled to act against his volition, but the circumstances in which he is placed are so adapted to his corporeal, his mental, and his moral constitution, as to excite the requisite volition.

The centrality of education in all this is plain, and we have already noted Smith's interest in schools. But his most important contributions were a much broader means of teaching men to conform to the great laws of nature, the conformity that was the precondition of human happiness: it was no accident that he became a dedicated popularizer of sound knowledge about health and hygiene. He lectured publicly on physiology – Crabb Robinson heard him in the Borough in 1827, and in 1832 he was lecturing on the 'animal economy' at the London Institution. He wrote the volumes on *Animal Physiology* for the *Library of Useful Knowledge*, published by the Society for the Diffusion of Useful Knowledge in 1829. In 1835, he expanded these efforts into *The Philosophy of Health*. He had, he said, three audiences in view: (l) individuals, who could be taught how longevity and happiness might be theirs through a clear knowledge of the human frame and the natural laws that govern it; (2) barristers, judges, and magistrates, who so often had to deal with questions of property, health, guilt, and innocence; and (3) legislators, who were not only ignorant of important distinctions, like that between infectious and contagious diseases, but who were incapable of 'detecting the loose statement, and the false induction of medical men on this subject...'.[33]

But the books were also intended to demonstrate the ingenuity of God's design and to expound a view of progress that is utopian in the extreme.[34] Civilization as we know it, said Smith – he was later to define it as marked by a sovereign authority, incorruptible administration, general diffusion of physical comfort and intellectual development, and the recognition of fundamental principles of religion and morality – is only a transitory state still dominated by selfishness and in which, for certain purposes, violence is still recognized. In time a new age will dawn, though in what mode or by what agency we cannot tell. 'But we are already in possession of the principle which will destroy the present and introduce a better social condition, namely...the maximum of the aggregate of happiness sought by the promotion of the maximum of individual happiness.' It is, of course, Bentham's greatest happiness principle, but the context in which it is set gives it a stunningly utopian twist, a utopianism with doubtful warrant in Bentham, but explicit in the principle of association, the example of a perfect, human Christ, and the overriding goodness of God.[35]

John Bowring displayed a similar utopianism with a gloss of Benthamite rhetoric. It is notably evident in *Minor Morals*, which he published at almost exactly the same time as Smith's *Philosophy of Health*, to teach children the principles set out in the *Deontology*, which Bowring published (or, more accurately, expanded) in 1834 from Bentham's manuscripts on ethics. One can also see it in Bowring's activities in East Asia in the 1840s and 1850s, when he prided himself on having more power over more people than anyone else in the world and was utterly confident that all the world could be made one through freedom of trade. In much the same way, Harriet Martineau was attracted to Auguste Comte and Positivism in the 1840s, but from a very early age she repeatedly evinced a degree of apocalyptic expectation that kept her on a constant lookout for Armageddon, the great war of opinion that her youthful recollections of Canning's oratory had led her to expect.[36] This apocalyptic strain is absent in Southwood Smith: the new state would come about by a natural evolution. I cannot resist the speculation, though I have no direct evidence for it, that if he found confirmation for this necessarian future in any non-necessarian source, it was not so much in Bentham as in the St. Simonians, who had close ties with the Foxite circle when they visited England on their missionary labours in the early 1830s.[37]

Beyond popularization, Smith's work as physician and government servant also followed from the ingenious methods by which God worked His will in man, methods that Hartley had explained. Smith was in a position to control some of the circumstances that governed the sensations men received and that thus underlay their volitions – not only so far as sanitation was concerned, but housing, hours of work, leisure, education, and political participation. He was certainly capable of sounding like the perfect Benthamite: 'What a dreadful accident near Durham,' he wrote in 1844, ' – nearly one hundred lives lost in a moment. I shall try to turn it to account to get a Registration of Accidents Bill.'[38] But he was not a compulsive centralizer like Chadwick and was himself deeply engaged in voluntary activity, notably in the founding of the Sanatorium, a middle-class nursing home in London in 1842, and in the establishment of the Metropolitan Societies for Improving the Dwellings of the Industrious Classes in the same year.[39]

His concern for wider political participation – of a piece with the ultra-radicalism of the London Unitarians in the 1820s – is reflected in the petition that he (with others) presented for a reduction in the sentence imposed on John Frost and fellow-Chartists involved in the Newport rising in 1839, on the practical ground that heavy sentences would have an adverse effect on both sympathizers with the rioters and those among their opponents who abhorred barbarous punishments; vindictive punishment would cause further estrangement and make more difficult the improvement of the working classes by the diffusion of useful knowledge and the acquisition of independence. But the petition advanced a theoretical ground that indicated that Smith was more than an amanuensis (the petition is in his handwriting): it was argued that enlightened policy calls for punishment that is not vindictive but preventive – the same theoretical position he had taken up in his sermon in 1818 and, more generally, in the *Illustrations*.[40]

There is, however, a more specific relationship between Smith's public work and his necessarian axioms; to understand it we must consider more fully some of Smith's views on the human mind. The *Illustrations* is a work of theology and metaphysics, the latter word carrying a special significance in the early nineteenth century: it had come to mean what we would call theory of knowledge.[41] It was as a metaphysician of this kind that Southwood Smith was proposed in 1827 for one of the two philosophy chairs at the new London University: the chair whose holder was to deal with 'that department of mental phenomena in which all that relates to action is concerned.' Smith might well have got the appointment, had not the Evangelical Zachary Macaulay happened to read the *Illustrations* and announced that he would withdraw his support from the University if so dreadful a heretic were appointed to teach moral philosophy.[42] Not for the last time did the blocking of an academic career lead to the enrichment of the public service.

On no subject did Southwood Smith insist so much as on the need to understand the workings of the human mind: such knowledge was prerequisite to both education and intelligent administration. He believed he knew, from Hartley and Belsham, the principles of the mind, and he tried to expand that knowledge. We have already seen the concern of his doctoral thesis with the health of the mind; and at the very end of his life he added nine chapters on the nervous system to his *Philosophy of Health*, a part of his plan (which he did not live to complete) 'of expounding the mental constitution with a view to the direction of the intellectual and moral faculties....'[43]

But he was as much or more concerned with the right rules for thought. In 1818, he was asked to preach at Ilminster before the Western Unitarian Society, a sermon subsequently published. His subject was *The Probable Influence on the Development of the Principles of the Human Mind on its Future Progress in Knowledge and Goodness*; his text was I Corinthians, 15:20: 'In understanding be men.'

> If in understanding we are men, in practice we shall be Christians; for knowledge and virtue are so entirely the same, that virtue is knowledge inspired with the attributes of life. Were we perfectly acquainted with our own nature, and the properties of all objects around us, our misconduct, and therefore our misery, would be nearly at an end. Every wrong judgment and every bad passion is the consequence of our not knowing the true nature of some object connected with us, or not understanding our own. The philanthropist rejoices therefore at the diffusion of knowledge, not only because it sheds a glory on his race, but because it affords the most favourable augury of its future fortunes. Discipline of the mind will impart to its possessor the true nature of the obligation of duty, give him a clear perception of the objects most calculated to produce solid and permanent happiness, teach him to control the passions, and build up proper associations – not adverse associations like honour, glory, or superstition, but rather that the greatest sum of enjoyment comes to him 'who thinks least of his own and most of others' good'

– a passage that suggests how well prepared he was for what Bentham had to say about emotive words and even for the felicific calculus. Moreover, a knowledge of the mind and the discipline that would flow from it will lead to the modification of existing institutions and to inculcating new attitudes towards the erring, who will be seen not as guilty men but as victims of circumstances, to whom our primary duty is enlightenment.

But let us narrow our gaze from these general goals to the more narrowly construed rules of reasoning, which also flow from a proper knowledge of the mind. Moral education, Smith said, would teach men that all opinions ought to be investigated freely and fully on the evidence and will make clear the true doctrine of authority – that we are right to extend confidence to the testimony of upright persons in matters of fact, but where the reasoning faculty is involved, a clear distinction must be made between argument and authority, and the judgement must not be swayed by names but only by clear evidence. Intellectual education will train the mind to keep away from things that are ultimately unknowable and so from questions on which so many philosophers have wasted their time; it will prove the Baconian method to be the best mode of conducting enquiries; and it will develop a habit of attention, teach the importance of precise meaning, of proper arrangement, and of generalization, and will teach, too, how to make a proper selection from the field of knowledge 'adapted to the natural bent and turn of the mind, and to that particular sphere in which it is probable its faculties will be asserted.' It is in these rules for philosophizing – commonplaces in textbooks of Unitarian dogmatics and remarkably paralleled in Harriet Martineau's 'Essays on the Art of Thinking'[44] that we can, I think, find important clues to the direction, emphasis, and temper of Smith's specifically medical researches, and in particular to his persistence in pursuing the 'sanitary idea'.

In her study of the attempts of the medical profession to understand and cope with cholera and that complex of diseases gathered under the term fever, Margaret Pelling has pointed out that Smith, with Chadwick following, was in a minority in the profession, that his medical career was entirely atypical. She traces his obligations to Sir John Pringle, John Armstrong, and Charles Maclean, as well as to the revived interest in Sydenham. But she overlooks the firm philosophical certainties that underlay his dogmatic adherence to the sanitary idea.[45]

Smith's *Treatise on Fever* of 1830 makes clear how skeptical he was about the general body of medical men; the ground of his suspicion was that they had not been trained to reason properly. Now medicine is an inductive science, and its practitioners are peculiarly susceptible to making hasty assumptions and holding to partial views; yet no one believes it necessary, he said, that they be trained in the art of induction or cautioned against sources of fallacy in making inferences. Whereas earlier writers on fever either assumed mere conjecture to be fact, or assigned to the genus what belongs only to the species, or characterized the disease by what belongs only to a stage of it, or mistook effect for cause, Smith sought in his own researches for indications of invariable concurrence, 'and the establishment of this relation of events, this constant connexion with each other, this uniform antecedence and sequence appears to me to be the only theory after which it is consistent with the principles of sound philosophy to search.'[46]

Good Baconian induction requires a proper respect for fact and a healthy skepticism about authority. So Smith searched and collated the factual evidence from past and modern observations, including his own intensive observations at the London Fever Hospital. These led him to isolate two categories of causes. The immediate or exciting cause he thought to be a poison formed by the corruption of animal or vegetable matter: in putrefying, they 'give off a principle, or give origin to a new compound, which when applied to the human body, produces the phenomena constituting fever.' There was much to be learned, and indeed he hoped to contribute to many secondary questions about that poison – how it was diffused, propagated, checked, diminished, or destroyed, and what conditions were favourable to its flourishing – all questions that would include 'the investigation of several exceedingly curious and important statistical questions,' with the object of leading to 'any useful principle of extensive application.' But

> what this principle or compound is, whether it be one of the constituent substances which enter into the composition of organized matter, or whether the primary elements of organized matter, as they are disengaged in the process of putrefaction, enter into some new combination, and thus generate a new product, we are wholly ignorant. Of the composition of the poison, of the laws which regulate its formation, and of its properties when generated, we know nothing beyond its power to strike the human being with sickness or death.[47]

The second order of causes is the predisposing causes. While they are not gone into deeply in the *Treatise* – he merely notes that heat and moisture are the most certain and perhaps the most powerful of these causes – a quarter century later he was categorical about what was important.[48] 'Every fact we have learnt respecting the great laws of nature, on our conformity with which our very existence depends, has taught us that the circumstances which produce excessive sickness and early death are preventable.' But about the primary or exciting cause, he knew no more than he did in 1830. Even with the predisposing causes, we are ignorant of much. Still, 'whatever may be the truth with respect to these points ... one thing is certain, that practically our concern is with the known causes, – the ascertained conditions. These are palpable, definite, and capable of complete removal and prevention.'

The terms of Smith's appointment to the Fever Hospital made it clear that collecting facts was a primary responsibility, and his *Treatise* is based on careful and extensive observation. Moreover, the sanitary idea had brought results. In so far as men understood how to deal with facts, facts bore out the conclusions of the General Board of Health at midcentury and certainly avoided the panicky, expensive, and inconvenient quarantine regulations against cholera, which the anti-contagionists, with Smith leading the charge, had fought in 1830 and for long thereafter.[49] It seems seriously unhistorical to criticize Smith and his colleagues for failing to make one particular imaginative leap when in fact he had been guided, implicitly if not explicitly, by rules he had stated in 1818. Every Unitarian philosopher of mind had urged the importance of avoiding the unknowable and concentrating on secondary causes; it was surely a small step to assimilate what was unknown and not likely soon to be discovered (a germ, say, as the 'principle' of the 'poison') to the unknowable, the more so when so much progress had been made by concentrating on what could be readily known.[50] In any event, one could not wait on more abstruse researches when men were dying through ignorance of the laws of nature. When Hackney College, in turmoil in the 1790s, was closed down, Thomas Belsham, the principal, wondered whether the skepticism of so many of his students might have grown from a desire for mathematical precision and clarity. That would not do: 'Often, while we are seeking after certainty, the time of action is lost,' and so conduct must be regulated by probability.[51]

In 1845, Southwood Smith's publisher asked him for a new edition of the *Illustrations*. He had no time to do it, as it turned out, and the book was not reprinted again until after his death in 1861. But what changes he would have made are clear from a letter he wrote in 1845 to the Rev. Charles Wellbeloved, who had retired a few years earlier as principal of Manchester College. Smith wanted to bring his book into line with the latest in biblical criticism, for a work written 'with the simple and sincere purpose of exhibiting the true meaning and spirit of Christianity ... as correct and worthy to influence the Christian mind as may be practicable' should contain nothing inconsistent with Scripture as the best authorities had come to understand it.[52] On the main arguments he had not changed his mind at all and saw no need to adapt the book to any system he had learned after 1822.

All Smith's published works bear out the assumptions and commitments set down in the *Illustrations*, his sermons, and in particular that sermon of 1818 on the human mind. All that is, but one: his oration over the body of Jeremy Bentham – a tribute to the usefulness of Bentham's theatrical gesture, a masterly exposition of the master's views, an assertion of Bentham's comparability to Newton. Gravitation was known before Newton, but Newton had shown how comprehensive the principle was. So Bentham had shown the comprehensiveness of the greatest happiness principle, 'the sole foundation of morals, the sole test of every thing that is good, and of everything that is evil, in individual or private conduct, in legislative enactment, in the forms or the measures of government – in a word, in the totality of human aims and actions.' Once prejudice was conquered and a few key intellects were converted, every institution, law, procedure, rule, and sanction would fall before that principle, while it would establish every institution, law, procedure, rule, and sanction shown by sagacity and experience to be productive of happiness. Surely here Smith was proclaiming his discipleship.

Perhaps we must make allowances for the emotional nature of the occasion and the demands of rhetorical balance; perhaps we must admit that of all pulpit oratory, a funeral sermon (which is what Smith was in fact delivering) is the most likely to be extravagant in praise of its subject. The oration cannot be dismissed so easily, but it can, perhaps, be read another way. That Bentham had discovered a principle – 'something which points out some external consideration as a means of warranting and guiding the internal sentiment of approbation and disapprobation' – was incontestable; the whole Unitarian intellectual enterprise was aimed at the discovery of laws or principles. The greatest happiness principle was a discovery of profound importance in the gradual revelation of physical and moral law, to which Smith devoted his life. But it was no more than a new, more penetrating formulation of an end already in view. I believe that Southwood Smith's career is related only incidentally, though importantly, to Benthamite principles and forms: whatever coloration Smith took on, and whatever specific devices or ideas he adopted from others, his career draws its force, consistency, and principal content from his mission as a Unitarian, necessarian philosopher.

In January 1853 there was an epidemic outbreak in Croydon. The Board of Health sent Southwood Smith and his colleague Dr John Sutherland to make a preliminary report on allegations from various sources that sewage works were responsible. After interviewing all the medical practitioners in the area, the two doctors concluded tentatively that the single point of general agreement was that the season had been unusually hot and damp. A more detailed investigation was conducted on behalf of the Board by Richard Grainger, the surgeon who had dissected Bentham's body two decades earlier; he came to the same conclusion.[53] Here, then, were three colleagues in the sanitary movement, united in defending the principles on which the Board of Health operated and convinced that they were right to concentrate on secondary causes of disease and their removal.

It happens that we can catch partial glimpses of the religious views of Richard Grainger.[54] His Hunterian Oration in 1848 emphasized the anatomical and physiological basis on which medical science must be founded; but he ended by drawing the attention of his audience to the ultimate bearing of these studies on the proof of design and the law that governed the physical universe. But for the moral law, he said pointedly, one must turn to the Bible, to which he himself devoted much study. On another occasion, he expounded the physical reasons that justified observance of the Sabbath, and when he founded the Christian Medical Society in 1854, his avowed purpose was the salvation of souls among his younger colleagues. He defended the Society against its critics on grounds that are a complete recapitulation of the classic concerns of Evangelicals.[55]

Grainger shared with Smith (and presumably with Sutherland) the same sense of overarching divine purpose and power, but there is a sharp disjunction between Grainger's acknowledgment of God's powers in nature and his gloomy assessment of man in his fallen state. For Grainger the glory of human reason, which gave access to the laws that governed the physical universe, did not reach to the origins of the universe and of life or to the mysteries of incarnation and resurrection. Smith rejected mystery and believed that the human mind, properly conducted, could over time approximate more and more to all but the ultimate in knowledge of the divine, and even in the ultimate things, man could know that God's beneficence and foreknowledge governed evil and misfortune. Revelation was thus confirmatory, not the sole source of knowledge for the moral law; Smith moved beyond dogma to place man firmly in the continuum of a divine economy directed to the attainment of ultimate happiness and perfection.[56]

In pursuit of these grand goals, Smith reflected the singleness of purpose and the seamlessness in thought that give a distinctive content to Unitarianism as the Priestleyan generations understood it. From his conversion to the end of his life, Smith was fixed in an all-encompassing explanatory system elaborated from a mid-eighteenth- century base and justified by all his subsequent experience.

There are two remarkable confirmations of this contention from authoritative sources. In a review of the *Philosophy of Health* in the *Monthly Repository*,[57] Southwood Smith was distinguished from other writers who had urged self-knowledge because he had provided the materials for cultivating it. Throughout all his work, the reviewer (probably Fox) said, he had shown 'the true attributes of a popular philosopher, the power of ascending from the particular to the general, from facts to principles, from phenomena to laws.' The *Illustrations* had shown that he had sounded the depths of the great moral questions, and the funeral oration for Bentham indicated, not a new departure, but the maturing and systematization of his speculations.

Two years earlier, Harriet Martineau had written to Lord Brougham to urge that Southwood Smith be appointed to the inquiry into the condition of factory children. She had refrained, she said, from recommending many people whom she knew better than she knew him; her proposal was 'for the sake of truth alone.' When he was appointed, she was sure it was her doing: she had put a necessarian philosopher into government.[58]

## Notes

Much of my original work on Smith was done during two sabbatical years in London, in 1959–60 and 1966–67. I am most grateful to the John Simon Guggenheim Memorial Foundation and the American Council of Learned Societies for their support. Earlier versions were presented as papers at the Victorian Studies Centre, University of Leicester, in the University Seminar on Political Thought at Columbia University, at the Institute for Advanced Study in Princeton, and at the Research School of Social Sciences in the Australian National University; comments made on those occasions have helped greatly to bring my interpretation to its present state. I am also much indebted to the librarians and staff at Dr Williams's Library and at Manchester College Oxford for assistance over the intervening years. The chapter was completed while I was a Christensen Research Fellow at St Catherine's College Oxford, and I wish to thank the Master and Fellows of the College, and in particular Dr José Harris, for making possible that stimulating and productive stay.

1. The principal disputants were Dr Oliver MacDonagh and Dr Henry Parris. For an authoritative review of the controversy, R. M. MacLeod, 'Statesmen Undisguised', *American Historical Review*, lxxviii (1973), 1386–405.
2. '"Statesmen in Disguise': Reflexions on the History of the Neutrality of the Civil Service"', *Historical Journal*, ii (1959), 19–39.
3. Without at all trying to make Unitarianism the great undiscovered key to the nineteenth century–it certainly was not, though it has been usually neglected or misunderstood – I have written about two other necessarians whose careers have substantial similarities to Smith's: *Harriet Martineau, a Radical Victorian* (London, 1960), and 'John Bowring and Unitarianism', *Utilitas*, iii (1992), 43–79. I have also noted what seem to me unmistakable Unitarian influences in the work of Elizabeth Gaskell: 'The Gaskells as Unitarians', in Joanne Shattock (ed.), *Dickens and Other Victorians: Essays in Honour of Philip Collins* (London, 1988), 144–71.

4. *New Statesman*, 16 July, 1938. It must be said in extenuation that Laski was reviewing Raymond V. Holt's *The Unitarian Contribution to Social Progress,* a work of appalling sectarian piety which suggests that the Unitarian nexus was central to a vast range of social reformers, among whom Holt includes some whose Unitarianism was at best tangential, while omitting others (like Harriet Martineau) for whom it was essential, though she later abandoned the connection.
5. Priestley, *Letters to a Philosophical Unbeliever*, Part I, in J. T. Rutt (ed), *The Theological and Miscellaneous Works of Dr. Joseph Priestley*, iv (1818), 368. For the emergence of Unitarianism within Dissent, C. G. Bolam, *et al.*, *The English Presbyterians, from Elizabethan Puritanism to Modern Unitarianism* (London, 1968), and R. K. Webb, 'The Unitarian Background', in Barbara Smith, (ed.), *Truth, Liberty, Religion: Essays Celebrating Two Hundred Years of Manchester College* (Oxford, 1986), 3 –30.
6. The term is sometimes written 'necessitarian', the ugly added syllable apparently preferred by those to whom the system was distasteful.
7. See, for example, Robert Aspland, *Causes of the Slow Progress of Christian Truth* (London, 1825)..
8. Instances are the extended reports of discussions in the Martineau family in Norwich, recorded in letters to the eldest brother Tom, who had gone to Madeira to recover his health; these letters, collected by Dr R. S. Speck, are in the Bancroft Library, University of California, Berkeley. The letters of William Roscoe, the Gregs, and the Rathbones in the University of Liverpool Library also reveal this style of thinking. In the University of Nottingham Library is preserved a minute book of a discussion society in the High Pavement congregation that indicates an informed and very serious approach to theological and metaphysical issues.
9. R. K. Webb, 'Flying Missionaries: Unitarian Journalism in Victorian Britain', in J. M. W. Bean (ed.), *The Political Culture of Modern Britain: Studies in Memory of Stephen Koss* (London, 1987), 11–31.
10. At present, biographical information on Southwood Smith is difficult to come by in the detail one would like, though this situation will be remedied by a biography now being written by Dr John Guy, whose advice in the latter stages of writing this chapter is gratefully acknowledged. In a badly flawed work of family piety, *Dr. Southwood Smith, A Retrospect* (London, 1898), Mrs C. L. L. Lewes failed to make any mention of Smith's Unitarianism – the Unitarian newspaper, *Christian Life* (15 April, 1899), called the book *Hamlet* without the prince – although Gertrude was raised as a Unitarian in Smith's household and was married in March, 1865 to the son of George Henry Lewes in Rosslyn Hill Chapel in Hampstead, with George Eliot in attendance – Gordon Haight (ed.), *The George Eliot Letters* (London, 1956), iv 184. Mrs Lewes's reticence about Southwood Smith's religion is no doubt explained by her subsequent conversion to

the Church of England. In this account, I have relied largely on F. N. L. Poynter, 'Thomas Southwood Smith – the Man (1788–1861)', *Proceedings of the Royal Society of Medicine*, lv (1962), 381–92. This was a first, and as it turned out, only glimpse into Dr Poynter's projected life of Smith, his notes having been destroyed before his death. The paper contains much of value, but it remains sketchy on many aspects of Smith's life and is defective on both the character and the effects of Smith's Unitarianism; the latter fault is common to much historical work touching on the denomination. Dr Poynter helpfully allowed me to see some of the Smith letters then in his possession.

11. Herbert McLachlan, *English Education under the Test Acts, being the History of the Nonconformist Academies, 1662–1820* (Manchester, 1931), 96–101.
12. Michael Neve (*Natural Philosophy, Medicine, and the Culture of Science in Provincial England: the Case of Bristol, 1790–1850*, Ph.D. thesis, University of London, 1984, 124–5, 137) makes the point that Unitarians in Bristol were not outsiders but an integral part of the elite culture of the town, a culture that, moreover, valued science as a means of strengthening that culture and maintaining its dominance.
13. So far Spencer has largely eluded me, but see Southwood Smith's deeply personal obituary notice of him in the *Monthly Repository*, xvii (1822), 767–9.
14. Andrew M. Hill, 'The Successors of the Remnant: A Bicentenary Account of St. Mark's Unitarian Church, Edinburgh, Part I: before 1776 until 1822', *Transactions of the Unitarian Historical Society*, xvi (1977), 101–23. L. Baker Short, *Pioneers of Scottish Unitarianism* (1963), 79–84.
15. The most prominent of these recruits was Robert Aspland, minister at the Gravel Pit Chapel in Hackney, founder of two major Unitarian journals – the *Monthly Repository* from 1806 and the *Christian Reformer* from 1815 – and the organizer and long-time secretary of the British and Foreign Unitarian Association, the only central body of the denomination down to the creation of the General Assembly in 1928. Others include the prominent missionaries William Vidler and Richard Wright.
16. James Yates, the minister at Glasgow, wrote to Richard Astley on 4 January, 1813 (Astley Papers, 1067/163, Shrewsbury Public Library) that Smith 'appears a sensible & intelligent man, tho' not furnished with the advantages of education'. The fine Unitarian historian Alexander Gordon (in 'Biographical Notes for the Centenary of the Edinburgh Congregation', Unitarian College MSS B.1, John Rylands University of Manchester Library) thought the reference in the *Monthly Repository* in 1813 to large crowds attending Smith's preaching was 'highly coloured'; Smith himself had told Gordon that at times there were only 20 in the congregation. But I do not think that either of these remarks invalidates the general point.

17. The book was published in Edinburgh.
18. The full title is *Elements of the Philosophy of the Mind and of Moral Philosophy, to which is Prefixed a Compendium of Logic* (London, 1801); note especially the section on madness on 178–80. Smith's reiteration of his obligations to Hartley and Belsham may appear to raise questions about my contention that Smith fits into a tradition descending from Joseph Priestley. Smith turned to Hartley, the originator of the entire line of argument, and to the most recent interpreter, but Priestley was omnipresent in the setting in which Smith wrote. Priestley died in 1804, just as Smith was undergoing his crisis of faith, and Unitarian periodicals and sermons over the next decade were full of references to the great martyr, as, indeed, are Smith's sermons. It is suggestive that a tract in which Smith argues against the Trinity, published by the Edinburgh Unitarian Fund and later reprinted in the *Christian Reformer*, v 1819, 361–8 and as a tract in Birmingham in 1820 bears the title *An Appeal to the Serious and Candid Professors of Christianity*, the exact title used by Priestley for a famous polemical piece addressed to orthodox believers in 1770: (J. T. Rutt (ed), *The Theological and Miscellaneous Works of Dr. Joseph Priestley*, ii (1817), 383–04). My use of the term Priestleyan is, to some degree, a shorthand reference, which I consider justified because of Priestley's centrality in transmitting the Hartleian philosophy and because of his pre-eminent place in the larger history of English Unitarianism.
19. She wrote enthusiastically to her brother James on 13 October, 1822, about a sermon by Smith, who he notes was almost certainly Southwood Smith, and early the next year she reported that there had been 'lively talk, both sympathetic and argumentative' in the Norwich household, 'joined in by Mr. Madge (the Norwich minister), W. Dawson, and dealing with the law of necessity, Southwood Smith's book, and Hartley, Harriet alone being completely necessitarian'. Following out her insistence that letters were 'written speech', Harriet Martineau insisted in the 1840s that her correspondents return her letters to her on pain of being deprived of future correspondence. James Martineau reluctantly complied but first made shorthand abstracts, which have been preserved in the library of Manchester College Oxford; the originals were presumably destroyed, so these abstracts, transcribed by Mr William S. Coloe, are all that remain. The critical notice of the *Illustrations* appeared in the *Eclectic Review*, n.s. x (1818), 336–50, 539–63. See also the highly favourable review of the first edition in the *Monthly Repository*, xi (1816), 473–6, and the poem, 'Lines occasioned by reading "Dr Smith on the Divine Government"', *ibid.*, xii (1817), 242–3.
20. In 1819, the young John James Tayler wrote to his brother (28 December, 1819, Dr Williams's Library, MS 24.102) about his intention to study medicine with a view to combining the two

careers. A minister's salary was insufficient to support a family, and he did not feel equal to the demands of teaching, so he consulted Southwood Smith, who advised him that the combination was quite practicable up to a point; 'the only question is, whether beyond that point, a physician, if we may say so, can arrest the course of his practice'. In the end Tayler did not pursue medicine and became a very great teacher indeed, at Manchester College.

21. There is a long, informative obituary of John Christie in *Christian Reformer*, n.s. (1858), 380–1.
22. On Gillies, *DNB.* Smith's wife died in 1858; see the brief obituaries in the *Inquirer*, (1858), 631, and *Christian Reformer*, 1858, 647. Smith's letters of 1844 in the Wellcome Library to Mary and Herman Smith about funds for Herman's entering a bookselling partnership in Frankfurt suggest that the family remained on relatively cordial terms. There are two charming recollections of the Highgate household (and of the circle) in Mary Howitt, *An Autobiography* (London, 1889), ii 30–1, 311–12.
23. Crabb Robinson Diary, 13 July, 1823, 23 April, 1851, Dr Williams's Library. Joseph Hunter's 'Thought Book', 20 November, 1856, British Library Additional MSS 39,818, f. 314. Abstracts of letters from Harriet to James Martineau, 26 January, 1830 and 30 January, 1834, Manchester College Oxford. The friend was a Mr Fisher, on whom see below, n. 37. Harriet conceded that her sister's unfavourable impressions of Smith were 'all derived from the Christie view of him'. It should be noted that this liaison, not at all uncommon at the time, was owing less to moral laxity than to the virtual impossibility of divorce: the most famous parallel is the relationship of Marian Evans (George Eliot) and G. H. Lewes.
24. Sarah Austin to Guizot, 18 December, 1861, in Janet Ross, *Three Generations of Englishwomen: Memoirs and Correspondence of Mrs. John Taylor, Mrs. Sarah Austin, and Lady Duff Gordon* (London, 1892), 381–4.
25. C. F. A. Marmoy, 'The "Auto-Icon" of Jeremy Bentham at University College London', *Medical History*, ii (1958), 1–10. Southwood Smith to William Munk, quoted in Munk's sketch of Smith in *The Roll of the Royal College of Physicians of London*, iii *1801–1825* (London, 1878), 237. Carlyle was reported to have made the comment to A. J. Scott in John Dunlop, *The Dunlop Papers*, Vol. I: *Autobiography of John Dunlop* (London, 1932), 168.
26. On permeation, S. E. Finer, 'The Transmission of Benthamite Ideas, 1820–1850', in Gillian Sutherland (ed.), *Studies in the Growth of Nineteenth-Century Government* (London, 1972), 11–32. For an assertion of Smith's Benthamism, J. B. Brebner, 'Laissez-Faire and State Intervention in Nineteenth-Century Britain', *Journal of Economic History*, Supplement, viii (1948), 59, 73. Brebner, arguing against A. V. Dicey's equation of Benthamism and laissez-faire, places

the blame on James Mill's advocacy of political economy. That Mill's work was well done is suggested by an editorial comment in the *Economist*, 10 April, 1847, about Smith, Dr Neil Arnott, and Edwin Chadwick: 'We respect (them) as physicians and philanthropists – we have no confidence in them as lawgivers. Dr. Southwood Smith, for example, in one of his most recent publications ... showed himself so misinformed on the subject that he has described Bentham, whose merit was that he exposed the error of legislation, as having reared the fabric of felicity by the hand of reason and of *law*.'

27. Smith's public health career is best followed in R. A. Lewis, *Edwin Chadwick and the Public Health Movement, 1832–1854* (London, 1952) and in M. W. Flinn's introduction to his edition of Edwin Chadwick, *The Sanitary Condition of the Labouring Population of Great Britain* (Edinburgh, 1965). Smith's own listing of his important accomplishments can be found in memorandums for Lord Brougham, 10 July, 1848, and 14 July, 1855, University College London. In the latter memorandum he suggests posts he would have been willing to accept in lieu of a pension and notes that he had declined appointment as officer of health of the City of London, a post taken by the celebrated Sir John Simon.
28. MS 12.60.
29. *Monthly Repository*, xvii (1822), 419–25, 767–9. *Christian Reformer*, iii (1817), 368–72. In 1825 Smith and Fox organized religious classes in Fox's chapel in Finsbury. There were about 60 over the age of 15 and 40 under, with Fox and Smith taking the seniors through the evidences of natural and revealed religion. Smith had written to Lant Carpenter in Bristol asking for recommendations for books and for his experience in his own school with separating the sexes, which some of the parents wanted very much, though Smith worried that it would double the work and have other disadvantages. Smith to Carpenter, 10 January, 1825, and Fox to Carpenter, 11 July, 1825, Manchester College Oxford. In the late twenties, Smith and Bowring were discussing 'an improved school' and wanted to talk to Bentham about it. Smith to Bentham, 22 August, 1828, British Library Additional MSS 33,546, f. 229. There is a suggestive parallel to the linkage of Smith's articles on the *Chrestomathia* and on Spencer's project in his influential article on 'The Use of the Dead to the Living', in the *Westminster Review*, i (1824), and his sermon, *The Wisdom and Benevolence of the Deity in the Ordination of Death* (London, 1821), on the death of the Rev. Thomas Howe, minister at Bridport, in which the 'Benthamite' language of pain and pleasure leads into a utilitarian explanation of death, rooted firmly in assumptions about divine benevolence and the glories of the future life.
30. Bentham to Smith, 19 January, 1830, University College London. Edward Livingston, *Project for a New Penal Code for the State of Louisiana* (London, 1824). In the Advertisement, Smith notes the

great interest of seeing 'how some of our institutions are viewed, and how when full liberty is allowed to change them, they are modified by an enlightened Legislator, who is uninfluenced by our prejudices, and unfettered by our customs....'

31. *Monthly Repository*, n.s., iii (1829), 17–21. See Belsham, *Elements* (1801), 350–3, 403-06; and John Prior Estlin, *Discourses on Universal Restitution* (1813), 110–19.
32. Compare the touching and revealing little book by Thomas Dixon, *The Sovereignty of the Divine Administration Vindicated; or a Rational Account of our Blessed Saviour's remarkable Temptation in the Wilderness; the Possessed at Capernaum; the Demoniacs at Gadara, and the Destruction of the Swine....* (London, 1766). There is a brief sketch of Dixon (1721–54) in the entry for his father of the same name, in *D.N.B.*
33. In a toast to the Royal Colleges of Physicians and Surgeons, c 1850, Smith said: '... from the medical body have come & constantly do come some of our most distingd. philosophers & ardent philanthropists – some who have enlarged the boundaries of science; others who have brought down science to the threshhold of the people & others whose sacred office it has been, not so much to alleviate the sufferings of their race, as to teach them how to raise and keep themselves above those sufferings.' British Library, Additional MSS 44, 919, f. 140.
34. A startling illustration of Smith's enthusiasm is a rapturous passage in the *Philosophy of Health* (11th edn., 295–7) about the functioning of the excretory system: '...how complete the absence of all note or sensible intimation that any such action is going on, yet how delicious the consciousness produced by its soundness and vigour; how pure the blood mantles in the cheek and diffuses its sparkling colour over all the transparent complexion; how the jocund spirits laugh from the eyes; how the intellectual and sympathizing mind beams forth from them with a higher and holier happiness!' This and much more. In 1861, George Eliot was more than once frustrated in her attempt to hear James Martineau preach. On one excursion, 'Mrs. Bodichon and I went to Little Portland St. Chapel, and lo, instead of James Martineau there was a respectable old Unitarian gentleman preaching about the dangers of ignorance and the satisfaction of a good conscience in a tone of amiable propriety which seemed to belong to a period when brains were untroubled by difficulties and the lacteals of all good Christians were in perfect order.' The lacteals carry chyle from the small intestine to the thoracic duct. George Eliot to Sara Sophia Hennell, 30 July, 1861, in Gordon Haight, (ed.), *The George Eliot Letters*, iii (New Haven, 1954), 441–2.
35. The criteria of civilization are set out in *Epidemics Considered with Relation to their Common Nature, and to Climate and Civilization....* (Edinburgh, 1856), 31. For the rest of this passage, *Philosophy of*

*Health*, end of chapter 3, at 105 in the 1834 edition, unchanged in the 11th, posthumous edition (1865).

36. Webb, *Utilitas*, 58–63, 70–6, and Harriet Martineau, *passim.*
37. Although Richard K. P. Pankhurst, *The Saint-Simonians, Mill and Carlyle*: *A Preface to Modern Thought* (London, n.d., c 1957) is primarily concerned with the two great figures, there are several mentions of Fox who was put in the way of the Saint-Simonians by Mill. The favourable review of the mission in the *Monthly Repository*, v (1831), 82–8, 181–9, 279–81, is by John Fisher, a member of Fox's congregation, and Fox himself comments in 194–5 and 481–2. Compare Harriet Martineau, *History of the Thirty Years Peace,* ii (London, 1850), 141–2.
38. To ? , 8 October, 1844. This was one of the letters that Dr Poynter showed to me, but it is not in the Wellcome Library and its whereabouts are now unknown.
39. The Sanatorium, which eventually did not succeed, was much discussed with Smith's friend Charles Dickens. See Madeline House and Graham Storey, *The Letters of Charles Dickens,* ii (1840–1) (Oxford, 1969), 164–5, 293–4; iii (1842–3)(Oxford, 1974), 5; and the oddly contrasting criticism in Kathleen Tillotson, (ed.), *Letters*, iv (1844–6) (Oxford, 1977), 515. The work of the Metropolitan Societies is summarized in Smith's *Results* of *Sanitary Improvement* ... (London, 1854). His granddaughter, Octavia Hill, became famous as a housing reformer.
40. British Library, Additional MSS, 44,919, ff. 131–2.
41. '*Mental Philosophy* is not uncommonly confounded with *Metaphysics*; and the absurdities and futile speculations, which have been classed under the latter, have been supposed by many to belong to the former. *Metaphysics* ... comprehends all investigations respecting those objects of human thought which, by sensation alone, could not be brought under the notice of the human mind; and it consequently includes the philosophy of the human mind; but it is obviously unjust to throw upon this department of metaphysics, the stigma which, if due to any, belongs to those branches alone, which have little or no relation to mental laws and operations.' William Shepherd, Jeremiah Joyce, and Lant Carpenter, *Systematic Education* (London, 1815), ii 241–2.
42. S. E. de Morgan, *Memoir of Augustus de Morgan* (London, 1882), 73. H. H. Bellot, *University College London, 1826–1926* (London, 1929), 57–8, 108. The very radical Dr John Elliotson was made a professor of medicine, so evidently the chair of moral philosophy was a touchier matter.
43. The psychiatric reformer Dr John Conolly, in *The Treatment of the Insane without Mechanical Restraints* (London, 1856), 162–3, notes the distressing lack of attention to education as a means of preventing nervous and mental disorders. Among the best of recent works

addressing the subject he singled out Southwood Smith's *Philosophy of Health*: 'From these works may be gathered many directions for the regulation of the life of children, conformable in principle and in object to the character of the non-restraint system applied to older and more disordered minds.'

44. *Monthly Repository*, iii (1829), 521–6, 599–606, 707–12, 745–57, 817–22. It seems likely that this is the sermon which Harriet praised to James in 1823; see above, n. 19.
45. Margaret Pelling, *Cholera, Fever and English Medicine, 1825–1865* (London, 1978), 8-9. Compare Norman Longmate, *King Cholera, The Biography of a Disease* (London, 1966), 160, 181, where Smith is scoffingly compared to Dr John Snow, who discovered in the 1850s that cholera was borne by the water supply. In an important article, 'Predisposing Causes and Public Health in Early Nineteenth-Century Medical Thought' *Social History of Medicine*, v (1992), 43–71, Christopher Hamlin proposes abandoning the contagionist-anticontagionist polarity as a structure for medical thought of the period and substituting the complementary categories of predisposing and exciting causes. My interpretation of Smith's position in this continuum differs somewhat from Hamlin's on the specifically medical question, but his learned setting of the context is invaluable. In his concentration on social context, however, it seems to me that Hamlin misses Smith's intense concern with housing (see above, p. 65) and, more important, the philosophical foundations of Smith's theoretical and practical work.
46. It must be recognized, of course, that Smith's decision to work on fever – that then still unravelled complex of diseases – was probably related to the death of his first wife from fever.
47. Compare *De morbis mente laesa* (1816), 26, where he argues that human ability can go no further to explain the effect of illness on the mind or the physical changes it entails. So subtle is the reality that the scalpel and eye of the anatomist will injure it, and the acuteness of the ethical philosopher cannot penetrate it. 'Perhaps only another Newton is wanting', though in the end the Newton he found, Jeremy Bentham, explained a different range of phenomena.
48. *Epidemics* (1856).
49. Southwood Smith, 'Contagion and Sanitary Laws', *Westminster Review*, iii (1825), 134–65; 'On Cholera', *Monthly Repository*, n.s. v (1831), 779–81. John Bowring, clearly drawing on Smith, criticized quarantine in his reports on Syria and Egypt and in publications as late as the 1860s; see Webb, *Utilitas*, 56. In 1860 a publisher sent Smith a brief memoir for review. He cut one sentence praising his extensive knowledge and practical views, but retained those about his sanitary work and his assistance to Shaftesbury in carrying the Ten Hours bill. He added his appointment to the Fever Hospital in 1825 and to the Eastern Dispensary somewhat earlier: 'Here it was that he learnt the

true sources of epidemics.' Smith to Messrs. Richard Griffin, 23 January, 1860, British Library Additional MSS 28, 512, f. 135–8.

50. Compare the obituary of another prominent sanitarian, Dr John Sutherland, *Lancet*, 25 July, 1891: 'Sanitation always had with him a direct and practical aim and object – viz., that of providing ... a healthy environment. In the army especially the range of modifiable conditions affecting health has first of all to be determined, and then the attainable conditions have to be secured. To a consideration of these subjects he gave great thought; they formed the occupation of his life. To say that some disease or other was solely attributable to contagion or depended upon a bacillus and to stop there as seems to be so much the tendency these days brought little satisfaction and no comfort to a practically minded man like Dr Sutherland.' In Smith's case, the practical impulse was underpinned by a firm philosophical and theological position.

51. Belsham to Theophilus Lindsey, 31 July, 1800, Dr Williams's Library, MS 12.57.17. See also the remarkable tribute by Dr Samuel Brown, *Westminster Review*, lvii (1852), 409–19 to the various pseudo-scientific enthusiasms of the 1840s: 'Cleanliness and temperance are the very religion of the materialist, and should be the complement of religion for all.'

52. 25 November, 1845, Dr Williams's Library, MS 24.81. The extensive biblical citations appear almost entirely in the final sections on universal restoration.

53. *Statement of the Preliminary Inquiry by T. Southwood Smith, Esq., M. D. and John Sutherland, Esq., M.D. on the Epidemic at Croydon, together with Reports by R. D. Grainger, Esq. and Henry Austin, Esq. to the General Board of Health* (London, 1853). Austin was an engineer.

54. Sutherland supplied extensive notes on the contemporary relevance of Jewish hygienic laws to a sermon preached in Manchester Cathedral in 1854, but it is not possible to proceed from that to any conclusions about Sutherland's religious position. Charles Richson, *The Observance of the Sanitary Laws, Divinely Appointed, in the Old Testament Scriptures, Sufficient to Ward off Preventable Diseases from Christians as well as Israelites* (London, 1854). On Richson, *D.N.B.*.

55. Richard D. Grainger, *Observations on the Cultivation of Organic Science, being the Hunterian Oration ...* (London, 1848); 'The Sabbath: Its Adaptation to the Physical Nature of Man', in *Seven Lectures on the Sabbath* (London, 1852); *An Address delivered to the Christian Medical Association on the Occasion of its first Meeting, November 10, 1854* (London, 1855).

56. In 1814, Smith had pointedly denied that the doctrine of the Trinity could be a mystery, 'for a mystery is that which is unintelligible, but which may be explained, but this is a direct contradiction, and is, therefore, incapable of proof even by miracles.... How little do they know of religion, who represent it as foolish and visionary in its

nature.... Can there be a more exalted pleasure, than that which the mind experiences when in moments of reflective solitude ... it dwells upon the thought, that there is seated upon the throne of the universe, a Being whose eye never slumbers nor sleeps, and who is perfect in power, wisdom, and goodness?... May we, ... exercising the faculties with which we are endowed, and worthily improving the Revelation which has been given us, at all times entertain such sentiments of our heavenly Father as will purify and elevate our minds, inspire them with sober but fervent devotion, console them under all the calamities of life, and lead them to anticipate with ardent hope, and to prepare with unwearied diligence, for the happiness of heaven.' *The Incompatibility of the Doctrine of the Trinity with that of the Divine Unity* (Glasgow, 1814), 8, 27–8.

57. n.s., ix (1835), 153–60.
58. Two notes to Brougham, April, 1833, University College London.

# 3

# Lyon Playfair and the Idea of Progress: Science and Medicine in Victorian Parliamentary Politics

*Anne Hardy*

*'The Progress of a country depends upon the progress of science'*
*Lyon Playfair, 1889*

Medicine and science have rarely contributed burning issues to popular debate and parliamentary politics in Britain, and doctors and scientists have relatively rarely sought to become actively involved in the business of politics. The late Victorian period was to some extent an exception to this generalization. The Second Reform Act of 1867 created a working-class electorate, and brought the liberal intelligentsia into the political arena.[1]

For the first time doctors and scientists became members of parliament and entered the House of Commons. In the following decade, three vigorous popular moral crusades exploded into that arena: the campaigns against the Contagious Diseases Acts, compulsory vaccination and animal experimentation. Each of these three campaigns presented its own challenge to the authority of the medical profession and, as each in turn reached the forum of the House of Commons, created a situation in which that authority might be conclusively demonstrated or disproved. Continuing concern for public health issues in the 1880s and 1890s provided further opportunities for the display of scientific authority, but the experience of the 1870s was critical in establishing that authority in the Commons.[2]

The scientific membership upon whom the defence of medical authority devolved was tiny. Between 1868 and 1874, when the issues of the Contagious Diseases Acts and of vaccination came before the House, there were just three scientific members. Two were doctors, John Alfred Lush, MP for Salisbury, and William Brewer, member for Colchester; the third was the chemist Lyon Playfair, who represented the universities of Edinburgh and St

Andrews. In the years up to 1900, there were never more than seven scientific MPs representing English and Scottish constituencies in the House at any one time.[3]

Within this small group, Lyon Playfair stands out as the central figure. He entered the House with an established reputation as a capable civil servant and an authority on sanitary matters, and it is clear from the debates on the Contagious Diseases Acts and on vaccination in 1870 that he was already the leading spokesman for medical and scientific interests. He continued in that capacity until his retirement from the Commons in 1892, although ably seconded in later years by Charles Cameron and Robert Farquharson. More than any other individual, it was Playfair who met and overcame the challenges of the popular crusades, and who established the authority of science in the House of Commons. In later years he used his authority to achieve important legislation on questions affecting the condition of people, and he was instrumental in finally resolving significant professional discontents among the doctors through legislation. While his intellectual and political concerns extended significantly into the areas of education and economics, his enduring contribution was to medicine and public health.

## The Making of a Politician

Lyon Playfair was born in Bengal in 1818, the son of George Playfair, chief inspector of hospitals for the province. The family was middle class, with a strong academic tradition, and roots in the Scottish university city of St. Andrews.[4] All George Playfair's four sons were sent back to Scotland early in their lives, to avoid the hazards of an Indian childhood, and were subsequently educated in Scotland. Lyon had initially intended to study medicine, but an allergy associated with hospital wards and dissecting rooms curtailed that ambition. Deflecting his father's wish that he should become a merchant, he turned instead to chemistry. While a medical student at Glasgow, he had become acquainted with Thomas Graham, and in 1838 he went to London as Graham's assistant at University College. In 1839, on Graham's advice, he proceeded to Giessen to study under Justus von Liebig, the founder of organic chemistry and one of the most influential teachers of the period.[5]

Playfair was an able and enthusiastic student, and was, besides, possessed of considerable personal charm. He became friendly with the sometimes difficult Liebig and translated the latter's seminal *Organic Chemistry* into English. At the 1840 meeting of the British Association for the Advancement of Science, Playfair presented a review of the state of organic chemistry which brought him to the attention of the geologists William Buckland and Henry de la Beche, who were at this time earnestly engaged in furthering the practical applications of their science. Playfair's familiarity with agricultural chemistry, his interest in its practical application, and his sympathetic character impressed both geologists. Over the next two years they evolved various plans for his employment, and eventually prevailed upon the Prime Minister, Sir Robert Peel, who was himself a leading exponent of scientific farming, to interest himself in Playfair's future.[6]

Through Peel's interest, Playfair found himself a member of the Royal Commission on the Health of the Towns in 1844, and a famine commissioner to Ireland in 1845. Thereafter he was never without some appointment on a royal commission or select committee, and pursued this work in tandem with his academic career. In 1858, he was appointed professor of chemistry at Edinburgh University, a position which he retained until his election to Parliament in 1868. Playfair's careers as civil servant and specifically as scientist are beyond the scope of this paper, but merit investigation as potentially contributing to our understanding of the world of Victorian science. Christopher Hamlin has graphically portrayed the internecine squabbles and bitter rivalries of analytical chemistry in this period, with particular focus on scientific lobbies and their machinations.[7] How far Playfair touched upon this world is not clear. It seems unlikely that he remained wholly unaffected, and it is possible that examination of his role as an expert witness and parliamentary commissioner may yet modify the conclusions presented here.

It seems likely, however, that his experiences as a civil servant contributed to his decision, in 1867, to stand for the newly-created parliamentary seat for the universities of Edinburgh and St Andrews. He had been an active campaigner for the establishment of Scottish university seats, and had supervised the campaigns to elect Gladstone as Rector of Glasgow University in 1859 and to elect him as Chancellor of Edinburgh University in 1868.[8] Perhaps these activities whetted his appetite for a higher political arena; it may be that his acquaintance with Gladstone inspired him to extend his political interests into the parliamentary sphere. Playfair left no personal political testament, and neither in his memoirs nor in his correspondence did he discuss his political career. The springs of his personal politics are therefore largely obscured, although something may be deduced from his parliamentary career and from his uncompleted memoirs.

One of the guiding forces of Playfair's whole career – both scientific and political – was the practical application of scientific knowledge. He himself claimed to have 'drifted' in this direction,[9] but it seems likely, from his early interest in organic chemistry, that he had a natural bent towards applied science. It may be that his friendship with Liebig was a formative experience intellectually, as well as opening the doors of employment in that direction, or it may be that the true spring of his interests lies yet deeper, in his Scottish heritage. His biographer, Wemyss Reid, onetime editor of the *Leeds Mercury* and a notable Victorian biographer, observed that 'rightly to understand' Playfair's life and character,

> One must understand something of the spirit which has led so many young Scotsmen to devote themselves to the service of their country .... To Lyon Playfair the good of his country was a thing to be pursued not merely in the Senate, or on contested fields, but in the laboratory and the council room, in social intercourse, in the humdrum round of daily life. It was a thing never to be lost sight of ... something calling ... for a patient and unremitting care, extending even to the most trivial tasks and incidents.[10]

This love of country may, however, have close ties to Playfair's Liberal politics, and may help to explain his somewhat maverick position within the public health movement, even though associated with it for much of his career.[11] Liberalism involves a deep commitment to the ideal of human liberty, and to the rights and opportunities of the individual,[12] but the state acts as guarantor of that liberty. If the state is prosperous, benevolent and powerful, the security of the individual is effected and provides the freedom within which social improvement, public education and economic progress, all of which enhance the opportunities of the individual, may be promoted. In this sense, Playfair's active politics were directed towards a comprehensive political ideal, and his advocacy of free trade, of science and medicine, and of education, sprang from his understanding that these disciplines were crucial to the achievement of his ideal. So it was that, in Reid's words, he was 'always more of a philosopher among politicians than of a politician among philosophers'.[13]

Playfair's commitment to this broad Liberal vision, far more than his training as a chemist or his espousal of active politics, set him apart from the mainstream of the Victorian public health movement, whose most prominent exponents had different – and narrower – political aims. Although friendly with Edwin Chadwick for over 30 years, Playfair was not influenced by Chadwick's ideas.[14] He evidently admired John Simon's work as Medical Officer to the

Privy Council, but there is no correspondence between them to suggest friendship or collaboration.[15] Nor are there any letters from Henry Rumsey among Playfair's papers, although Rumsey was a politically active member of the British Medical Association. The eminent sanitarians do not feature in Playfair's memoirs, and although he commonly pre-fixed the words 'my friend' when naming, for example, Angus Smith or Sir John Lubbock in public speeches, he did not do so for either Rumsey or Simon.[16]

Playfair's concern for public health appears not to have been driven by any burning sense of social injustice, or moral outrage at the waste and tragedy of human life taking place daily among the poorest of his country's citizens; his writings carry none of the passionate lucidity of moral outrage that make memorable those of Chadwick and Simon, and of other, lesser, sanitary figures. Rather, his speeches on sanitary reform reveal how fundamentally public health was just one component of his wider political vision. Addressing the medical students of King's College London, for example, his theme was the 'benefits which the public may in future enjoy from the application of your knowledge to the purposes of the State'. He urged his audience to encompass both curative and preventive medicine as 'a sort of religion, and on himself as a priest of humanity, bound to spread the sphere of his usefulness to all within his range'.[17] In this way doctors could help to maintain the prosperity of the state. It was a point which Playfair had made yet more explicit in his address to the Social Science Association in 1874:

> When the rate of mortality is too high, that is, when the individuals of its population, which constitute the particles of the State, waste too rapidly, the State suffers from public maladies. Hence the State medical officer and the private physician work on like principles; for to the former the community, to the latter the individual, is the patient.... The health of the country – and that governs the productive power of its people – depends as much upon the applications of medical science as the working of a machine depends upon a good application of mechanical laws.[18]

And on the productive power of the people depends the prosperity, and hence the power, of the State. In the final event, for Playfair, individual liberty depended on the health of the individual, and so medicine and physicians became important contributors to the wider welfare of society. It was the social and political significance which Playfair attached to the practical application of medical knowledge that led him to defend and to promote the interests of medicine and public health, and of their practitioners, within the walls of the House of Commons.

## A Parliamentary Career

By the time Playfair entered parliament he had 25 years experience as a civil servant behind him. He was to serve in the Commons for a further 25 years, before, being considered too old for office, he was translated to the House of Lords. Like all but one of the medical and scientific MPs elected to English and Scottish constituencies before 1900 he was a Liberal; and in common with all but one of the medicals, he had a Scottish background.[19] His early prominence in the House derived from several factors. Between 1868 and 1885, his position as representative of Edinburgh and St Andrews universities, the largest medical constituency in the country, gave him a special authority in medical affairs. It was presumably for this reason, and perhaps because of his friendship with Sir Robert Christison, that he acted as spokesman for the British Medical Association's parliamentary bills committee until Robert Farquharson entered parliament in 1880.[20] If these circumstances were not sufficient to establish a position, Playfair's experience as a civil servant had given him a wide familiarity with social questions, and with techniques of marshalling evidence, and these circumstances added to the authority with which he spoke.

Playfair possessed considerable gifts as a speaker, and it seems likely that these confirmed his standing in the House. Robert Farquharson recalled how the Commons 'always used to fill when Playfair was up': his wide knowledge and unique powers of clear exposition made him a pleasure to listen to.[21] Playfair was one of only four individuals whom Farquharson considered to have made a mark on entering the Commons over the age of 40; the others were Joseph Chamberlain, Sir Henry Fowler and John Morley. There can be little doubt that it was Playfair's ability as a speaker that won him eminence: his 'lucid and up-to-date disquisitions on science were always eagerly followed by a crowded house'.[22] However, Farquharson himself became a recognized authority on medical and scientific affairs, and was always listened to with respect, and Sir Charles Cameron likewise occupied a position as a recognised medical authority.[23] Indeed the readiness of the late Victorian Commons to listen to medical men and scientists discussing subjects in their specialist fields contrasts sharply with the impatience of French non-medical deputies at the same period.[24] Nor was Playfair's influence limited to the debating chamber, and he may have been exceptional in this regard, at least in the early years. He had the ear of the government on scientific questions, and was recognized to do so by the scientific community. 'You are the only scientific man the Govt (sic) cares to listen to', observed Joseph Hooker in 1873, 'and perhaps the only powerful one'.[25]

Playfair's political standing was such that it enabled him to continue his parliamentary career when his relationship with his Scottish constituency fragmented in the later 1870s. His own political sympathies were Liberal, but the constituency was essentially Conservative. Playfair knew this, and in the early 1870s confined his parliamentary energies to social questions and avoided politics.[26] However, as tensions within the Liberal Party mounted, he found this more and more difficult, and could clearly be seen to be identifying himself with measures to which the Conservatives were strongly opposed.[27] He only narrowly retained his seat in the 1880 election, and his decision to stand down in 1885, on the grounds that he disapproved of government proposals to separate the Scottish and English educational systems, probably marked deeper problems with his constituents.[28] He had no difficulty in securing another seat, and was eventually elected for South Leeds, where the local Liberals wanted 'a man who would confer distinction on us'.[29]

Throughout his parliamentary career Playfair remained a convinced Liberal. In the early 1870s, he formed one of a group of semi-radicals who were, in the words of J. P. Parry, happy with the liberating, up-lifting time of Gladstone and the Liberal Party at this time, who were 'warm friends' to the common man, and who wished that the government would go further in attacking entrenched orthodoxy and in infusing spiritual feeling into politics.[30] Within this group, Playfair was one of the few whose allegiance to Gladstone survived the division over Irish Home Rule in 1886. His Liberalism moved along 'the old historic lines', and he was never tempted into sympathy with socialism or any of the post – 1886 factions within the Liberal Party.[31] In this respect Playfair's politics were clearly shaped both by the basic liberal ideal of civil and intellectual liberty, and by its later extension to encompass freedom from poverty, illness, bad housing and inadequate education.[32] His principal political concerns were public health, education and free trade, which he saw as the three necessary elements of social progress.[33] The three concerns were linked by this ideal of progress, but progress dependent on the proper development and utilization of science. For Playfair, medicine was the key to human well-being just as scientific education and scientific progress were essential to the economic success on which further social progress depended.[34]

Although Playfair's standing as a scientific authority remained unquestioned in the Commons, his political career – like his scientific one – was only moderately successful in terms of professional recognition.[35] That he enjoyed parliamentary life seems indisputable: he wrote to his prospective wife in 1878 that he had 'no vehement desire' to remain in parliament and would only stand again if his seat were uncontested, yet he fought several contested elections at Edinburgh, and sought another seat when his position there became untenable.[36] It is also likely that he was ambitious for office, although this is not revealed in his fragmented memoirs. Farquharson recalled that he was 'much aggrieved' at being excluded from office in 1892;[37] it is clear that he entered the House of Lords reluctantly. 'I am anxious,' he wrote to Gladstone, 'to be of use to your Government in or out of office. The Lords do not make use of men, even when they are Masters of a subject.'[38] In the event, Playfair's time in office was minimal: he was Postmaster-General in Gladstone's first ministry, 1873–4; between 1880 and 1885 he was Chairman of Committees and deputy speaker; in 1886 he spent five months as vice-president of the Council.

In terms of personal political success, Playfair's parliamentary career may have been a disappointment to him. In terms of the contribution which he was able to make to the future of British medical science and of the British medical practitioner, and to the health and welfare of the British people, his career in the Commons must be seen as highly influential.

### Subjects of Parliamentary Concern

In parliamentary debate, Playfair contributed on three broad fronts: health and medicine, education, and economic policy. As suggested above, his personal philosophy associated the three subjects as crucial forces shaping an improved future for his country and its people. Constraints of space here dictate a focus on his contributions to medical issues, yet even this limited approach reveals the interdependence of his ideas on health, medicine, education and political economy.

### The Moral Crusades

The three contentious issues of the Contagious Diseases Acts, vaccination and vivisection, together with the 'woman question' constituted the great moral crusades of late Victorian England. All four subjects reached the forum of the Commons during the 1870s, and Playfair contributed to the debates on all four.[39] The agitations over the first three were closely linked both inside and outside parliament. They appealed to the same fears of and hostilities to science, and within the Commons the same spokesmen performed consistently on the different issues.[40] Playfair, of course, was ranged in defence of science.

Playfair's position as the professional defender of science was first spelt out in his speech in defence of the Contagious Diseases Acts in May 1870. He began by refuting in detail the charge that the Acts had been passed hastily, and proceeded to deal with the arguments against them – that they were opposed to religion, justice, morality and public liberty – one by one. He emphasized that where disease could be prevented by the enforcement of judicious legislation, then it should be, and in conclusion stressed the public-health benefits accruing: 'the undoubted result has been largely to mitigate disease and to lessen immorality'.[41] As Paul McHugh has pointed out, it was one of the few attempts to defend the acts in terms as comprehensive as those in which they were attacked.[42] Playfair's marshalling of evidence, and his use of statistics supplied by Dr Balfour of the Army Statistical Department, were especially notable: Sir Alexander Grant, Principal of Edinburgh University, considered them to be 'perfectly unanswerable'.[43]

The theme of disease prevention, with the recognition that the liberty of the individual should be restricted in the interests of the community, became a recurrent motif of Playfair's career. This was particularly the case with the arguments over compulsory vaccination, of which he was a wholehearted supporter, but it also informed his approach to public health in general and to vivisection. For Playfair, disease prevention and science were closely linked, and the conjunction represented one of the most positive features of Victorian society. In his speech on the Contagious Diseases Acts, for example, he declared,

> It is a very old notion that diseases should not be combated because they are Divine punishment for sins, relevant or irrelevant. Such views have become rare in modern times, because we are constantly reminded, in the progress of science, that there is far more of mercy than of wrath in Divine arrangements.[44]

This motive clearly operated also in Playfair's battle to retain and reinforce the laws of compulsory infant vaccination in Britain. In this battle, he was highly successful,[45] despite being accused of inconsistency by the anti-vaccinationists because his views on necessary parliamentary measures changed with changing circumstances.[46] Once again, his most telling speeches on the vaccination issue made devastating use of statistics.[47]

In the case of both the Contagious Diseases Acts and vaccination, Playfair was defending existing legislation in the face of relatively new forces of organized opposition.[48] He fought these issues on ground familiar to him from his long-standing acquaintance with public-health issues, and his more recent experience of dealing with cattle plague in 1866. The controversy over the desirability of legislation on vivisection which broke in 1875 brought him a different challenge; that of modifying proposed legislation in a hitherto unregulated and highly controversial area.

The background to the 1876 Cruelty to Animals Act, and the political procedures by which it was achieved, have been admirably detailed by Richard French, who has shown how medical scientists, working through Playfair as their representative in the Commons, succeeded in modifying an Act which most of them deplored and which many of them believed unjustified.[49] Playfair himself may have had some sympathy with the humanitarian case, but, as his biographer stressed, his overriding belief was in the greatest good of the greatest number, and thus in the right of scientists to further the interests of humanity and widen the bounds of medical knowledge by animal experiments.[50] It is clear, in any case, that this was one issue of critical concern to the medical community who made up Playfair's parliamentary constituency: he claimed to have received some 3,500 letters on the subject, and his papers contain a number of letters from eminent scientists on the issue.[51] Whatever Playfair's own humanitarian convictions, they could not be allowed to obtrude on an issue of such central concern to his political constituency.

Playfair's own views on the vivisection issue are not illuminated by his speeches in the Commons, for it is clear that many of his arguments had been suggested by his friend Robert Christison, who was a wholehearted opponent of any attempt to regulate laboratory practice through legislation.[52] Thus the parallel between animal experiments and blood sports, which Playfair used with telling effect, originated with Christison. 'If the cry be listened to of "Down with the Doctors!", we must be prepared to couple it with "Down with Sport",' Christison had written in May 1875, at the beginning of the episode.[53] He also advised Playfair to demonstrate the beneficial results of such experiments:

> What a golden opportunity, – if the H(ouse) of Commons or the Peers meddle at all with the subject, – for pointing out the discoveries which vivisection has unfolded in all branches of medicine as a science and practical art![54]

The overwhelming pressure from the medical community and his own political interests determined Playfair's position on vivisection, although it seems certain that his commitment to the principle of progress aligned his sympathies on the scientists' side. He was not, however, simply the funnel of pro-vivisection medical pressure groups: his parliamentary standing and skilled oratory made him invaluable to the physiologists. The Home Secretary's fear for his bill in the Commons, which Richard French has contrasted with Playfair's similar anxiety for the medical case in that House,[55] was at least in part a tribute to the influence which Playfair commanded in the lower House.

The dominant theme of Playfair's attitude towards all three contentious issues was the same: a conviction that progress – scientific progress as it contributed to improving the welfare of mankind – should not be obstructed. This position was consistent with his advocacy of educational reform, which would enable the public to appreciate the benefits of science and recruit more scientists to the service of their country, and with his adherence to the tenets of the political economy he had learned as a young man.[56] For Playfair, social improvement and economic progress depended on advances in science and medicine.

## Public Health

On public-health issues in general, Playfair's attitude was equally determined by his belief in political economy, and tempered by his faith in education, by his assessment of the best interests of the medical profession, and by his passionate commitment to free trade. The public-health legislation which came before the Commons during the period of Playfair's membership was of two types. First there were the classic sanitary measures: water supplies, housing, viral registration, infant welfare, sanitary administration and disposal of the dead. Secondly, there were measures affecting food supply, on which Playfair's views were generally in sympathy with the free trade interest.

As regards the classic sanitary concerns, Playfair's attitude was progressive and consistent. He approved public health legislation in general, and was anxious that it should establish a sufficiently powerful and effective administration.[57] Associated with this anxiety was his concern to create an informed and effective body of public health officials. 'The appointment of medical officers of health is one of the most important parts of the measure', he noted of the 1872 Public Health Bill. He attacked the suggestion that the

MHOs should be drawn from the ranks of the Poor Law medical officers, because the new officers should be specialists (and qualified as such) in the health of communities rather than of individuals (and he later deplored the Local Government Board's failure to make use of the expertise of John Simon's department in framing the administrative provisions of the 1872 Act: 'I am certain that their experience could not have guided the utter confusion of organisation in regard to medical officers of health').[58] But Playfair also advanced the interests of science generally, and the prospects for scientists, by combating the 'metropolitan focus' of the Bill, which had proposed to establish the Local Government Board as analytical chemist for the whole country. Centralization was always injurious, he argued, because it weakened local administration. He continued:

> Centralisation in science is pernicious, because it prevents the diffusion and stunts the development of science in all provinces ... the diffusion throughout the provinces of the science bearing on the health of the people should be the object of the central Board.[59]

Several factors were obviously at play here, including the non-metropolitan bias of a Scottish professor, but the argument was absolutely consistent with Playfair's promotion of employment opportunities for scientists, and his understanding of the wider economic implications of public health measures.

The same considerations are evident in Playfair's discussion of the Artisans Dwellings Bill in 1875. Again, he stressed the necessity for central government support for medical officers, if the measure was to be effective.[60] Although he agreed with Cross, the Bill's promoter, that local government should not be subject to too much interference from central government, he went on to emphasize the costs of ill health: the annual cost of sickness in Liverpool, for example, amounted to £370,000. Money invested in sanitary improvement, Playfair declared, 'is productive taxation'. Government, reinforced if necessary from the centre, was the prerequisite of savings in human capital[61]

This position was not simply the result of a need to play to a constituency. In 1889, years after he had severed his connection with the demanding university constituency, Playfair acclaimed the 'zealous labour' of doctors against disease, and took the government to task for failing to involve them properly in the processes of health administration. To entrust that administration to lawyers and Poor Law officials was, he declared, 'an amazing example of unbelief in the first principles of the laws of health'. Doctors alone could administer the existing law efficiently:

> The well being of the people depends upon physical causes, which when intelligently understood mean physical science, and the trained physician is the natural and the most intelligent agent for extending its knowledge and application to the prevention of disease.[62]

The practical benefits of applied science were a constant point of reference in Playfair's vision of social progress.

On the classic concerns of public health, Playfair was thus progressive, and had a clear view of how progress was to be achieved in health and sanitation. None the less, his arguments and perspectives fell within the existing spectrum of discourse on the subject and commanded respect, as carrying the authority of science, without provoking adverse reaction. He was not, however, without the courage to extend his arguments to unpopular progressive ideals; indeed the Scottish scientific members were remarkable in this respect. The outcry over cremation which erupted in 1884 demonstrated the singular progressiveness of the Scots, both in terms of the application of scientific authority, and in their willingness to challenge established social tradition.

The advocacy of cremation in place of burial as a means of disposing of the dead dated, in England, from the surgeon Henry Thompson's visit to Vienna in 1873, which resulted in the founding of the Cremation Society in the following year.[63] It was, however, the cremation on a Welsh hillside of the young son of the eccentric physician and self-proclaimed druid William Price, and Price's subsequent prosecution at Cardiff Assizes in February 1884, that opened the subject for public discussion. Medical concern at the forensic implications of the practice led to the introduction of a bill to regulate the practice in April 1884. The bill was sponsored by Charles Cameron, Robert Farquharson and Lyon Playfair. It was thrown out, by 149 to 79 votes, after what one Irish member termed a 'rollicking Scotch morning', in the course of which Farquharson had produced a phial of ash from a cremated cow for the education of the House.[64] The susceptibilities of opposing members were clearly deeply affected by this Scottish transgression of a central tenet of Victorian Protestant culture.[65] The member for Bridport, indeed, declared that while the opinions of the scientific trio on vaccination and vivisection had hitherto been received with respect, this was less likely to be extended to them in future.[66] It was perhaps a measure of the standing which Cameron, Farquharson and Playfair had achieved in the House that their pronouncements appear to have been received with undiminished respect subsequent to the cremation vote.

Sanitary orthodoxy and sanitary radicalism can thus both be found in Playfair's attitude to classic public health issues. His ideas were largely fixed, determined by his liberal principles and scientific commonsense.[67] By contrast, his treatment of questions relating to food supply, a relatively new field of sanitary concern after 1870, reveal how his ideas developed with the extension of scientific knowledge.

Three specific food supply issues commanded parliamentary attention in the later decade of the century: the adulteration of food and drugs, the introduction of margarine, and, with growing urgency, the problem of animal diseases. The character of the great Food and Drugs Adulteration Act of 1875, which forms the basis of modern legislation, was transformed during its passage through the Commons by the joint efforts of Playfair and Charles Cameron.[68] From being a discretionary bill with enough loop-holes to permit continued widespread adulteration, the final act ensured the appointment of public analysts and so created a new professional organization; the prerequisite for the enforcement of standards of safety and purity in the retail food and drugs trades.[69] Once again, the interests not only of the public but also of science were served in this new sanitary legislation.

The subject of margarine first came before the Commons in 1881, when Sir Herbert Maxwell, MP for Wigtownshire, introduced a motion recommending that its sale be regulated. Margarine (also known as oleomargarine and butterine at this time) had been developed by a Frenchman, Hippolite Megè-Mouriès, in 1869. During the 1870s, its manufacture became widespread, notably in the Netherlands and in North America. By the early 1880s, the Dutch were mixing it with the butter which they exported to Britain.[70] Despite rising butter sales and rising butter imports, it seems likely that English agriculturists viewed the arrival of margarine with apprehension, but that they dared not admit it in the face of the prevailing free trade ethos. Maxwell certainly represented agricultural interests, but he denied any protectionist motive for restricting the sale of margarine, and claimed a concern for the interest of the consumer. However, the very wording of his resolution, that 'such of these compounds as are harmless shall only be sold under distinctive names, and that the importation or sale of those which are hurtful or dangerous to health be prohibited altogether', carried an implicit threat.[71]

Playfair acted quickly to counter the implication that margarine could be dangerous. In essence, he argued, both butter and margarine were animal fats; in terms of taste and flavour margarine was no competition for butter; and that the poorer classes generally ate butter whose nutritional value had been reduced by added water and salt and which quickly went rancid. Margarine had 'little tendency' to become rancid: it could only displace bad butter to improve the health of the working classes.[72] Playfair's scientifically based nutritional argument reinforced the unspoken argument for the primacy of free trade: the question of prohibiting margarine was not re-opened. There remained only the need to ensure that it was not fraudulently marketed as butter, which was dealt with some years later.[73]

Playfair's intervention in favour of margarine may, however, have been crucial. His biographer noted that his share in 'making "the poor man's butter" ... easily procurable was not a small one'.[74] Without Playfair's informed defence of the qualities of margarine, it is possible that the case for restricting its sale on health grounds would have met with greater success. In the United States at the same period the butter protection lobby made dramatic use of such arguments in their campaign to undermine the margarine industry.[75]

The adulteration and margarine questions were of social importance, and were argued as such by Playfair. They were also essentially static questions, in which the terms of scientific argument went unchanged. In the case of animal diseases, however, developments in scientific knowledge forced Playfair to restructure his arguments in the years between 1878 and 1890. Playfair was no stranger to the problems of animal diseases, for he had been a member of the Royal Commission on Cattle Plague in 1866, and had been an influential advocate of the stamping out policy then imposed.[76] When the question of regulations for the control of foot and mouth disease emerged in 1878, Playfair was strongly opposed to proposals for restricting the import of cattle from abroad. Although there can be little doubt that his free trade principles were involved, he based his case on social issues:

> Do not let us impose unnecessary and heavy restrictions on the meat markets, when we know that all restrictions augment the price of a commodity. Surely this is a disastrous policy at a time when the working classes are poor, and when trade shows no signs of revival?[77]

Playfair's argument may have been effective, in that the Contagious Diseases (Animals) Act as passed contained only the briefest of clauses regarding imported cattle, and concentrated on measures to control herd movements within Britain.[78]

The problem of foot and mouth did not go away, however. In 1884 the matter came before the House again. By this time scientific discoveries had sharpened the issues involved: foot and mouth, which had been thought to spread by immediate contagion, was now known to travel by mediate infection through the agency of men and articles. Secondly, the physiologists were just beginning to recognise the serious effects of milk in the production of human disease.[79] Both these scientific discoveries aggravated the seriousness of the preventive problem, as Playfair was well aware. None the less, he continued to argue the free trade case, insisting that until energetic domestic measures were taken to stamp out the disease there was little point in restricting imports: statistically speaking, imports were a 'very minor evil', while the agricultural community had done little to stamp out the disease at home.[80] It was a powerful speech, but for once Playfair made little impact on the House. The 1884 Amendment Act considerably strengthened the hand of the Privy Council in prohibiting the import of diseased cattle.[81] Indeed, Playfair's position was the more irregular, in that provision for the monitoring and exclusion of cases of human infectious disease coming from abroad had recently been augmented.[82]

Playfair was, however, right in his assessment that it would take much more than the prohibition of imports to resolve the problem of epizootics. By the 1890s, bovine pleuro-pneumonia, swine fever, and foot and mouth were all continuing to cause concern. A last straw was added by the recognition that tuberculosis in cattle had implications for the health of man.

In March 1890, the MP for Salford, which was home to one of the country's largest cattle markets, called for urgent consideration of the matter. Once again, it was a free trade issue: the condemnation of British meat was in accordance with the views of individual magistrates, but there were no checks on imported foreign meat.[83] Both Farquharson and Playfair registered their concern, and the latter specifically criticized the newly-established Board of Agriculture. Playfair was by now moving – as he had 15 years earlier over adulteration – towards a specialized administrative solution; the matter had reached a point where it was no longer primarily a free trade issue. Playfair had already drawn attention to the desirability of a scientifically based agricultural department, such as existed in other countries, notably in North America.[84] He now reiterated the point, and called for a scientific enquiry into the question of bovine tuberculosis.[85]

The debate on bovine tuberculosis was the last in which Playfair participated in his scientific capacity. The recognition that the problem of animal disease could no longer be fought from a free trade perspective suggests pragmatism; his proposed resort to scientific expertise was consistent with his solutions to other public-health problems, and with his faith in the power of science ultimately to resolve problems associated with the human condition.

### Reform of the Medical Profession

One of the most wearisome topics to occupy parliamentary time in the years after 1869 was that of the reform of the medical profession. In the nineteenth century, the profession was evolving from its medieval to its modern form, and the process of evolution was painful.[86] As physicians, surgeons and apothecaries transformed themselves into consultants and general practitioners, inter-collegiate rivalries and intra-professional resentment blossomed. The Medical Act, 1858, had established the Medical Register and the General Medical Council, but the general practitioners were not represented on the latter, and were besides anxious to obtain a 'single portal' of entry for the whole profession, whereby all its branches would at least start equal in terms of qualification and status. Between 1870 and 1886, no fewer than 22 bills to amend the 1858 Act were introduced into the Commons. Despite general consensus on the need for further reform, all these bills failed.

As long as Playfair represented the universities of Edinburgh and St Andrews, he could not help but be closely concerned with the issue of medical reform. Although he was not without sympathy for the discontents of 'this long-agitated profession', he plainly regarded 'medicals' as a difficult, quarrelsome lot.[87] He described his disappointment, in his memoirs, at finding his medical colleagues in Edinburgh in a state of chronic war with each other.[88] His letters to Edith Russell, who became his third wife, also testify to his detached view of a profession which he once intended to make his own. 'On Saturday I dined with about two hundred doctors at Greenwich,' he wrote to Edith in 1878, 'they were certainly a frigid assembly'.[89] His position was complicated by his position as a Liberal MP in a Conservative constituency: during elections he was vulnerable to opposition insinuations that he was not sufficiently active in the cause of medical reform.[90]

It was, however, Playfair who finally succeeded in resolving the 'angry controversies' of the medical profession. In 1886, Gladstone appointed him Vice-President of the Council – the Victorian equivalent of the Minister of Education. In this role he was instrumental, with the support of his colleagues in the House, in pushing through the Bill which became the Medical Act

Amendment Act 1886. Although it did not fully meet the desires of the general practitioners, it did accomplish two significant reforms: the ordinary practitioners gained representation on the General Medical Council, and it was provided that every practitioner should be qualified in medicine, surgery and midwifery before being admitted to the Register. Voicing some reservations, Sir Walter Foster, representing the British Medical Association, commended the Bill for its 'simplicity and modesty', while Farquharson noted that a 'difficult and perplexing' question had at last been placed on a sound legislative basis.[91]

The interests of the wider medical profession were not the only professional issues with which Playfair concerned himself. He was alert to the needs and problems of doctors in the services,[92] and early in his parliamentary career was instrumental in obtaining superannuation provision for Poor Law medical officers.[93] Once again, the efficiency of medical officers in the interest of public health, whether in the services or among the civilian population, formed a central theme in his arguments. Thus in the 1884 debate on conditions in the East India Medical Service, he stated explicitly:

> The improvements in public health, introduced by a skilled Medical Service, have produced vast economies in our Indian Government. You cannot keep up that efficiency without tempting the best men to enter the service.[94]

This remark echoed his 1870 justification for offering Poor Law medical officers superannuation: it would encourage the retention of only younger and more efficient men in service. Using a classic Chadwickian argument, he noted that it was cheaper to prevent than to support pauperism in Britain:

> If they properly paid and organised their medical combatants, whose profession it was to fight disease, so that they had a right to count upon their services and efficiency, economy to the country would be great.[95]

The consistency of Playfair's argument, after an interval of 14 years, supports his biographer's contention that he was a political economist 'of the orthodox type'; that he was 'unswerving and inflexible in his adherence to the doctrines of political economy which he had learned as a youth'.[96] In Reid's view, it was Playfair's good fortune to be able to draw the 'true economic lessons' from the changing conditions of human life through which he lived. While this was certainly true of Playfair's support for public health personnel, and his insistence on the proper employment of medical and scientific advice where circumstances required it,[97] it seems clear that Playfair's good fortune lay in the political conditions of the 1870s and 1880s, which favoured the constructive survival of the old political economy. By the 1890s, the insidious advance of socialism was opening the way for new interpretations of old problems, and Playfair's political economy was revealed not as constructive but as reactionary.

This shift in values and perspectives was made plain with the abortive Royal Commission on the Aged Poor of 1893–5, when Playfair's career in the Commons was over. Playfair's achievement of the 1886 Medical Act Amendment Act, by contrast, represented a triumph for the old political economy in its defence of professional standards and professional content as the best guarantee of efficient professional performance.

**The Aged Poor Commission**

Although returned for South Leeds in 1892, Playfair's Commons career came to an end in that year. His translation to the House of Lords did not end his career as a civil servant, however. In February 1893 he started work with the Royal Commission on the Aged Poor. The Commission's brief was to examine and reconsider public provision for the old. The question of state assistance for the old had recently become a focus of popular attention, following on social developments in Germany, and the Commission found itself considering a number of schemes for implementing similar provision in Britain. The political divisions which were fragmenting the Liberal Party soon became apparent, and created fundamental disagreements within the Commission. The final report, presented in 1895, was divided. The majority report, for which Playfair was largely responsible,[98] reaffirmed faith in the existing Poor Law provision; a minority report, activated by Joseph Chamberlain, dissented.[99] Chamberlain himself had presented a scheme for state assisted pensions, and the Minority Report was strongly critical of the main Report, condemning it as inadequate, over-optimistic and unrepresentative of public opinion on the central issue. It was perhaps a charge on Playfair's direction that the Minority Report concluded by calling for a special Royal Commission, 'better able to deal with the complicated technical details of the subject in an impartial and scientific spirit'.[100]

For Playfair, the idea of state assistance was quite incompatible with the traditions of political economy by which he had set his political conviction. Writing to his son George in March 1895, he observed that the Aged Poor Report had given him much trouble, and had brought him into 'active conflict' with Chamberlain. None the less, Playfair declared,

> All will be repaid if the public see how rapidly his scheme of public pensions would have degraded the working classes, and taken away their motives for thrift and dignified independence of public charity.[101]

The trend of political thinking lay away from Playfair's mid-Victorian traditionalism, although sympathizers like Wemyss Reid praised the 'frankness and courage' with which Playfair and Aberdare had 'vindicated those doctrines of political economy upon which the wealth of nations depends'.[102]

It may have been the last gasp of the old political economy. The Commission had no immediate outcome, and 14 years later, Lloyd George introduced the old age pension.

### Conclusion

The course of Playfair's political career from 1870s to the 1890s appears to follow a classic curve from progressive beginner to reactionary retirement. Yet this impression, created by the division over the Aged Poor Commission, is too simplistic. Playfair believed in progress even if he retained traditional ideals of the value of independence and self-sufficiency for working people, and in the 1890s he was far from alone in standing by these ideals. In 1895, after all, they remained sufficiently strong to defeat Chamberlain's plan for state aid by a majority which included Joseph Arch and C. S. Loch.

The significance of Playfair's political career lies not in the unswerving nature of his personal political convictions, but in the position of scientific authority which he acquired in the Commons. It is a measure of his authority that, where the central issues of legislation before the House concerned medicine or public health, Playfair's influence was almost invariably decisive. His success in arguing the case for vaccination, for vivisection, and for the Contagious Diseases Acts demonstrates the willingness of the Commons to be influenced by cogent, scientifically-based reasoning in areas recognized to fall within the special authority of science. Where other interests were involved, however, the scientific perspective commanded less influence; the history of the animal disease acts shows it to have been overshadowed by the concerns of agriculture.

However well respected, scientific authority was strongest where it took a stand against essentially moral assaults on scientific issues. The pattern of parliamentary response to scientific argument clearly demonstrates the truism that a receptive climate of opinion is necessary for advocacy to be successful. Lyon Playfair, who arrived in the House with an established scientific and political reputation, was responsible for securing the authority of science and medicine in the Commons, but educated Victorian opinion had already accepted the principle of scientific authority on issues recognized to fall within the competence of scientific and medical expertise. The cremation episode, no less than Playfair's failure to convince successive governments of the importance of proper provision for scientific education, indicates the limits of scientific influence.

**Table 1: Medical men and scientists in the House of Commons, circa 1868–1910•**

| **Name** | **Party** | **Constituency** | **Commons Career** |
|---|---|---|---|
| Lyon Playfair FRS (1818–1898) | Liberal | Edinburgh & St Andrews; Leeds South | 1868–1892 |
| J.A. Lush FRCP (1815–1888) | Liberal | Salisbury | 1868–1880 |
| W. Brewer FRCP (d.1881) | Liberal | Colchester | 1868–1874 |
| Sir J. Lubbock FRS (1834–1913) | Liberal | Maidstone; London University | 1874–1900 |
| Sir C. Cameron (1841–1924) | Liberal | Glasgow | 1874–1900 |
| R. Farquharson FCRP (1836–1918) | Liberal | West Aberdeenshire | 1880–1906 |
| Sir W. Foster FRCP (1840–1913) | Liberal | Chester; Ilkeston | 1885–1910 |
| Sir H. Roscoe FRS (1833–1915) | Liberal | Manchester South | 1885–1909 |
| G.B. Clark FRCS (1846–1930) | Radical | Caithness; Edin. | 1885–1900 |
| Sir G. Stokes FRS 1819–1903 | Conservative | Cambridge University | 1887–1891 |

• This list does not include Irish medical MP, and may not be exhaustive, since it has not been compiled by systematic analysis of House of Commons records.

## Notes

1. Peter Clarke, *Liberals and Social Democrats*, (Cambridge: Cambridge University Press, 1978), 5
2. The term 'science' is here used in its widest sense, as also embracing medicine.
3. See Table 1. I have omitted consideration of the Irish medical MPs, whose political and social background and concerns I judge to have been significantly different from those of the mainland representatives.
4. Wemyss Reid (ed.), *Memoirs and Correspondence of Lyon Playfair* (London: Cassel & Co, 1899), 3–4.
5. *Ibid.*, chapter 3.
6. Reid, *Playfair*, 43; Peel Papers, British Library Additional MSS 40517, F08; 40518 f. 3, 311, 313, 317, 350. For Peel's agricultural interests see Norman Gash, Sir *Robert Peel*, (London: Longmans, 1972), 678–9.
7. Christopher Hamlin, *A Science of Impurity* (Bristol: Adam Hilger, 1990).
8. Gladstone Papers, British Library Additional MSS 44280 f 143, Playfair to Gladstone 12 November, 1859; *ibid.* f. 149, Playfair to Gladstone 18 May, 1868.
9. Reid, *Playfair*, 98.
10. *Ibid.*, 6–7.
11. Playfair's earliest explicit sanitary concern dates from his voluntary service in the 1848 cholera epidemic; in 1874 he recalled his experience of 30 years of sanitary work: Reid, *Playfair*, 103; *B MJ* 1874, ii 461.
12. Ian Bradley, *The Strange Rebirth of Liberal Britain*, (London: Chatto, 1985), 9.
13. Reid, *Playfair*, 10.
14. Letters from Chadwick to Playfair written between 1855 and 1887 are in the Playfair Papers, Imperial College 154–7. Playfair did not take up either Chadwick's enthusiasm for re-cycling sewage, or his conviction that cattle plague was 'typhoidal' in character.
15. For Playfair's recognition of Simon's work see *B.M.J.* (1874), ii 461. There may have been deep personal differences between the two men. Dorothy Porter points out that Simon was opposed to the extension of the Contagious Diseases Acts, which Playfair supported.
16. See *B.M.J.* (1874), ii 455–61; (1875), i 735.
17. *Ibid.*, 1875, i 736.

18. *Ibid.*, 1874, ii 461.
19. The only scientific Conservative was Sir George Stokes (1819–1903), MP for Cambridge University 1887–91. A further partial exception was Gavin Brown Clark (1846–1930), MP for Caithness 1885–1900, an Independent who 'practically always' voted with the radical wing of the Liberal Party: *B.M.J.* (1930), ii 126. By Scottish background I mean that they were either Scots or had been educated in Scotland. The exception was Walter Foster (1840–1913), MP for Ilkeston, Derbyshire 1887–1910.
20. J. Brand, *Doctors and the State,* (Baltimore: Johns Hopkins Press, 1965),161. Christison was President of the BMA in 1875, the year in which Playfair was elected to honorary membership of the Association: Imperial College, Playfair Papers 1147. For the friendship see Reid, *Playfair,* 40, 182; Robert Christison, *The Life of Sir Robert Christison* (Edinburgh: Blackwood & Sons, 1886), vol. 2, 34–5
21. Robert Farquharson, *The House of Commons from within* (London: Williams and Norgate, 1912), 103. Buckland also testified to Playfair's communication skills; Peel Papers, British Library Additional MSS 40517 f. 108.
22. *Ibid.*, 66.
23. *Munk's Roll of Fellows of the Royal College of Physicians,* iv 246 (Farquharson); *B.M.J.* 1924, ii 692; Farquharson, *House of Commons,* 116 (Cameron).
24. Jack D. Ellis, *The Physician Legislators of France* (Cambridge: Cambridge University Press, 1990), 134.
25. Playfair Papers, IC 358. Hooker to Playfair 4 October, 1873.
26. Reid, *Playfair,* 206.
27. Christison, *Life,* 34–6.
28. Reid, *Playfair,* 337.
29. Playfair Papers, IC 1103, James Gozney to Playfair, 5 June, 1885.
30. J. P. Parry, *Democracy and Religion,* (Cambridge: Cambridge University Press, 1986), 149.
31. Reid, *Playfair,* 286.
32. Bradley, *Rebirth of Liberal Britain,* 25–6.
33. These concerns are mirrored in the structure of his one volume of collected essays and speeches, *Subjects of Social Welfare* (1889), which is divided into three parts under these headings.
34. See *Subjects of Social Welfare,* 37–42, and his 1869 speech on scientific education: Hansard, Parliamentary Debates, third series, cxcviii 203–10.
35. Playfair's standing as a research scientist was not high. He appears to have done little original research: see his *D.N.B.* entry.

36. Reid, *Playfair,* 268. Playfair's reluctance to fight contested elections was in fact financial: see Playfair Papers, IC 1103, James Gozney to Playfair 5 June, 1885.
37. Farquharson, *Commons,* 103–4. Playfair visited Gladstone to ask why he had not been given office: 'You are too old for office' was the reply. 'But, sir, I am much younger than you.' – 'That may be, but I am the exception to all rules.'
38. Gladstone Papers, British Library Additional MSS 44280 f. 232: Playfair to Gladstone 1 November, 1892.
39. One of his attractive features to the female historian must be his thorough-going advocacy of the political and educational rights of women. See in particular his speech on the Women's Disabilities Bill 1870 which concluded that 'the time has arrived when all capable citizens, whatever may be their sex or position in society, should have equal laws and equal rights':Parliamentary Debates, third series, ccl 230–4.
40. Richard D. French, *Anti-vivisection and Medical Science in Victorian Society* (Princeton: Princeton University Press, 1975), 228–9.
41. *Parliamentary Debates,* third series, ccl 1234 –337
42. Paul McHugh, *Prostitution and Victorian Social Reform* (London: Croom Helm, 1980), 58–9.
43. Playfair Papers, IC 334, Grand to Playfair 12 June, 1870.
44. *Parliamentary Debates,* third series, ccl 1330.
45. See R. M. McLeod, 'Law, medicine and public opinion: the resistance to compulsory health legislation 1870-1907', *Public Law* (1967), part 1, 121; part 2, 194. The pro-vaccination position began to crumble at around the time that Playfair retired from the Commons. He was still hotly defending the position in his memoirs: Reid, *Playfair,* 297–300.
46. *Parliamentary Debates,* third series, ccxii 934.
47. McLeod, 'Law, medicine and public opinion', part 2, 194.
48. *Ibid.,* part i 113–14; McHugh, *Prostitution,* 55 *et seq.*
49. French, see n. 40 above.
50. Reid, *Playfair,* 325.
51. *Parliamentary Debates,* third series, ccxxi 926; see also Lyon Playfair, list of correspondence in the Imperial College Archives, 1967.
52. cf Christison to the Lord Advocate, 15 June, 1876, copy in Playfair Papers IC 177; 'I look upon the proposed Bill, and any Bill at all like it, with absolute dismay.'
53. Christison to Playfair, 12 May, 1875: Playfair Papers, IC 176.
54. *Ibid.*
55. French, *Vivisection,* 128.
56. On education see *Parliamentary Debates* third series, cxcvii 203–10; ccii 558–65; for his economic convictions, Reid, *Playfair,* 9–10.

57. Brand, *Doctors and the State,* 14, 19: *Parliamentary Debates,* third series, ccx 856–8; ccxxiii 1245–55.
58. *Parliamentary Debates* third series, ccx 856–8. For Playfair's defence of Simon see *B.M.J.* 1874, ii 461, and Royston Lambert, *Sir John Simon 1816–1904 and English Social Administration* (Bristol: McGibbon & Kee, 1963), 545, 551.
59. *Ibid.,* 859–60.
60. *Ibid.,* ccxxii 379–82.
61.. *Ibid.,* 382.
62. Speech to the Social Science Association, Glasgow, 1874, reprinted in Lyon Playfair, *Subjects of Social Welfare* (London: Cassell & Co., 1889), 38.
63. Peter Jupp, *From Dust to Ashes: the replacement of burial by cremation in England 1840-1967* (London: Cremation Society , 1990), 14–16.
64. *Parliamentary Debates,* third series, cclxxxvii 996. The Scottish scientists were supported by a fourth Scotch member, Sir George Campbell, MP for Kirkaldy.
65. Jupp, *Dust to Ashes,* 14. See also James Stephens Curl, *The Victorian Celebration of Death* (Newton Abbot: David & Charles, 1976).
66. *Parliamentary Debates* third series, cclxxxvii 995.
67. He argued the sanitary case for cremation in the popular paper, *Good Words* in July, 1885. The article was reprinted in *Subjects of Social Welfare,* 96–104.
68. John Postgate, 'Sticky breches and poisoned lozenges', *New Scientist,* 128 (1990), 32; P. J. Rowlinson, 'Food adulteration. Its control in 19th Century Britain', *Interdisciplinary Science Reviews,* 7 (1982), 69; *Parliamentary Debates,* third series, ccxxii 593–610.
69. *Food and Drugs Adulteration Act* 1875, 38 & 39 Vict. ch. 63.
70. W. G. Hoffmann, '100 years of the margarine industry' in J. H. van Stuyvenberg (ed.), *Margarine; an Economic Social and Scientific History 1869–1969* (Liverpool: Liverpool Universtiy Press, 1969), 9–15.
71. *Parliamentary Debates,* third series, cclx 494.
72. *Ibid.,* 513.
73. *Margarine Act* 1887, 50 & 51 Vict. ch. 29.
74. Reid, *Playfair,* 372.
75. James Harvey Young, '"This greasy counterfeit": Butter versus oleomargarine in the United States Congress, 1886', *Bulletin of the History of Medicine,* 53 (1979), 403–10.
76. Reid, *Playfair,* 202–03.
77. *Parliamentary Debates,* third series, xxli 335–44.
78. *Contagious Diseases (Animals) Act* 1878, 42 & 43 Vict. ch. 74, section 35. The Privy Council was empowered to forbid the import of live cattle or

carcases, and to slaughter or quarantine animals in port, as necessary.

79. *Parliamentary Debates,* third series, cclxxxv 174.
80. *Ibid.,* 177–80.
81. *Contagious Diseases (Animals) Amendment Act,* 47 Vict ch. 13, sections 1, 2.
82. Anne Hardy, 'Smallpox in London: factors in the decline of the disease in the 19th century', *Medical History,* 27 (1983), 127–30.
83. *Parliamentary Debates,* third series, cccxlii 1555.
84. He had done so in the debate on the establishment of the Agricultural Board in the previous year: *Ibid.,* cccxxxii 1783.
85. *Ibid.,* ccxlii 1563. A Royal Commission was set up later that year, and further Commissions followed in 1894 and 1901: F. B. Smith, *The Retreat of Tuberculosis 1850–1950* (London: Croom Helm, 1988), 176–8.
86. See i S. L. Loudon, *Medical Care and the General Practitioner: 1750–1850* (Oxford: Oxford University Press, 1986); Ivan Waddington, *The Medical Profession in the Industrial Revolution* (Dublin: Gill & Macmillan, 1984); Jeanne Peterson, *The Medical Profession in Mid-Victorian London* (Berkeley: University of California Press, 1978).
87. *Parliamentary Debates,* third series, ccvii 40; clxxxix 1263.
88. Reid, *Playfair,* 181. The colleagues in question were Robert Christison, James Young Simpson, and James Syme: the two former became Playfair's good friends.
89. *Ibid.,* 282.
90. *Ibid.,* 286, 288.
91. *Parliamentary Debates,* third series, ccv 244.
92. *Parliamentary Debates,* third series, ccxii 1801; ccxxvii 1799; ccl 1435; ccxc 1622–5
93. *Ibid.,* ccii 722–4; *Medical Officers' Superannuation Act 1870,* 33 & 34 Vict. ch. 94.
94. *Ibid.,* ccxc 1265.
95. *Ibid.,* ccii 724.
96. Reid, *Playfair,* 440, 9.
97. See for example his contributions to the debates on the Arctic Expedition of 1875 and on the threat of Colorado Beetle in 1877: *Parliamentary Debates,* third series, ccxxxiv 1975, ccxxxvi 781.
98. Playfair replaced the ailing Lord Aberdare as Chairman of the Commission in December, 1894.
99. *Royal Commission on the Aged Poor, British Parliamentary Papers* 1895 xiv part 1.
100. *Ibid.,* 95.
101. Lyon Playfair to George Playfair, 31 March, 1895: Playfair Papers, IC 563.
102. Reid, *Playfair,* 400.

# 4

# Désiré Magloire Bourneville and French Anticlericalism during the Third Republic

*Bernard Brais*

## Introduction

The first four decades of the Third Republic (1870-1914) were for the new medical élite of Paris a period of substantial social gains. This cohort, which took control of the Paris Medical Faculty and many of the key hospital services of the capital during the late 1860s and 1870s, saw their association with reformist republican politicians rewarded by the construction of numerous new facilities for the scientific transformation of French academic medicine. Though the association of republican ideology and science had been long standing in France, it was following the 1848 Revolution that part of this young group of Germanophile medical men joined republican ranks.[1] However, disillusioned by Napoleon III's 1851 coup, and prevented from political activism by the repressive police state of the first decade of the Second Empire, most turned away from politics to concentrate on scientific research and on pursuing the different positions essential for an academic career in Paris.[2]

When the Imperial Regime became more liberal, during the 1860s and in particular after the passing of the 1868 laws on freedom of expression and of association, many proclaimed their republican inclination and joined the chorus of social and political reformers who challenged the Empire. Following the Prussian victory over the imperial forces in early September 1870, key leaders of this new medico-scientific élite, like Paul Bert (1833–86) and Charles Robin (1821–85), joined the charismatic Léon Gambetta (1838–82) in the interim government of National Defense which opposed the Prussian troops until the end of January 1871. This older group of medical reformists were joined by many of their younger medical trainees, such as Désiré Magloire Bourneville, in the fostering of medical reform as an integral part of the republican political platform. Some got involved in politics, while others used the lay or professional press to promote their demands.

This article reviews the life and works of one of the most controversial physician–politicians and medical journal editor of the Third Republic: Désiré Magloire Bourneville (1840–1909). Bourneville's career is a remarkable illustration of key features of medical politics in Paris during the early Third Republic: first, how closely the medical reform movement which sprang during this period reflected national political concerns, in particular the secularization of French society as a whole; second, it stresses the importance municipal and intraprofessional politics played in the functioning of the medical world of Paris; and lastly, it supports the claim that human networks based on friendship and shared interests played an even larger part than party membership in campaigns to ensure the implementation of reforms.

Bourneville's place in the history of medicine in France during the nineteenth - century has been largely ignored until recently. His involvement in medical and national politics, according to his friend Henri Thulié, had a lot to do with the 'conspiracy of silence' which shrouded his work up to the 1970s.[3] However, recent works in the history of nineteenth century French medicine, in particular Jacques Léonard's capital book *La médecine entre les savoirs et les pouvoirs*, have started to expose Bourneville's importance during the last three decades of the century.[4] This renewed interest in the famous editor of *Le Progrès Médical* explains the recent flurry of works completed on Bourneville. These include a book on his contribution to the treatment of mentally handicapped children,[5] five theses on different aspects of his life,[6] and a collection of papers presented at a 1990 symposium on Bourneville organized by the *Société Française d'Histoire de la Neurologie*.[7]

## Youth and Militancy

Bourneville was born on 20 October, 1840 in the village of Garencières, Normandy. His father, a humble property owner, made his living from the transformation of sewage from septic tanks into agricultural fertilizer.[8] A cholera epidemic prevented Bourneville from completing his secondary education. However, on the recommendation of a family friend, the alienist Louis-Jean-François Delasiauve (1804–93), he entered the Paris Medical Faculty in 1860.[9] During medical training, he spent much of his time on Delasiauve's psychiatric wards at Bicêtre, the Salpêtrière and at the country asylum of Vallée. He acquired the prestigious position of *interne des Hôpitaux de Paris* in 1865. In 1868, he spent his third year of internship in Jean-Martin Charcot's service at the Salpêtrière. This was the begining of a very rich and complex relationship between the two men. However, the fact that Charcot accepted the young Norman as his intern is somewhat surprising, because Bourneville did not fit the stereotype of Charcot's previous five interns. Bourneville was academically much weaker than his predecessors, having finished only 31st of the 42 successful interns in 1865, while all of Charcot's prior interns ranked in the top third of their promotion.[10] Furthermore, Bourneville was interested in psychiatry, while all of Charcot's previous trainees, except for Jules Cotard, were studying to become medical internists. It is possible that Bourneville's established journalistic skills may have swayed Charcot to take him as his assistant.[11]

Prior to 1868, Bourneville collaborated on numerous medical publications. He published his first scientific article in 1861.[12] The same year, he started writing papers for Delasiauve's *Journal de Médecine Mentale*, and soon became the publication's unofficial editor.[13] In 1862 he wrote articles for *La Médecine Contemporaine*, a journal devoted to hydrotherapy.[14] In 1865, he and his friend Noël Pascal (1825–89), having left this journal after a disagreement with its editor, founded *Le Mouvement Médical*.[15] This journal was written mostly by medical students and young graduates who actively promoted medical and social reforms. Noël Pascal, who was the editor of the journal until 1873, was a well-known opponent of the Imperial Regime. His vocal opposition to Louis Napoléon's 1851 coup forced him to leave France for many years, like Victor Hugo and a cohort of democrats. Undoubtedly, it was the progressive liberalization of the Empire during the 1860s which allowed a boom in the publishing of such militant republican medical journals as *Le Mouvement Médical* or its suggestively named allied publication *La Réforme Médicale.* This trend paralleled the creation of numerous new political papers during this period. Bourneville was one of *Le Mouvement Médical's* most prolific contributors. He filled the pages of the journal with articles and course transcripts. He was such an inveterate writer that one of his fellow interns wrote an acrimonious letter to the journal denouncing Bourneville's repeated and unauthorized writing up of material from various hospital services, and asking that a meeting should be arranged physically to settle their contentions![16] Bourneville ultimately became the co-editor of the publication from 1871 to 1873. Bourneville's genuine interest in publishing made him keep abreast of new reproductive techniques.

In 1868, he founded the first Parisian medical journal which included photographs: *La Clinique Photographique de l'Hôpital Saint-Louis.* This journal would be named *La Revue Photographique des Hôpitaux* in 1869, and *L'Iconographie de la Salpêtrière* in 1876. Concurrently with his extensive medical journalistic activities, Bourneville also wrote for the political press.

It was in 1867, that Bourneville joined the chorus of republicans who in new publications challenged the Second Empire.[18] He contributed to two extreme-leftist publications of Charles Delescluze (1809–71). In 1867, he published nine short articles in *Le Panthéon de l'Industrie et des Arts.*[19] Though they were reviews of medical and surgical novelties, Bourneville managed to include some political and in particular anticlerical statements.[20] Bourneville's contribution to Delescluze's *Le Reveil, Journal de la Démocratie des Deux Mondes* is more controversial. His name does not appear on any article, though contemporary biographies usually state that he wrote for the paper.[21] Jacqueline Lalouette makes a strong case that he was probably the author, under the pen-name of 'Chevalier Crédulin de la Bigottièrre des Moines', of 12 columns during the summer of 1870, entitled: 'Annales diaboliques. Fragments pour servir à l'étude de l'Eglise infaillible'.[22] Therefore, Bourneville, while continuing his medical education, acquired, during the 1860s, a broad journalistic experience which he used extensively during the 1870s and 1880s, under the patronage of Jean-Martin Charcot, to build a huge medical publishing empire, of which *Le Progrès Médical* was the most successful venture.

Bourneville's medical training ended with the fall of the Second Empire. The Third Republic was in sight, and republicans closed ranks. Unfortunately, true republicans had to wait until the definite installation of the Third Republic in 1875, and their progressive take-over of all echelons of state administrations during the following ten years or so, to see some of their cherished reforms implimented.[23] The reforms demanded by the medical élite of the capital since the 1840s had to be postponed to a large extent until the second half of the 1870s. The various levels of government had to change hands before substantial funds could be granted for the construction of a new medical faculty, numerous research laboratories and modern hospital services. As Bourneville once wrote: 'Money is the sinew of science as of war.'[24] For example, plans for the construction of a new Paris Medical Faculty had been studied by the Imperial Government but nothing had come of it.[25] The association of some of the leaders of the new medico-scientific élite of the capital with republican policy makers was to ensure a better promotion of this project. In 1878, the first stone of the new Medical Faculty was laid. Moreover, the new medical élite went further than just mingling with republican politicians, some of its leaders engaged in active politics.

Jack Ellis, in his book on French physician-legislators, provides a detailed study of the increasing political involvement of doctors during this period.[26] At the national level, for example, physicians who had accounted for 4.9 per cent of the members of Napoleon III's *Corps Législatif*, averaged 10 to 12 per cent of the new Republic's legislative assemblies.[27] As to their political affiliation, it is clear from Ellis's work, that most were on the left of the political spectrum, being members in most cases of either the Republican left, the Republican Union, the Radical Left or the Extreme Left.[28] The great majority of this new breed of physician-legislators did not come from Paris.[29] However, the few representatives of the Parisian medico-scientific élite were to have the most significant influence. Their republicanism, which was clearly tainted with scientism, corresponded to a widespread belief shared by the so-called heroic generation of republicans. In fact, many historians agree that republicans of the early Third Republic wholeheartedly endorsed the same scientific values as the progressive medical élite of the capital, and 'replaced religion by the worship of science'.[30] This was particularly true of the more radical republicans with whom, as we will see, Bourneville engaged in political campaigns, and whose merits he defended in his *Progrès Médical*.[31]

### *Le Progrès Médical;* Medical Journalism and Politics

Bourneville founded *Le Progrès Médical* in 1873. It soon achieved considerable popularity and influence. Bourneville's weekly was not only devoted to the publication of original articles on cutting-edge medical science, its editorial policy was also actively to promote progressive reforms whether medical, social or political in nature. A study of the first 30 years of the *Progrès'* existence enables one to identify Bourneville's political positions, to establish his circle of allies, and, furthermore, to discover how Bourneville used *Le Progrès* to promote his own and his friends' interests.

In his history of *Le Progrès Médical*, Marie René Loeper states that the idea of the journal came from Charcot, who in fact set out its objectives, planned its organization and also supplied Bourneville with many of the original collaborators. Charcot, to borrow Loeper's words, was 'the star who had shown the way and guided the journal'.[32] Some have even suggested that Charcot owned the journal, but there is no evidence to support this claim.[33] Though many of Bourneville's first group of collaborators were also Charcot's students, a large number came from *Le Mouvement Médical*. In fact, *Le Progrès Médical* was in many ways a continuation of this journal. Not only did the new journal take over the office of *Le Mouvement Médical* at 6, rue des Ecoles in the Latin Quarter, it also adopted the same layout. Furthermore, *Le Progrès Médical* benefited from a tremendous brain drain from the older publication. Fifteen of *Le Mouvement Medical's* contributors joined Bourneville's new team, while just five stayed with the weakened journal which survived only until the end of the decade. Noël Pascal, who sold the former publication in 1873, happily left most of the infrastructure of *Le Mouvement Médical* to his friend Bourneville. Pascal was proud of the affiliation between the two journals: 'The sweetest reward is that *Le Mouvement Médical* has given rise to *Le Progrès Médical*'.[34] Though Charcot undoubtedly played a key role early on in the creation of the journal, the editorial policy was left entirely to his pupil.

Bourneville claimed the purpose of the journal was the promotion of 'new ideas ... its only bias being to always defend truth, justice and freedom'.[35] Politically, *Le Progrès* made no attempt, from its inception, to conceal its militant republicanism heavily tainted with anticlericalism. The first editorial made its position very clear. Though the Republic was under conservative monarchist control, the journal vigorously denounced the composition of the new *Conseil Supérieur de l'Instruction Publique*, because it included religious leaders. It saw in the new Council an undesirable 'hybrid association of science and religious faith'.[36] When the Third Republic was more firmly established, after 1877, *Le Progrès* could make its position even clearer: ' ... in our opinion, radicalism must be seen as a disinfectant, truly the only one powerful enough to cleanse what has been infected by the clerical plague'.[37] As we will review, Bourneville's political platform was dominated by the same anticlericalism his journal advocated. Surprisingly, the journal rarely discussed issues related to public health; it had a clear preference for the promotion of institutional reform. Continuous promotion of medicine as a science, and defence of radical socio-political reforms, ensured that by the late 1870s *Le Progrès* was seen as the voice of the medical avant-garde of the capital.[38] This image was reinforced by the journal's own publicity, as one can judge from an 1882 advertisement in

Merlet's *Annuaire de la Presse Française:* 'Republican journal with substantial medical and scientific advertising. Its editor is a physician at the Bicêtre hospice. Journal of the avant-garde of the scientific movement, its editorial staff is composed of the medical élite who for the most part belong to the *internat des hôpitaux*'.[39] *Le Progrès Médical* was the only publication to flag its political colours among the 98 French medical journals listed in the 1882 catalogue.

*Le Progrès* apparently rapidly became one of the most widely read medical weeklies in Paris. When the first issue of *Le Progrès* appeared on 14 June, 1873, over 60 medical journals were published in France.[40] *La Gazette des Hôpitaux Civils et Militaires* (*Le Lancette Français*) had the largest readership, followed by *La Gazette Médicale de Paris, Le Journal des Connaissances Médicales Pratiques, La Tribune Médicale, L'Union Médicale* and *Le Journal de Médecine et de Chirurgie*.[41] Except for *La Tribune Médicale* which had been founded in 1867, all of these general medical publications were created before Napoleon III's 1851 coup.[42] The creation of *Le Progrès Médical* should be seen as part of a medical journal publication boom which started with the liberalization of the Second Empire and accelerated during the Third Republic. The repressive police state of the early Empire prevented not only the creation of political papers but also of more reformist medical journals. It was only with the liberalization of the regime during the 1860s that one notes the creation of a new breed of militant journals like *Le Mouvement Médical* founded in 1865, and a few others which did not survive the tumultuous year of 1870. Furthermore, this new freedom of speech compounded by both technological innovations which reduced the cost of printing, and the removal in 1867 of a deontological ban on advertising by pharmaceutical companies, fuelled this tremendous boom in medical publications.[43] *La Tribune Médicale* was the first true success of this boom, but it was soon overtaken by *Le Progrès Médical*. Though *Le Progrès* was undoubtedly one of the greatest success stories of this rapid growth in medical publishing, it was soon in competition with new weeklies for this lucrative market. *Le Paris Médical* which was founded in 1875 and *La Semaine Médicale*, founded in 1881, were to become its biggest rivals for the next decades, while the older general medical publications would, in most cases, not survive much past the turn of the century.[44] Unfortunately, as opposed to the political press, there are no circulation statistics available for medical journals during this period. Therefore, one has to rely on indirect sources to establish the popularity of *Le Progrès*. Léon Daudet (1867–1942) in *Les Morticole* his 1894 satirical parody of the medical world of Paris, stigmatizes

Bourneville as Cloaquol, the all-powerful and crafty proprietor of *Le Tibia Brisé*, the most popular and influential journal of the imaginary country.[45] From non-fictional sources, it is clear that Daudet's caricature of Bourneville and the influence of his journal was only a slight vindictive exaggeration. For example, Maxime Laignel-Lavastine and M. Fosseyeux, in their review of the history of French medical journalism during the nineteenth and early twentieth centuries, single out *Le Progrès Médical* and *La Presse Médicale*, founded in 1893, as the two French medical journals which achieved the largest circulation before 1936.[46]

The key to understanding the influence Bourneville derived from the popularity of his journal in the medical world of the capital is to realize that the journal had become, to borrow Léonard's words: 'a sort of monitor of the medical Latin Quarter'.[47] Evidence to support this claim, besides Charles Richet's account of the early days of the journal, is that *Le Progrès Médical* is the only medical journal mentioned in secret police reports on student agitations in the 'quartier des Ecoles' during the 1870s and 1880s.[48] Significantly, in October 1878, while the undercover agent reported that the student quarter was quiet because classes had not yet started, he felt it was his duty to mention that a recent article in *Le Progrès*, on the possible creation of a Catholic medical school in Paris, was widely discussed.[49] The fact that *Le Progrès Médical* was the only medical journal mentioned in the thousands of police reports testifies to the great popularity of the journal with medical students. One needs to recall that medical students, over two thousand strong, were by far the most turbulent in the Latin Quarter. The daily activities of the Faculty were often disturbed by student rioting through the 1870s, which caused repeated closure of the institution. Though *Le Progrès* never officially approved of these manifestations, the journal constantly defended student rights whenever possible.[50] To further increase the journal's popularity with trainees, it also published, as of 1874, a yearly student guide to medical teaching in France. This detailed listing of all lecture series given in the capital and in the provinces soon became a must for all students. Bourneville's recommendations to students, in his introduction to the first edition of the guide, underlined the ideological beliefs he wanted his journal to instil in the medical youth of France: ' ... you should not fear to impassion yourself for science because it will make excellent physicians of you, but also impassion yourself for everything concerning humanity, because this will make you worthy of the title of *citoyen.* To witness your dedicated work will fill us with pride, because it will thrust our country in the direction of progress and freedom'.[51] The extent of *Le Progrès'* popular appeal with medical students can be appraised by the accusation of a right-wing newspaper that Bourneville coerced students to read his journal by making it somehow compulsory for their education.[52] However, the ultimate popularity of *Le Progrès* with the wider medical public was clearly the product of many other successful editorial strategies used by Bourneville, the most significant of which was to give, from the outset, a progressive image to his journal.

Bourneville's success in portraying his journal as the one of the French medical vanguard rested on a dual strategy of providing ample space in his journal for the publications of promising young medical men, while at the same time actively promoting them as leaders of medical science and reform.[53] Bourneville used various schemes to foster the reputation of certain of his medical allies. He generously publicized their lectures and books. The journal also published laudatory reviews of the teaching of its contributors and friends,[54] while printing captious reports on the works of rivals.[55] Bourneville's dedicated promotional efforts were rewarded by a tremendous fidelity on the part of the scientists his journal supported. Moreover, Bourneville in an 1873 editorial presented those men whom he wanted his readers to see as the leaders of the scientific movement in the capital. He singled out the hospital physicians Charcot, Jules Parrot (1829–83), Aristide Verneuil (1823–95) and Alfred Vulpian, and the laboratory researchers Louis Ranvier (1835–1922) and Victor Cornil (1837–1908).[56] Obviously all were frequent contributors to his journal. Furthermore, Bourneville in this editorial presented his mentor and the chief patron of the journal, Jean-Martin Charcot, as the prime medical reformer in the capital.

Charcot's visibility was greatly enhanced by the increasing readership of *Le Progrès*. It is clear that *Le Progrès*' deliberate campaign to promote Charcot's medico-scientific stature was needed at the time of the journal's foundation. Charcot was still a minor figure in the rising medical élite of the capital. Full professor at the Faculty since 1872 only, Charcot's lectures at the school and at the Salpêtrière did not yet attract the large audiences that they would during the late 1870s and 1880s.[57] Symbolically, the cover article of the first issue of *Le Progrès* was a transcription of a lecture delivered by Charcot at the Salpêtrière.[58] Furthermore, beside providing an increasingly large readership for Charcot's writings, the journal actively sought to enlarge the audiences of his lectures by printing rave reviews of his teaching and generously advertising his books.[59] For example, Charcot's name and the subjects of his upcoming lectures were placed in larger and more eye-catching print at the top of the weekly list of lectures in Paris than any others.[60] The close association of *Le Progrès Médical* with Charcot ensured that the journal was seen as the 'official spokesman of Charcot's school'.[61] The basic role played by the editor of *Le Progrès Médical* in Charcot's school was later summarized by *Le Bulletin de la Société Française d'Histoire de la Médecine*, as: ' ... Charcot had a school, and who says a school implies a coterie. To exist a coterie needs influence and publicity. We know the influence Charcot held with such imperious authority. At the time, without the support of either Charcot or (Charles) Bouchard, there was no salvation. As for the publicity, the mentor entrusted his pupil Bourneville who made it his speciality.'[62] Bourneville was clearly Charcot's publicist, but in exchange Charcot provided his uncompromising pupil the needed support of a powerful network of allies.

On studying the School of the Salpêtrière in more detail, one is struck by its complexity and political ramifications. Though one can find no clear reference to Charcot's political beliefs in his own writings, his convictions apparently were known to all. A contemporary biography stated that 'Charcot's greatest faults are to have renounced his faith and to be a Jacobin ... '[63] His close relationship with Léon Gambetta (1838–82) is often used as evidence of his republicanism.[64] Charcot's 'hegemony' over the medical world of the capital during the 1880s was clearly not due only to his scientific achievements.[65] His power was also based on an extensive network of friends and pupils active in academic and political arenas. Bourneville, his chief publicist, was a key figure of Charcot's network, but other individuals were also staunch political supporters of both mentor and pupil.

Henri Liouville (1837–87) and René Waldeck-Rousseau (1846–1904) were surely the closest to Charcot. Liouville was the son of a famous French barrister, head of the Paris bar at one time.[66] He was an intern of Alfred Vulpian's at the Salpêtrière in 1867. He entered Parliament in 1877 as a member of Gambetta's *Union Républicaine*, and married Charcot's stepdaughter the following year. From Jack D. Ellis's study, it is clear that he was one of the most influential physician-legislators until his premature death in 1887.[67] He was one of the leaders of the *Groupe Médical Parlementaire*.[68] He was a prime promoter of a law on compulsory smallpox vaccination,[69] and a vocal advocate of reform of French public health.[70] He contributed to *Le Progrès Médical* during the 1870s, and was called 'a friend of the journal' by Bourneville.[71] Liouville's close friend and colleague from the *Union Républicaine*, René Waldeck-Rousseau, would marry his widow. Though Waldeck-Rousseau, like Charcot, was implicated in the Panama Canal scandal in 1892, he still managed to have a successful career, which culminated in his becoming prime minister in 1899.[72]

Apart from Bourneville, Victor Cornil, an intern at the Salpêtrière in 1865, was Charcot's most powerful and successful political ally.[73] He, like Liouville, came from a wealthier stock than most physicians in the National Assembly during the Third Republic.[74] Though Cornil was close to Gambetta during the late 1860s, he chose to join the more centrist Republican Left when he entered the National Assembly. He served as a deputy from 1876 to 1882, and as a senator from 1885 to 1903.[75] Furthermore, Cornil was made full professor of the Medical Faculty of Paris thanks to the unconditional support of Charcot, taking over Charcot's Chair of Pathological Anatomy in 1882.[76] Cornil acknowledged his debt to his mentor in 1892: 'It is not only in medicine that we have learned from his contact, but also intellectually, politically and philosophically ... I owe him what I am today.'[77] As mentioned above, Cornil was promoted by *Le Progrès* as one of the leaders of progressive medicine in Paris. He was also a frequent contributor to the journal until he took over his stepfather's *Le Journal des Connaissances Médicales Pratiques* in 1876. *Le Progrès* also actively supported the reform of leading physician-legislators who were also leading academics, and with whom Charcot shared reformist ideas about scientific medicine. The journal was particularly keen in supporting the reforms proposed by Paul Bert (1833–86), Charles Robin (1821–85) and Paul Broca (1824–80).[78] Though undoubtedly, much of Bourneville's power was based on Charcot's network of students and friends, Bourneville's own political allies were also important in increasing his own and his mentor's sphere of influence.

Bourneville, not only in the various elected assemblies but also in the columns of his journal, would forcefully support the reforms proposed by some of his closest political associates, many of whom, like himself, had joined the free masonry.[79] Among this legion of republican politicians, two particularly stand out: Georges Clemenceau (1841–1929) and Louis Blanc (1811–82). Clemenceau was also a physician who trained during the turbulent 1860s.[80] His political career was long and impressive. He was a close friend of Bourneville, serving as his witness when Bourneville was challenged to a duel in 1883 by Georges-Marie Félizet (1844–1908).[81] Bourneville would support Clemenceau's political campaigns in *Le Progrès*. For example, he would present and support Clemenceau's repeated efforts to have the 1838 Law on insanity abrogated.[82] Clemenceau would do the same in his newspaper *La Justice* or in the National Assembly.[83] For instance, during the weeks prior to Bourneville's 1883 election to the Chamber of Deputies, *La Justice* published no less than six articles where 'their friend Bourneville' was singled out as the best candidate in this race.[84] Bourneville's friendship with the famous radical politician Louis Blanc was also significant. Bourneville was one of Louis Blanc's political organizers for years before his death in 1882.[85] He then took over Blanc's seat in the National Assembly. As Bourneville got more involved in active politics, his own and his mentor's circle of contacts obviously increased.

## Municipal Councillor

I shall turn now to Bourneville's involvement in municipal politics. As was common at the time, Bourneville first became a municipal politician prior to entering into the national arena.[86] He was elected municipal councillor on 30 May, 1876, for the Saint-Victor district of the fifth *arrondissement* of Paris.[87] He represented this part of the Latin Quarter for seven years. He also sat as general councillor in the Departmental Legislature of la Seine from 1879 to 1883.[88] It is important to know that the Municipal Council played a key role in the administration of Paris hospitals. The budgets of the *Assistance Publique*, a suprastructure managing most of the hospices and hospitals of the French capital, were reviewed by commissions of the Council. These commissions then made recommendations in the form of reports to the Municipal Council and the *Préfet de la Seine*. The Prefect could ask the director of the *Assistance Publique* to alter previous decisions or to implement changes suggested by the commissions. The reports were written by the *rapporteur*. During his mandates, Bourneville was by far the most prolific *rapporteur*. In 1877 alone, he produced eight of the ninety-three reports, which represented a substantial literary output of more than four hundred pages.[89] Most of these reports concerned medical subjects, in particular on improvements to buildings and facilities of different institutions. Bourneville's medical training and obvious interest in medical reforms ensured that soon after his election he was made responsible for the writing of the report on the 1878 budget of the welfare agency.[90] Without apparent second thought, Bourneville published its recommendations in *Le Progrès*.[91] It is striking that many of the proposals put forward seem to serve Bourneville and his friends' own interests. First and foremost, it requested what would become the reform most associated with his name: the laicization of the personnel of hospitals under the control of the *Assistance Publique*. It also requested minor and major improvements to the two hospitals Bourneville knew best: Bicêtre and his mentor's Salpêtrière.[92]

Bourneville's 1877 report marks the beginning of an effective campaign by the editor of *Le Progrès* to reform Parisian hospitals.[93] I will now review four reforms Bourneville was able to have implemented as a municipal councillor. The first two will display his militant anticlericalism, while the others will show how advantageous his political position was for him and his mentor.

Anticlericalism as a political movement flourished in France during the 1860s and 1870s. To borrow Theodore Zeldin's words: 'anticlericalism was originally a protest much less against religious belief than against the political pretensions of the Church'.[94] It soon polarized French society into two opposing camps. To understand anticlericalism, one has to remember that France constitutionally remained a Catholic State until the passing of the 1905 law on the separation of State and Church, and that ' ... anticlericalism is a social and cultural phenomenon peculiar to Catholic societies; it is a complement to the history of the Roman Catholic Church'.[95] René Rémond, in his splendid history of French anticlericalism, puts forward a convincing argument that when the Church prospered so did anticlericalism.[96] Therefore, it comes as no surprise that a new and more militant anticlericalism flourished during the Second Empire. During the first years of the Imperial Regime, there was a close collaboration between Church and State. Religious communities made rapid strides during the early 1850s, by increasing in number, wealth and membership.[97] Furthermore, 'the second half of the nineteenth century was also the heyday of miracles', the most famous being the ones of La Salette in 1846 and Lourdes in 1858.[98] To the increased political power of clericals, intellectuals and republicans voiced their discontent. French scientific and medical communities became bastions of this opposition.[99] In 1868, when Bourneville joined Charcot's service, his chief was singled out as a materialist by clericals.[100] In fact, science became a sort of 'republican spiritualism'.[101] Bourneville in the 1860s did not hide his radicalism, a label which at the time implied a staunch anticlerical stand.[102] As a child of Catholic Normandy, and a medical student during these conflictive times, it is not surprising to see that when he became a politician, his platform was dominated by his desire to oppose religious authority. He and his journal clearly supported Léon Gambetta's 1877 famous declaration: 'clericalism, that is the enemy!'[103]

The first successful campaign Bourneville launched took place during his first year as a municipal councillor. The *Assistance Publique* had asked the Prefect's permission to place placards at the head of hospital beds. This apparently insignificant policy spurred Bourneville's indignation, because the name of the patient was to be followed by his or her religion, the name of the chaplain, whether sacraments had been received, and lastly if the patient had changed religion during his or her hospitalization. Bourneville vociferously opposed at Council meetings what he saw as another example of infringement of the sacred freedom of belief, while publicly denouncing the proposed policy in *Le Progrès.*[104] As many secret police reports corroborate, students joined Bourneville in denouncing the administration's project by often verbally abusing hospital chaplains.[105] The general uproar forced the welfare agency to drop its plans. The significance of this incident resides in the conclusion Bourneville drew from this victory: 'This small reform demonstrates that by persevering in its request, the press can obtain if not all, at least some of the reforms it demands.'[106] Bourneville had learned that his privileged position as both politician and editor of *Le Progrès* entrusted him with quite an influence. This rekindled his desire to push forward with his most ambitious reform: the laicization of Paris hospital and hospice personnel.

In 1875, Bourneville started publicly to demand the laicization of hospital personnel and the creation of nursing schools to supply the *Assistance Publique* with lay workers to replace nuns.[107] Most hospitals in the capital had been in the hands of religious orders for centuries.[108] Bourneville felt this had to change, so that religious propaganda would stop in these institutions, and doctors could be supplied 'with servants' rather than nuns who only had to answer to the head of their order.[109] Over the next 25 years, *Le Progrès* published numerous editorials pressing for these reforms.[110] Furthermore, the journal seemed to relish in reporting various news items on priests' and nuns' failings as healers of body and soul.[111] For example, the story of a chaplain and a nun, who after having tried to encourage religious fervour on the part of a patient for an entire evening, found the poor young man hanging from the ceiling in the morning.[112] At a more intellectual level, Bourneville, Charcot and many other students of the *maître* published articles and books suggesting that most saints and demoniacs were simply mad, epileptic or hysterical.[113] Bourneville went as far as starting in 1883 a collection of such historical works: *La bibliothèque diabolique*.[114] Charcot's *Les démoniaques dans l'art*,[115] and Bourneville's *Science et miracle; Louise Lateau, ou la stigmatisée belge* stand out as prime examples of this medico-anticlerical output.[116] This pathologizing of possession was, as Jan Goldstein suggested, another manifestation of their shared anticlericalism.[117] *Le Progrès* would go as far as reporting Valentin Magnan's (1835–1916) statement that: 'prophets of biblical times and sorcerers of the Middle Ages correspond exactly to the messiahs and emperors seen in our asylums'.[118] Contemporary medicine was therefore thought by Bourneville and his acolytes to provide a scientific explanation for all mystical events. Clerics were well aware of the political nature of this theorizing. Following Charcot's death, the clerical paper *La Croix* would write: 'Charcot used his explanation of miracles as a stepping stone to rise above the Church ... and for this he was bestowed a halo by the masses'.[119]

Bourneville, as soon as he became municipal councillor in 1876, actively embarked on a campaign for the laicization of hospital personnel. His first victory came with the granting, in 1878, of 2,000 francs by the Municipal Council for the creation of two nursing schools.[120] The Salpêtrière school was opened in 1878 and another at Bicêtre in 1879. His second success came in 1878 with the removal of some of the Salpêtrière's chaplains from the payroll of the welfare agency.[121] However, his reforms soon prompted a large opposition. Between 1879 and 1881, two petitions started to circulate against the removal of nuns.[122] By 1881, close to half of the hospital physicians had signed.[123] The rival journal, *La France Médicale*, became the spokesman for physicians opposed to Bourneville,[124] with Armand Després (1834–96) as his most vocal opponent.[125] Després, also a hospital physician, pursued Bourneville first in the Municipal Council and then in the National Assembly. He accused Bourneville of all possible evils, and denounced his growing influence over the *Assistance Publique*.

However, by 1880, not only was the Municipal Council firmly in the hands of republicans, but the new Prefect, Ferdinand Hérold (1828–82), and Charles Quentin (1826-1903), the new Director of the *Assistance Publique*, were both republicans. This completed what Bourneville referred to as the 'républicanization' of the administration of the welfare agency.[127] The first symbolic reform of the new order was to replace the names of saints for hospital services by names of 'illustrious scientists' in 1880.[128] The same year, the Prefect Hérold forced the *Assistance Publique* to secularize the

Hospices des Petits Ménages and La Rochefoucauld.[129] *Le Conseil de Surveillance* of the welfare agency resented this decision because it had not been consulted, and a series of resignations followed.[130] Bourneville went further, and demanded that conservative members of the Council who supervised asylum administration, *Le Conseil Supérieur des Asiles de la Seine*, be also replaced by true republicans.[131] Ensuing changes in the composition of the two councils turned the scale in favour of anticlericals. Bourneville could confidently write: 'It seems that the campaign we have supported for so long, will shortly deliver all the desired results'.[132] His statement was over enthusiastic, because most new laicization had to be fought for.[133] Albeit, the personnel of many hospitals was secularized during the 1880s, the reform was only completed during the 1960s.[134] Though Bourneville's status gained much from this relative success, as 'the man behind the laicization of hospitals', he became the target of much slandering.[135] Després continued to charge Bourneville, even accusing him of being the 'occult director' of the welfare agency.[136] In 1887, it was alleged in the Senate that Bourneville had made money from the nursing schools he directed, a situation that placed him in conflict of interest.[137] Bourneville got his friend Victor Cornil to defend him in the Senate, while many republican newspapers expressed their support.[138] The backing of the director of the *Assistance Publique* during the investigation, ensured his victory. However, Bourneville's growing influence as a politician, and the numerous advantages he seem to derive from his elected positions, would continue to ensure a fair share of controversy.

Bourneville personally benefited from his position as municipal councillor. In 1879, a new competition for the selection of *aliénistes des hôpitaux* was created unilaterally by a decree of Prefect Hérold.[139] Bourneville was chosen following an animated *concours* as psychiatrist of the Hospice of Bicêtre. Apparently, Charcot actively fostered some backing for his pupil as one can assess from a letter he sent to an unidentified colleague: 'Bourneville talked to me about his problem. As it could have been expected, much opposition has appeared, though he is surely the most deserving. Because of the circumstances, could you provide him with your support'.[140] The jury was apparently hostile to Bourneville's selection, and had to be swayed by Prefect Herold himself.[141] Later Després denounced these manipulations.[142] Bourneville had to defend himself in the Municipal Council, and send letters to various newspapers to vindicate himself.[143] Though his critics would often return to this possible illegitimate favour, the slandering campaign rose one notch in 1881. Bourneville was then accused of negligence when a lay employee of his service was found guilty of having sodomized four young patients and having transmitted syphilis to three of them.[144] Bourneville defended himself vigorously with some success, stating that he was on holiday at the time the aggressions were performed. Though he was never prosecuted, this scandal again raised the issue of the quality of lay personnel.

Bourneville's professional ambitions did not stop with his appointment to Bicêtre. On a yearly basis, starting in 1877, he had asked that the *Assistance Publique* create a special pediatric unit at the hospital.[145] In 1883, he presented the Municipal Council with a detailed report on the construction of a vast new service for the treatment of mentally retarded and epileptic children at Bicêtre.[146] The funds were approved, and Bourneville was appointed its director.[147] When the construction of his service was completed in 1892, it had over four hundred beds, an extensive educational programme, a library and a large pathological museum.[148] Though the service was seen as one of the better equipped and most progressive in the world, it continued to be criticized because of its cost and its unproven therapeutic success.[149] However, Bourneville's contribution to pediatric neuropsychiatry was significant, to the extent of being considered as the father of this discipline by some.[150] Though his expensive ***médico-pédagogique*** programme never had much international following, his anatomo-pathological research on mental retardation was considered first-rate. His most significant contribution was the original description of tuberous sclerosis in 1880, a condition which is still often referred to as Bourneville's disease.[151]

Charcot who backed his pupil in every possible way, owed much to Bourneville's dedication. In fact, Bourneville's relentless promotion of Charcot's interest at the *Assistance Publique* ensured that, even before his mentor was made Professor of the Diseases of the Nervous System at the Faculty in 1882, his service at the Salpêtrière had grown into a large fully-equipped Neuropathological Institute.[152] Between 1878 and 1882, Bourneville in seven different reports asked for substantial improvements to the Salpêtrière.[153] He claimed that the hospital was in critical need of these improvements because it had been completely neglected during the Second Empire.[154] Bourneville's key role in ensuring the improvements to Charcot's service was known to all, as can be appraised from an 1889 article in the *B.M.J.*: 'Mr Bourneville's assistance has been of great use in aiding Mr Charcot to develop some of these departments. His position in the Municipal Council, which largely controls the hospitals of Paris, and the Chamber of Deputies giving him influence which has been energetically employed in this and in many other cases to secure ameliorations in the construction and installation of various hospitals.'[155] To Charcot's old hospital service, with the financial backing of the *Assistance Publique*, were added over the years: a library, a pathological anatomy museum, an ophthalmology consulting room, a casting workshop, a photography workshop, a pathological anatomy laboratory, a psycho-physiological laboratory, a large amphitheatre, an electro-diagnostic laboratory, and a large out-patient clinic with a 60 bed short-stay ward.[156]

By the early 1880s, Bourneville, by accumulating the positions of hospital psychiatrist, municipal councillor and editor of *Le Progrès Médical*, had attained a social position of considerable power. His interest in medical, and in particular hospital reform, ensured him quite an influence on the *Assistance Publique*, to his own and his mentor's great benefit. It is clear that the accusation that Bourneville was the 'director *in partibus*' of the welfare agency was only a moderate exaggeration.[157] The magnitude of funds Bourneville was able to have unlocked for his own and his mentor's services was considerable.[158] However, Bourneville, as many other politicians at the time, elected to leave the Municipal Council, known as 'the purgatory of the national deputation', and in 1883 enter the national political arena.[159]

**Deputy**

Bourneville's career in national politics was less impressive. His first electoral success came on 4 February, 1883, again in Paris' fifth *arrondissement*. He took over the seat in the National Assembly of his friend Louis Blanc. He campaigned as a radical-socialist in the ranks of his friend Georges Clemenceau's Extreme Left. The latter had jumped into the national political arena with a vengeance a few years earlier. Bourneville's general political programme was the one of the *Comité républicain radical de la démocratie sociale*.[160] The group's militant anticlericalism is shown in their demand for the urgent separation of State and Church. During the campaign, Bourneville declared: 'I have set my heart on one thing more than any other, it is the laicization of the *Assistance Publique* by the elimination of nuns and chaplains.'[161] Therefore, it is clear that Bourneville wanted to continue to demand the secularization of hospital personnel in the National Assembly. However, he was less successful in promoting his cherished reform than as a municipal councillor. He presented two bills in 1887 to remove chaplains from the payroll of two hospitals, but both were rejected.[162]

He was elected for a second mandate on 18 October, 1885, again as a candidate of the Extreme Left, which was still a minor political party at the time. He voted consistently along party lines through both mandates.[163] He rarely participated in debates, and when he did, it was mostly on medically - related topics as he had done in the Municipal Council. However, one notes that he again used the dual strategy of promoting reforms both in a public assembly and in *Le Progrès Médical*. This scheme was well known to Clemenceau and other politicians, also newspaper editors. Therefore, Bourneville was not truly original in the use of this strategy, but his innovation lay in using a medical publication for political propaganda. This was logical, if one remembers that Bourneville was mostly interested in promoting medical reforms and the interests of medical allies. It then comes as no surprise that his major campaigns in the National Assembly were to denounce the prolonged vacancy of certain chairs of the Medical Faculty,[164] promote a bill to force old university professors into retirement,[165] request the continued laicization of hospitals,[166] and demand that sufficient funds be granted to complete the construction of the Ecole Pratique of the Medical Faculty. His June 1889 outcry in the Assembly about the delays in the construction of the Ecole Pratique is a good example of Bourneville's dual approach for the promotion of reform.[167] While he publicized in *Le Progrès* the grievances of Louis Hubert Farabeuf (1841–1910), the Professor of Anatomy who was the most affected by the slow construction, at the same time he echoed his concerns in the Assembly.[168] Farabeuf later recognized the importance of Bourneville's support, which had tightened the bonds between the two men.[169] Bourneville, through such service to fellow physicians, considerably extended his web of influence.

Though Bourneville's stature as a deputy was never prominent, his literary output was acknowledged in the production of reports, as it had been in the Municipal Council. His report on the agricultural use of Paris sewage was apparently seen as a standard for its thoroughness.[170] However, political turmoil would make him lose his seat in 1889. The election of 1889 was dominated by popular support for General Boulanger (1837–91). In his constituency, Bourneville faced Alfred Naquet (1834–1916), a well-known republican physician who had joined the ranks of the Boulangists. Furthermore, the laicization of hospitals was a major issue in the election.[171] Public resentment towards the 'man behind the laicization of Paris hospitals' and electoral support to Boulangist candidates were largely responsible for Bourneville's defeat.[172]

Bourneville, though having supported the suppression of the Senate in previous campaigns, would later try his luck at senatorial elections. He ran four times for a senatorial seat in 1896, 1897, 1899 and 1900, but always failed to be elected.[173]

## Bourneville's Fall

With the loss of his seat in the National Assembly, Bourneville's influence in the medical world of the capital started to decline. More than any other factor, Charcot's downfall in the early 1890s as the 'caesar of the Faculty' was responsible for the rapid lapse of his publicist into the darkest period of his life.[174] Charcot's authority was formally contested by his ambitious pupil Charles Bouchard (1837–1915) during the 1891 competition for associate professorship.[175] Bouchard, who was president of the jury, used various dubious means to ensure the success of his pupils and prevent the selection of Charcot's star candidate: Joseph Babinski (1857–1932).[176] Furthermore, social and political manoeuvring were extensively used by both camps. Bourneville tried to defend his mentor as forcefully as he could. The competition was not yet over that *Le Progrès Médical* pointed out the numerous procedural irregularities.[177] When the winners were finally announced, Bourneville complained: 'It is not exactly the results that the medical public expected for the Medical Faculty of Paris'.[178] This marked the beginning of the mobilization of the entire Charcot-network. While Bourneville continued to publish articles in his journal,[179] his friend Clemenceau printed an overt attack on Bouchard in his newspaper *La Justice*.[180] Following this article, the political press got interested in 'The Tempest at the Medical Faculty'.[181] Because only the Ministry of National Education could overturn the results of the *concours*, political and social pressure was applied on the Minister, Léon Bourgeois (1851–1927). From the correspondence between Charles-Edouard Brown-Séquard (1817–94), who supported Charles Bouchard, and his assistant, Arsène d'Arsonval (1851–1940), one discovers that politicians, newspapers and socialites were recruited to defend Bouchard.[182] Meanwhile, Victor Cornil fought for his mentor in the corridors of the Senate.[183] Cornil also charged his brother-in-law, the barrister Lesage, to defend the case of the unsuccessful candidates at the Ministry.[184] However, the efforts of Charcot's coterie failed, and this defeat, to borrow d'Arsonval's words, signalled that: ' ... the reign of Charcot at the Faculty was over'.[185]

Charcot, who suffered from a heart condition, died in 1893 in the middle of this controversy. His school was left in disarray, and as Loeper stated: 'with Charcot's death, Bourneville had lost his strongest backing, and a good deal of his power'.[186] The cards were reshuffled in the medical world of Paris, and Bourneville lost most of his stature. *Le Progrès Médical*, the 'officiel de Charcot', was soon in financial straits.[187] Bourneville left the editorial control of the publication in 1898.[188] He continued his work at Bicêtre though criticism from Alfred Binet (1887–1911) and other psychologists became relentless.[189] He died in poverty in 1909 at the age of 69.[190] Eleven years later, his pride, his service of Bicêtre, was closed down because it was believed to be too expensive and educationally outmoded.[191]

## Conclusion

Bourneville's career is a remarkable example of a man who straddled the realm of medical and national politics. His political success until 1889 rested on two pivotal factors: influence and publicity. It is clear that Charcot and his friends served as the power-network which protected Bourneville when he boldly sailed through troubled waters. This group of republicans, who shared a faith in French scientific medicine, did not, however, belong to the same political parties, their private ties transcended party lines. Furthermore, their ambitions being primarily medical, the purpose of their forays into municipal and national politics was above all to increase their influence in the medical world of the capital.[192] Bourneville's main function in this network was that of publicist, not to say propagandist. Bourneville's genius resided in his use of a medical journal to sway medical opinion on political issues. He was not the first nor the last journal editor to do so, one just needs to recall Amedée Latour's vigorous campaigns to promote the interest of his *Association Générale des Médecins de France* in the pages of his *Union Médicale*, or across the Channel, the career of Thomas Wakley (1795–1862) the founder of *The Lancet*.[193] However, Bourneville's ability to give his journal a vanguard republican image ensured that when fellow republicans took over the different elected assemblies during the late 1870s and early 1880s, some of the institutional reforms he had been campaigning for over the years could be carried out. Furthermore, the crafty editor of *Le Progrès Médical*, by providing his allies with a privileged means to sway medical opinion, increased his own realm of influence in the capital. However, Bourneville did not limit himself to promotion and publicity. As a municipal councillor, he also succeed in having some of his own and his network's demands implemented. In the final analysis, Bourneville's unequivocal ascendency on the *Assistance Publique* was the most profitable outcome of his political career.

Lastly, Bourneville's anticlerical campaigns illustrated how intricately medical and political reform movements were intertwined. The laicization of hospital personnel epitomizes this reality. Bourneville would defend this reform in political arenas in these terms: 'It is in the name of the freedom of conscience that, as a true republican, we have always asked for the secularization of education. It is in the name of the same freedom of conscience... that we demand the laicization of the *Assistance Publique.* These two reforms are so intimately linked that we cannot accomplish one without the other.'[194] On the other hand, Bourneville would insist on a different purpose when fostering support from a medical audience: 'We wish to provide heads of services with servants, who can be promoted or fired according to their skills or incompetence. Some seem to forget that a man's home is his castle.'[195] Therefore, this anticlerical reform was both one of trying to decrease the power of the Church in the field of public welfare, but also one to ensure a new dominance of physicians over nurses and a greater influence of the medical profession on hospital administration. Hence, concurrently with the victories of militant and triumphant anticlericalism during the 1870s and 1880s, one discerns the strides of triumphant French medicine.

## Notes

1. For a full discussion of the relationship between science and republican ideology, see: C. Nicolet, *L'idée républicaine en France* (Paris: Gallimard, 1982). Though Nicolet underlines that the ties between science and republicanism go back to the times of Condorcet (1743–94) (*ibid.*, 209), it is clear from his work that the Third Republic was to see a very extensive blending of science and republican ideology (*ibid.*, 209-311). For an analysis of the rise to power of a new French médical élite during the 1860s and 1870s, see: B. Brais, *The Making of a Nineteenth Century Neurological Celebrity: Jean-Martin Charcot* (London: M. Phil., University College London, 1990).
2. In 1873, Bourneville deplored the 'intellectual atony' of the medical community during the period spanning the years 1850 to 1868 as due to ' ... a fear that by asserting too freely one's opinions, ... one may offend powerful men, and by doing so, compromise one's career', D. M. Bourneville, 'Situation scientifique', *Le Progrès Médical*, i (1873), 137. For an example of this refraining of political activism during this period by a future star of the medico-political élite, see: P. Broca: *Correspondance*, 1841–57 (Paris: Typographie Paul Schmidt, 1886).

3. H. Thulié, 'Le docteur Bourneville', *Revue Philanthropique*, xxv (1909),177.
4. J. Léonard, *La médecine entre les savoirs et les pouvoirs: histoire intellectuelle et politique de la médecine française au XIXe siècle* (Paris: Aubier Montaigne,1981), 197.
5. J. Gateaux-Mennecier, *Bourneville et l'enfance aliénée* (Paris: Editions du Centurion, 1989).
6. J. F. Piera, *Histoire de la laïcisation des hôpitaux de Paris vue à travers Le Progrès Médical de 1873 à 1893* (Paris: Thèse de Doctorat en Médecine, Université de Paris XII-Créteil, 1979); M. C. Louis, *Histoire de la laïcisation des hôpitaux de Paris vue à travers Le Progrès Médical de 1893 à 1909* (Paris: Thèse de Doctorat en Médecine, Université de Paris XII-Créteil, 1979); J. Gateaux-Mennecier, *Les médecins aliénistes, les psychopédagogues et la déficience mentale à la fin du XIXe siècle, étude du service des enfants idiots de Bicêtre* (Paris: Thèse de Doctorat, Université Paris-V, 1986); M. Poisson, *Désiré Magloire Bourneville et les écoles municipales parisiennes d'infirmiers et d'infirmières, un regard sur les origines de la profession d'infirmière en France, ou l'histoire d'un rendez-vous manqué avec les femmes* (Paris: Mémoire de Maîtrise, Université Paris-VIII, 1990); and J. Plaisant, *Le Docteur Bourneville et les élections sénatoriales*, (Paris: Thèse de Doctorat en Médecine, Université de Paris XII-Créteil, 1991).
7. J. Poirier, J. L. Signoret (eds.), *De Bourneville à la sclérose tubéreuse* (Paris: Flammarion,1991).
8. J. Gateaux-Mennecier, *op. cit.*, (1989), 39.
9. J. Poirier, P. Ricou, J. L. Signoret, 'Bourneville (1840-1909): repères chronologiques', in J. Poirier and J. L. Signoret (eds.), *op. cit.*, 3.
10. *Annuaire de l'Internat en médecine et chirurgie des hôpitaux civils de Paris* (Paris: Librairie Arnette, 1964).
11. J. Gateaux-Mennecier, *op.cit.*, (1989), 39.
12. D. M. Bourneville, 'Mémoire sur le poids relatif entre les hémisphères cérébraux des épileptiques', *Journal des Connaissances Médicales Pratiques*, xviii (1861), 225–6, 239–41, 253–4.
13. J. Gasser, 'Bourneville, journaliste et éditeur', in J. Poirier & J. L. Signoret (eds.), *op. cit.*, 67.
14. J. Poirier, P. Ricou, J. L. Signoret, *op. cit.*, 3.
15. D. M. Bourneville, 'Noël Pascal', *Le Progrès Médical*, ix (1889), 363.
16. A. E. Louvet, 'A. M. Bournville', Le Mouvement Médical, i (1085), 222
17. *Ibid.*, 67.
18. J. Lalouette, *Le citoyen Bourneville, militant républicain et libre-penseur*, in J. Poirier and J.L. Signoret (eds.), *op.cit.*, 40.
19. J. Gasser, *op. cit.*, 40.
20. *Ibid.*, 41.
21. For example: 'Bourneville, D. M.', in P. Larousse (ed.), *Le grand dictionnaire universel du XIXe siècle* (Paris: Administration du grand dictionnaire universel, 1877), xiii 406.
22. J. Lalouette, *op. cit.*, 41.

23. G. Weisz, *The Emergence of Modern Universities in France, 1863-1914* (Princeton: Princeton University Press,1983), 116–17.
24. D. M. Bourneville, 'La Faculté de Médecine de Paris en 1886', *Le Progrès Médical*, v (1887), 10.
25. J. Rohr, *Victor Duruy, ministre de Napoléon III* (Paris: Librairie générale de droit et de jurisprudence, 1967), 96.
26. J. D. Ellis, *The Physician-Legislators of France* (Cambridge: Cambridge University Press, 1990).
27. *Ibid.*, 4, and T. Zeldin, *France, 1848–1945* (Oxford: The Clarendon Press, 1973), 23.
28. J. D. Ellis, *op. cit.*, 119.
29. *Ibid.*, 20.
30. R. Rémond, *L'anticléricalisme en France de 1815 à nos jours* (Bruxelles: Editions Complexe, 1985), 126; and G. Weisz, *op. cit.*, 116.
31. R. Rémond, *op.cit.*, 44.
32. M. Loeper, 'Histoire du journal', *Le Progrès Médical*, l (1922), 585.
33. F. Platel, *Les hommes de mon temps* (Paris: Bureaux du Figaro, 1890), 387. However, there is no mention of Charcot on Bourneville's request to publish *Le Progrès Médical* filed to the Paris police headquarters on 13 May, 1873, nor is there in the police report authorizing the printing of the new journal (Archives de la Préfecture de Police de Paris: B^ 906[Bourneville]).
34. N. Pascal, 'A nos lecteurs', *Le Mouvement Médical*, viii (1873), 674.
35. D. M. Bourneville, '1873-1883', *Le Progrès Médical*, iii (1883), 6.
36. 'Composition du Conseil Supérieur de l'Instruction Publique', *Le Progrès Médical*, i (1873), 4.
37. 'Une facétie cléricale', *Le Progrès Médical*, vii (1880), 321.
38. C. Richet, 'Au temps héroïque de la médecine', *Le Progrès Médical*, l. (1922), 589.
39. E. Merlet, *Annuaire de la presse française* (Paris: Merlet, 1882), 162.
40. V. Gébé, *Catalogue de journaux publiés ou paraissant à Paris* (Paris: O. Lorenz Librairie-Commissionnaire, 1877).
41. M. Loeper, *op.cit.*, 585; J. Gasser, *op. cit.*, 69; P. Le Gendre, *Un médecin philosophe: Charles Bouchard* (Paris: Masson, 1924), 50; and 'Bourneville', *Bulletin de la Société d'Histoire de la Médecine*, xvii. (1923), 142.
42. Year of foundation of the top medical publications of the early 1870s: *La Gazette des Hôpitaux Civils et Militaires* (1828), *La Gazette Médicale de Paris* (1830), *Le Journal des Connaissances Médicales Pratiques* (1833), *La Tribune Medicale* (1867), *L'Union Médicale* (1848) and *Le Journal de Médecine et de Chirurgie* (1830). Note that *Le Progrès Médical* was published until 1987.
43. J. Léonard, *op.cit.*, 197.
44. 'Bourneville', *Bulletin de la Société d'Histoire de la Médecine*, vii. (1923), 142.
45. L. Daudet, *Les Morticoles* (Paris: Charpentier, 1894).

46. M. Laignel-Lavastine, M. Fosseyeux, 'Le journalisme médical en France aux XIXe et XXe siècles', *Acta Medica Latina*, lii. (1936), 381–2.
47. J. Léonard, *op. cit.*, 197.
48. C. Richet, *op. cit.*, 589.
49. Archives de la Préfecture de Police de Paris, 25 (Etudiants, Surveillance Générale des Ecoles, 1876-1881), report dated 10 October, 1878.
50. G. Weisz, *op. cit.*, 22. For examples of the journal's defence of student rights, see: D. M. Bourneville, 'Les bureaucrates de l'Ecole de Médecine', i (1873), 101–2; 'Bulletin du Progrès Médical: aux étudiants', iii (1875), 247; 'Les bibliothèques des Facultés: nouvel impôt sur les étudiants', ii (1874) 31; and 'Le secrétariat de la Faculté de médecine', iii (1875), 245. *Le Progrès* 'commitment to medical students' concerns is illustrated by H. C. de Boyer's statement: 'It is to abide by *Le Progrès*' motto, and to carry on its tradition that we report on the recent projects drafted by the student Congress ('Sur le Congrès International et sur les Cercles Scientifiques entre étudiants', *Le Progrès Médical*, iv [1876], 469).
51. D. M. Bourneville, 'Le Numéro des étudiants', *Le Progrès Médical*, i. (1874), 674.
52. A. De Quesnay, 'Les bourreaux', *Le Pilori*, 192 (1882), 3.
53. A study of the number of leading articles published in *Le Progrès* by the top ten collaborators between 14 June, 1873 and the end of 1874 (number in parenthesis), reveals the extensive space provided for their works: Charcot (34), Cornil (19), Bourneville (14), Chouffe (13), Ferrier (13, translation from English), Parrot (9), Peltier (8), Richet (8), Ranvier (7), and Rosapelly (7).
54. For examples of positive reviews printed in *Le Progrès Médical*, see: 'Clinique médicale de l'Hôtel-Dieu: M. Béhier', i (1873), 274; and 'Asile Sainte-Anne: ouverture du cours de M. Magnan', vii (1880), 65.
55. For examples of negative reviews printed in *Le Progrès Médical*, see: 'Ouverture du cours de M. Brown-Séquard au Collège de France', vi (1878), 940–1; and 'Cours de clinique de pathologie mentale: M. le professeur Ball', xi (1891), 383.
56. D. M. Bourneville, 'Situation scientifique: l'association française pour l'avancement des sciences', *Le Progrès Médical*, i (1873), 137.
57. B. Brais, *op. cit.*, 90–2
58. J. M. Charcot, 'De la compression lente de la moelle', *Le Progrès Médical*, i (1873), 1–2.
59. D. M. Bourneville, 'Cours d'anatomie pathologique: M. Charcot', *Le Progrès Médical*, iii (1875), 192.
60. 'La chronique des hôpitaux', *Le Progrès Médical*, i (1873), 314, 341.
61. A. Corlieu, *Centenaire de la Faculté de Médecine de Paris* (Paris: Imprimerie Nationale, 1896), 564.
62. 'Bourneville', *Bulletin de la Société Française d'Histoire de la Médecine*, xvii (1923), 139.

63. Point-Calé, 'Le Professeur Charcot', *Les Hommes D'aujourd'hui,* ccxiii 2.
64. J. Goldstein, 'The Hysteria Diagnosis and the Politics of Anticlericalism in Late Nineteenth Century France', *Journal of Modern History,* 54 (1982), 223.
65. L. Daudet, 'Le professeur Charcot ou le césarisme de faculté', in *Les oeuvres dans les hommes* (Paris: Nouvelle Librairie Nationale, 1922), 197–8.
66. J. D. Ellis, *op. cit.*, 25.
67. *Ibid.*, 5 and 25.
68. *Ibid.*, 141.
69. *Ibid.*, 184.
70. *Ibid.*, 172.
71. 'Agrandissement de l'Ecole de médecine', *Le Progrès Médical,* iv (1876), 430. For praises of Liouville's political work printed in *Le Progrès,* see: 'Rétablissement des cours cliniques dans les asiles d'aliénés', iv (1876), 559; and 'Le budget de l'Instruction Publique', iv (1876), 569.
72. J. Y. Mollier, *Le scandale de Panama* (Paris: Fayard, 1991), 429.
73. J. D. Ellis, *op. cit.*, 55 and 118.
74. *Ibid.*, 24–5.
75. *Ibid.*, 245
76. 'Banquet offert à M. le Professeur Charcot', *Les Archives de Neurologie,* xxiii (1892), 447.
77. *Ibid.*, 447.
78. *Le Progrès* supported Bert's 1873 plan to reform medical education: 'Le budget et l'enseignement médical', i (1873), 340–50; 'Rapport de M. Bert à l'Assemblée Nationale: situation médicale', ii (1874), 298–9; 'Rapport de M. Bert à l'Assemblée Nationale: répartition des étudiants entre les facultés et les écoles secondaires', ii (1874), 332; 'Rapport de M. Bert: du nombre des facultés nouvelles qu'il convient de créer', ii (1874), 378–9; and 'Rapport de M. Bert: du choix des villes où il convient de créer des facultés; écoles de plein exercice', ii (1874), 410–11. Bert was an official collaborator of *Le Progrès Médical* in 1875. He would refer to *Le Progrès* as Bourneville's 'excellent journal' ('Le laboratoire de physiologie de la Sorbonne', *Le Progrès Médical,* v [1877], 916). For support of Robin, see: 'Rétablissement des cours cliniques dans le asiles d'aliénés, iv (1876,), 559.
79. J. Lalouette, *op. cit.*, 48.
80. J. B. Duroselle, *Clemenceau* (Paris: Fayard, 1985).
81. Bourneville, who had actively promoted, in the Municipal Council, the creation of a competition for the selection of obstetricians (accoucheurs) of the Paris hospitals, was personally attacked by many surgeons who saw obstetricians as professional rivals. Georges-Marie Félizet was the most vocal surgeon to oppose Bourneville. Following a letter from Bourneville to *Le XIXe Siècle* to

denounce Felizet's accusations, the latter sent two witnesses to challenge Bourneville to a duel. The matter was settled amicably by Bourneville's two friends, Georges Clemenceau and Sigismond Lacroix, both fellow radical politicians and newspaper editors (D.M. Bourneville, 'Le service médical des hôpitaux de Paris', *Le Progrès Médical*, iii (1883), 398–40).

82. 'Le budget de l'Instruction publique', *Le Progrès Médical*, iv (1876), 569; and 'Réouverture des cours de clinique mentale à l'Asile Sainte-Anne', *Le Progrès Médical*, v [1877], 47–8.
83. 'Laïcisation de l'Assistance Publique: renseignements sur le laïcisation des hôpitaux, interpellation de M. Després à la Chambre des Députés', *Le Progrès Médical*, x (1890), 429.
84. Bourneville is called a 'friend' in the following articles of *La Justice*: 'Election du Ve arrondissement, première circonscription', 1095 (1883), 2; and 'Election du cinquième arrondissement', 1117 (1883), 1. Other articles published in *La Justice* in 1883 to support Bourneville's candidacy, were: 'Discours du candidat Bourneville', 1092, 1; 'Election du V^e^ arrondissement', 1095, 3; 'Election du V^e^ arrondissement', 1099, 3; and 'Election du V^e^ arrondissement', 1100, 3.
85. D. M. Bourneville, *Inauguration de la statue de Louis Blanc* (Paris: Lucotte et Cadoux, 1887).
86. J. D. Ellis, *op. cit.*, 84.
87. J. Cadeaux-Mennecier, *op. cit.*, (1989), 112.
88. *Ibid.*, 112.
89. Except for the years of his 1876 election and in 1879, when he was preparing for the competition to select a hospital psychiatrist, Bourneville wrote the greatest number of reports of all municipal councillors: 1877 (8 of the 93 reports), 1878 (8/131), 1879 (6/159), 1880 (12/212), 1881 (5/111), and 1882 (9/123).
90. D. M. Bourneville, 'Budget de l'Assistance Publique pour l'exercice 1878; Budget de la Ville de Paris pour le même exercice: chapitre XXI, art. 1^er^ (subventions pour les dépenses annuelles des hospices et hôpitaux)', *Rapports et documents du Conseil Municipal de Paris*, 87 (1877).
91. D. M. Bourneville, 'Budget de l'Assistance publique', *Le Progrès Médical*, v (1877), 896.
92. Bourneville recommended that the salaries of the pharmacists and accountants of Bicêtre and the Salpêtrière be increased, the creation of new pediatric sections at the two hospices, and major improvements in the baths and water supply of the Salpêtrière (*ibid.*, 896).
93. Bourneville was responsible for the reports on the annual budget of the welfare agency from 1877 to 1881: *Rapports et Documents du Conseil Municipal de Paris*: 87 (1877); 84 (1878); 54 (1879); 190 (1880); and 85 (1881).
94. T. Zeldin, *op. cit.*, 1025.
95. R. Rémond, *op. cit.*, 57–8.
96. *Ibid.*, 13–16.

97. *Ibid.*, 160.
98. P. Guillaume, *Médecins, église et foi depuis deux siècles* (Paris: Aubier, 1990), 62.
99. R. Rémond, *op.cit.*, 49.
100. *Ibid.*, 9 and 164; B. Brais, *op. cit.*, 62; and J. D. Ellis, *op. cit.*, 38–9.
101. R. Rémond, *op.cit.*, 172.
102. *Ibid.*, 207.
103. J. Chastenet, *Gambetta* (Paris: Fayard, 1968), 262. Gambetta's famous statement was later reproduced in *Le Progrès Médical*: D.M. Bourneville, 'La laïcisation des hôpitaux devant les électeurs de Paris et le Conseil d'Etat', xiii (1893), 382.
104. Bourneville published the following editorial in *Le Progrès Médical* in 1876: 'L'Assistance Publique: les nouvelles pancartes des hôpitaux', iv 657–8. His collaborator E. Teinturier wrote: 'Les pancartes', iv (1876), 669; and 'Encore les pancartes', iv (1876), 681.
105. Archives de la Préfecture de Police de Paris: 25 (Etudiants, Surveillance générale des Ecoles), reports of 22 September, 3 October and 26 October, 1876.
106. D. M. Bourneville, 'L'Assistance Publique: les nouvelles pancartes des hôpitaux', *Le Progrès Médical*, iv (1876), 658.
107. D. M. Bourneville, 'Assistance publique: Les infirmiers des hôpitaux', *Le Progrès Médical*, iii (1875), 449–50.
108. J. Imbert (ed.), *Histoire des hôpitaux en France* (Toulouse: Privat, 1982).
109. D. M. Bourneville, 'L'Assistance Publique: les nouvelles pancartes des hôpitaux', *Le Progrès Médical*, iv (1876), 658; and D. M. Bourneville, 'Religieuses et laïques', *Le Progrès Médical*, i (1881), 215.
110. Bourneville published in *Le Progrès* over ten editorials on the subject between 1875 and 1881.
111. For examples published in *Le Progrès Médical*, see: 'Un curé accoucheur', iv (1876), 509; D. M. Bourneville, 'Religieuses et laïques', vi (1878), 238–9; 'Comment l'enfant faillit mourir et la soeur manquer ses vêpres', vi (1878), 529; and 'Une facétie cléricale', viii (1880), 321.
112. 'Les soeurs des hôpitaux', *Le Progrès Médical*, viii (1880), 359.
113. J. Goldstein, *op. cit.*, 209–39.
114. H. Thulié, *op.cit.*, 175. Nine volumes were published in this collection between 1883 and 1893.
115. J. M. Charcot, C. Richer, *Les démoniaques dans l'art* (Paris: A. Delahaye,1887).
116. D. M. Bourneville, *Science et miracle: Louise Lateau, ou la stigmatisée belge* (Paris: A. Delahaye, 1878).
117. J. Goldstein, *op. cit.*, 236–8.
118. 'Clinique mentale: ouverture du cours de M. Magnan', *Le Progrès Médical*, iii (1883), 87.
119. Le Moine, 'Charcot', *La Croix*, 3150 (1893), 1.
120. *Procès-verbaux du Conseil Municipal de Paris*, 6 August (1878), 10.

121. D. M. Bourneville, 'Chapitre XX des dépenses du projet de budget pour 1879 (Assistance Publique; aliénés; enfants assistés; etablissement de bienfaisance)', *Rapports et Documents du Conseil Municipal de Paris,* 119 (1878), 83.
122. These petitions were also published in *Le Progrès Médical:* D. M. Bourneville, 'Religieuses et laïques', i (1881), 210; and 'Laïcisation des hôpitaux', i (1881), 248–9.
123. Seventy-seven of the 150 physicians holding a hospital appointment in Paris in 1881 signed either of the two petitions against laicization. Victor Cornil was the only pupil of Charcot's to sign, with seven other colleagues, the only petition in support of hospital laicization. Though Charcot did not sign any of the petitions, he, his wife and his rich father-in-law financially supported the nursing school of the Salpêtrière [A. Brichon, 'Laïcisation de l'Assistance Publique', *Le Progrès Médical,* i (1881), 439].
124. *Le Progrès Médical* refers in these terms to the rival journal: '*La France Médicale,* the official mouth-piece for the physicians and surgeons whose protest against laicization has brought warm congratulations from right-wing municipal councillors and newspapers hostile to the Republic, has published a new petition...' ['Laïcisation des hôpitaux', i (1881), 249].
125. In 1881, Després published, in various newspapers seven letters attacking Bourneville and his reform. Transcripts of these letters can be found in *Le Progrès Médical:* D. M. Bourneville, 'Soeurs et laïques', i, 178–81; 'Laïcité de l'Assistance Publique', i 186; 'Religieuses et laïques', i 212; 'Laïcisation des hôpitaux', i, 244; 'Lettre de M. Després au Temps', i 248; and 'Laïcisation de l'Assistance Publique: septième lettre de M. A. Després', i 265–6.
126. 'Lettre de M. Després au Temps', *Le Progrès Médical,* i (1881), 248.
127. 'Réunion du Conseil Municipal de Paris, séance du 19 décembre', *Le Progrès Médical,* i (1881), 1035.
128. 'Laïcisation de l'Assistance Publique sous la monarchie et de nos jours', *Le Progrès Médical,* ix (1880), 413; and 'La direction de l'Assistance Publique et le recruitement des infirmiers', *Le Progrès Médical,* i (1881), 1035.
129. *Procès-verbaux du Conseil de Surveillance de l'Assistance Publique,* 2 December (1880), 98.
130. The heated debate between the discontented councillors, Hérold and Quentin occupied much of the meetings of 2, 16 and 30, December (*ibid.,* 98–100, 108–18, and 155–60). The two councillors to resign were: Duvillier and Léan de Saint-Gilles (*ibid.,* 110 and 230).
131. 'Une question à M. Hérold', *La Lanterne,* 4 February, 1385 (1881), 1.
132. D. M. Bourneville, 'Laïcisation de l'Assistance Publique', *Le Progrès Médical,* i (1881), 134.
133. P. Sollier, 'Revue de l'année', *L'Année Médicale,* xi (1888), 393.
134. Between 1878 and 1887 seventeen hospitals and hospices in Paris

were laicized. L'Hôtel-Dieu was the last of the major hospitals to have its personnel secularized in 1908. However, the reform was only completed in the 1960s (N. Simon-Dhouailly, *La leçon de Charcot: voyage dans une toile* [Cahors: Imprimerie Tardy Quercy, 1986], 114).

135. Pierre and Paul 'Le Dr. Bourneville', *Les Hommes D'Aujourd'hui*, clii. 4.
136. 'Laïcisation de l'Assistance Publique: réponse de M. Peyron à M. le Dr. A. Desprès, nouvelle lettre de ce dernier', *Le Progrès Médical*, vii (1887), 279.
137. *Ibid.*, 279.
138. The newspapers which supported Bourneville's campaigns over the years were: *Le Siècle, Le Rappel, La Justice, La République Française* and *La Petite République Française* ('Laïcisation de l'Assistance Publique: nouvelle lettre de M. Desprès', *Le Progrès Médical*, ii [1882], 767).
139. 'Un arrêté relatif au mode de nomination des médecins aliénistes de Bicêtre et la Salpêtrière', *Procès-verbaux du Conseil Municipal de Paris*, 4 March (1879), 224.
140. Wellcome Library for the History of Medicine, Autograph Letters Collection: Charcot, letter 65659. Unfortunately the letter is not dated and the name of the correspondent is not indicated. It is likely, however, that it was written in 1879 at the time when Bourneville was competing in the *concours des aliénistes de la Seine.*
141. Bourneville wrote in these terms about the opposition to his selection as *aliéniste des hôpitaux de Paris:* 'In spite of the relentless opposition by the score of judges who reproved of my political opinions, I was selected' ('Lettre de Bourneville', *Le Pilori*, 194 [1890], 2).
142. Desprès raises the possible intervention of the Prefect Hérold in: 'Lettre de Desprès', *Le Clairon*, 705 (1883), 1.
143. 'Conseil Municipal de Paris, séance du 10 mai', *Le Progrès Médical*, ii (1882), 371.
144. 'La direction de l'Assistance Publique et le recrutement des infirmiers', *Le Progrès Médical*, i (1881), 1033–6.
145. *Procès-verbaux du Conseil Municipal de Paris*, 20 January (1877), 1216. For his repeated requests, see: *Rapports et Documents du Conseil Municipal de Paris*: 119 (1878), 84; 154 (1879), 77; 190 (1880), 82; and 85 (1881), 82.
146. D. M. Bourneville, 'Sur la création d'un quartier spécial pour les enfants idiots et épileptiques à l'hospice de Bicêtre', *Rapports et Documents du Conseil Municipal de Paris*, 65 (1883).
147. *Procès-verbaux du Conseil Municipal de Paris*, 29 June (1883), 1317.
148. J. Cadeaux-Mennecier, *op. cit.*, (1989), 126, 186.
149. *Ibid.*, 198, 205, 238.
150. *Ibid.*, 263.
151. D. M. Bourneville, 'Contribution à l'étude de l'idiotie', *Archives de Neurologie*, ix (1880), 81–91. M. Bonduelle,'L'histoire de la sclérose tubéreuse; des circonvolutions cérébrales ou l'enfant trouvé de Bourneville', in J. Poirier and J. L. Signoret (eds), *op.cit.*, 129.

152. J. M. Charcot, 'Leçon d'ouverture', in J. M. Charcot, *Oeuvres complètes de J.-M. Charcot* ( Paris: Lecrosnier et Babé, 1890), iii 1.
153. *Rapports et Documents du Conseil Municipal de Paris*: 25 and 119 (1878); 3 and 154 (1879); 51 and 190 (1880); and 60 (1882).
154. D. M. Bourneville, 'Sur la construction d'un service balnéo-hydrothérapique à la Salpêtrière', *Rapports et Documents du Conseil Municipal de Paris*, 60 (1882), 6.
155. E. Hart,'Medical Paris of today: M. Charcot at the Salpêtrière', *B.M.J.* i (1889), 322.
156. J. M. Charcot, *op. cit.*, (1890), 2.
157. S. Nivette, 'Balance des comptes', *Le Soleil*, 336 (1889), 1.
158. It is very difficult to assess from the official documents the exact amounts Bourneville was able to have voted for his nursing schools and the hospices of Bicêtre and Salpêtrière. What is clear, is that much of the money came as 'extraordinary subsidies' voted by the Municipal Council. For example, the Salpêtrière benefited from 22 per cent of the *subvention extraordinaire* of 6,000,000 francs voted in 1881 for improvements to Paris hospitals. The Salpêtrière was the most privileged institution of the 12 hospitals and hospices subsidized (D. M. Bourneville, 'Sur la création d'un quartier spécial pour les enfants idiots et épileptiques à Bicêtre', *Rapports et Documents du Conseil Municipal de Paris*, 25 June, 65 [1883], 27–8). Furthermore, Bourneville was able to have a third of the 3,000,000 francs from the subvention extraordinaire voted in 1883 allocated to the construction of his pediatric unit at Bicêtre (*ibid.*, 26).
159. R. Martin, 'Les candidats du V^e^', *Le National*, 5 (1883), 2; and J. D. Ellis, *op. cit.*, 84.
160. The main items of this programme for radical political and social reforms were: the immediate creation of a Constituent Assembly with all powers, the drafting of a new constitution, the suppression of the Senate and of the Presidency of the Republic, the absolute freedom of the press and of unions, the universal freedom of access to a secular education, the separation of State and Church, the profound revision of the criminal code, the institution of compulsory military service, the design of a new income tax system, the decentralization of the national bureaucracy, the recognition of the right to work and welfare, the creation of a national pension plan, and the reorganization of the Central Bank ('Election du V^e^ arrondissement, première circonscription', *La Justice*, 1095 [1883], 2). With such a programme it is not surprising that a right-wing newspaper considered that: 'Bourneville represents this faction of the Municipal Council of Paris which wants to bring us back to the *Commune* by promoting anarchy' (P. Foucher, 'L'élection du V^e^ arrondissement', *Le National*, 5068 [1883], 1).
161. R. Martin, 'Les candidats du V^e^: chez M. Bourneville', *Le National*, 5070 (1883), 2.

162. F. Delrieu, J. Poirier, 'Bourneville, député', in J. Poirier and J. L. Signoret (eds), *op. cit.*, 64.
163. *Ibid.*, 62.
164. *Annales de la Chambre des députés*, 3 (1884), 882–3.
165. Bourneville proposed to impose a retirement age for university professors in the National Assembly on 15 December, 1884 ('Chambre des Députés; séance du 15 décembre', *Le Progrès Médical*, iv [1885], 14). Bourneville again used *Le Progrès Médical* to promote this reform: 'La limite d'âge pour les professeurs des facultés', iii (1884), 1034–5; 'Limite d'âge des professeurs des facultés: mise à la retraite de Gavaret, Hardy et Sappey', vi (1886), 626; 'Limite d'âge des professeurs de l'enseignement supérieur', x (1890), 68; and 'A la Faculté de Médecine: enseignement clinique, limite d'âge', xii (1892), 279. Bourneville went further in this campaign, he singled out for forced retirement professors he despised: Gavaret, Hardy and Sappey in 1886, Brown-Séquard in 1890, and Benjamin Ball and G. Sée in 1892.
166. *Annales de la Chambre des députés*, 3 (1884), 943–4.
167. *Annales de la Chambre des députés*, 2 (1889), 717–18.
168. *Ibid.*; and 'Chambre des députés (séance du 13 juin): Etat des travaux de l'Ecole Pratique de la Faculté de Médecine; de la limite d'âge des professeurs de l'enseignement supérieur', *Le Progrès Médical*, ix (1889), 480–4.
169. L. H. Farabeuf, 'A propos de l'article nécrologique sur Bourneville', *La Presse Médicale*, xxx (1909), 515; and M. J. Imbault-Huart, 'L'institution médicale à l'époque de Bourneville', in J. Poirier and J. L. Signoret (eds), *op. cit.*, 35.
170. J. D. Ellis, *op.cit.*, 138. D. M. Bourneville, *Rapport fait au nom de la commission chargée d'examiner le projet de loi ayant pour objet l'utilisation agricole des eaux d'égout de Paris et l'assainissement de la Seine* (Paris: Imprimerie A. Quantin, 1885).
171. S. Nivette, *op. cit.*,1; R. Rémond, *op. cit.*,174; and V. Leroux-Hugon, 'La laïcisation des hôpitaux de Paris et la création des écoles d'infirmières laïques', in J. Poirier and J. L. Signoret (eds), *op.cit.*, 75.
172. R. Rémond, *op. cit.*, 197.
173. J. Plaisant, *op. cit.*
174. L. Daudet, 'Le professeur Charcot ou le césarisme de faculté', in *Les oeuvres dans les hommes* (Paris: Nouvelle Librairie Nationale, 1922), 197; Loeper, *op. cit.*, 586; and P. Cornet, 'Echos d'un columbarium', *Le Progrès Médical*, xxx (1909), 308.
175. For more details on Charcot's decline see the last chapter of B. Brais, *op. cit.*, 171–203.
176. V. Iraque, 'The Charcot-Bouchard Controversy', *Archives of Neurology*, 43 (1986), 290–5.
177. 'Les incidents du concours d'agrégation', *Le Progrès Médical*, xii (1892), 57.
178. D. M. Bourneville, 'Le concours d'agrégation en médecine', *Le Progrès Médical*, xii (1892), 223.

179. D. M. Bourneville, 'Le concours d'agrégation en médecine', *Le Progrès Médical*, xii (1892), 239–40; D. M. Bourneville, 'Le concours d'agrégation en médecine d'après les journaux politiques', *Le Progrès Médical*, xii (1892), 248–9; and D.M. Bourneville, 'A propos des concours d'agrégation', *Le Progrès Médical*, xii (1892), 458.
180. P. Degouy, 'Un concours d'agrégation', *La Justice*, 4445 (1892), 1.
181. 'La tempête de la Faculté de Médecine', *Le Matin*, 2946 (1892), 1. For examples, see: D. M. Bourneville, 'Le concours d'agrégation en médecine d'après les journaux politiques', *Le Progrès Médical*, xii. (1892), 248–9.
182. L. Delhoume, *Dr Claude Bernard à d'Arsonval* (Paris: Baillière et Fils, 1939), 439–43.
183. D. M. Bourneville, 'Le concours d'agrégation en médecine d'après les journaux politiques', *Le Progrès Médical*, xii (1892), 248.
184. *Ibid.*, 248.
185. L. Delhoume, *op. cit.*, 443.
186. M. Loeper, *op. cit.*, 586.
187. A. Corlieu, *op. cit.*, 268.
188. M. Loeper, *op. cit.*, 586.
189. J. Cadeaux-Mennecier, *op. cit.*, (1989), 262. Alfred Binet stigmatized Bourneville's médico-pedagogique method as 'pompous' (A. Binet and T. Simon, 'Langage et pensée', *L'Année Psychologique*, 14 [1908], 284).
190. H. Thulié, *op. cit.*, 180.
191. J. Gateaux-Mennecier, *op. cit.*, (1989), 262.
192. As discussed by Christophe Charle, this type of self-interested political practice by academics was not uncommon (*Les élites de la République* [Paris: Fayard, 1987], 420).
193. M. Gille, 'Amédée Latour, journaliste et membre de l'Académie de Médecine', *Bulletin de la Société Fançaise d'Histoire de la Médecine*, 31 (1937), 127–8. M. Bostetter, 'The Journalism of Thomas Wakley', in J. H. Wiener (ed.), *Innovators and Preachers: The Role of the Editor in Victorian England* (Westport, Greenwood Press, 1985), 275–92.
194. 'Question de M. Bourneville au sujet de la laïcisation des établissements hospitaliers', *Procès-Verbaux du Conseil Municipal de Paris*, 17 March, (1881), 241.
195. D. M. Bourneville, 'Religieuses et laïques', *Le Progrès Médical*, i (1881), 215.

# 5

# The Demographic Argument in Soviet Debates over the Legalization of Abortion in the 1920s

*Susan Gross Solomon*

In November of 1920, the Soviet Commissar of Health N. A. Semashko and the Commissar of Justice M. Kurskii signed an edict legalizing abortion on social as well as medical grounds.[1] This decree, whose content had been discussed in medical circles for over a year,[2] made it legal for a licensed physician to perform an abortion on a patient who cited adverse social (read 'economic') conditions as the justification for her request. With the passage of the 1920 edict, the Soviet Union became the first Western nation to de-criminalize the voluntary termination of pregnancy on non-medical grounds.

When the legalization of abortion had been proposed a decade earlier in Russia, it had evoked some intense opposition in medical circles.[3] According to the official Soviet presentation of events, the 1920 decree put an end to that opposition: whereas many Soviet physicians initially greeted the new decree with hostility, by the mid-1920s, 'it was impossible to find an opponent of the legalization decree.'[4] The written record tells a very different story. Far from ending opposition to the legalization of abortion, the passage of the 1920 decree seems to have added new impetus to the medical criticism of legalization.

Of particular interest is the critique levelled by the two groups of Soviet physicians whose day-to-day practice was directly affected by the 1920 edict: specialists in obstetrics and gynaecology and specialists in maternity and infant care. An analysis of this substantial body of criticism shows that, for most of the 1920s, the demographic argument (i.e., the contention that decriminalizing abortion had a negative impact on the growth of population) played a relatively insignificant role in the case against legalization. Those physicians who opposed the new policy confined their attention almost exclusively to the medical consequences of decriminalizing abortion. The demographic (as indeed the moral) consequences of legalizing abortion remained a minor theme until the early 1930s.

To the comparativist, the lack of attention by Soviet physicians in the 1920s to the impact of the legalization of abortion upon the growth of the population is striking. In the post-war decade, many countries of Europe, notably France and Germany, were gripped by a 'fear of depopulation'.[5] In Germany, where the proposal to decriminalize abortion was being hotly debated, the impact of legalization upon the birth rate was a key issue in the medical discussions.[6]

To be sure, the demographic situation of Russia in the 1920s was fundamentally different from that of Germany or France. Russia had traditionally enjoyed a high birth rate.[7] While she had experienced a population implosion as a consequence of the War, her recovery was quite rapid. The restoration by late 1922 of the Russian birth rate to its pre-war level *could* explain the virtual absence of a demographic argument in the medical debate over abortion. *But for one fact*: in the first post-war decade, the fear of declining population figured prominently in the discussions of contraception by many of the same Soviet physicians who were involved in the debate over abortion. The puzzle, then, is the selective appearance of the demographic argument in medical discourse on fertility.

The puzzle is sharpened when we read Soviet medical discourse on abortion against the background of two other bodies of literature: first, the works on population growth written by Soviet demographers in the 1920s; and second, the assessments by foreign demographers of the implications of the decision to decriminalize abortion for the growth of population in Russia.

### The Edict of 1920 and the Medicalization of Abortion

The removal of criminal penalties for the performance of abortions made Russian physicians, rather than judges, the authorities over the artificial termination of pregnancy. But the fact that abortion was medicalized says nothing in itself about the terms of that medicalization. Critical questions remain to be answered. What was the scope of the state's grant of authority to doctors on the issue of abortion? What claims to authority did Russian physicians themselves make on the abortion issue? Were physicians ready to issue the kinds of social judgements necessitated by the new edict or were they inclined to confine themselves to judging the medical aspects of abortion?

An accurate understanding of the terms under which abortion was medicalized in the Soviet Union requires that we strip away three widely held myths. To begin with, radical though it was, the edict of 1920 was far from an unqualified endorsement of abortion.[8] In fact, the text of the edict opened with a statement that abortion was an evil to which women were driven because economic conditions made it impossible for them to care for their children. So dire was the economic need that legal punishment had proven ineffective in curbing the recourse of women to underground abortions which endangered their health and, occasionally, their lives. The only way to prevent women from harming themselves, so ran the argument, was to legalize abortion and to require that the operation be performed under sanitary conditions by a licensed physician. Further, the 1920 edict did not reflect a lack of commitment on the part of the state to a policy of pro-natalism.[9] Indeed, the Women's Division of the Party saw nothing inconsistent in supporting the 1920 abortion decree and in agitating for the preservation of maternity.[10] For those who signed the new decree, as indeed for those who supported it, there was no contradiction here. In the dire economic conditions that followed the revolution, the perceived choice was not between abortion and the maintenance of high birth rates; rather, the choice was between legalized (read 'safe') abortions and underground abortions. As soon as economic conditions improved, however, the signatories of the decree envisaged that abortion would be unnecessary.

The 1920 edict and the regulations for its implementation cast physicians – in particular obstetricians and gynaecologists and specialists in maternity and infant care – in the role of guardians of the safe performance of abortions. Physicians were to fulfil this mandate not only by conducting the operation under sanitary conditions, but also by administering the abortion system itself. While overall responsibility for monitoring the functioning of the abortion law rested with the Commissariat of Public Health and its Division for the Protection of Maternity and Infancy,[11] it was practising physicians who were charged with making the system work.

Over the course of the 1920s the administration of the abortion system became increasingly complex. In response to the flood of women seeking cost-free abortions, in January, 1924 a priority list for access to cost-free abortions was established and, in November of that same year, regional abortion commissions were set up to hand out permissions for free abortions and to oversee that the much-publicized priority list was being followed.[12] In their day-to-day practice, physicians could be called upon to supply the abortion commissions with medical certificates attesting to such matters as the length of pregnancy, the health of the patient, etc.[13] But many physicians were also involved more directly in the functioning of the commissions. The *troiki*, as the commissions came to be called in the vernacular, were staffed by an obstetrician/gynaecologist, a specialist in maternity and infant care, and a representative of the Women's Division of the Communist Party.[14] As members of the *troiki*, physicians were engaged in vetting requests for cost-free abortions. To that extent, they were routinely judging social entitlement.

Finally, appearances notwithstanding, the state's grant of authority to physicians on the abortion issue was limited in important respects.[15] To be sure, the implementation of the 1920 edict required physicians to make social judgements, but those judgements turned on questions of individual entitlement. As they assessed the merit of individual claims, Soviet physicians found themselves hedged about with a battery of rules on entitlement that had been issued by government ministries. Under these circumstances, the mandate of Soviet physicians was to make the abortion system work; their role was not to question the implications of the policy of legalization for society as a whole.

## Medical Discourse on Abortion

The physicians most directly affected by the passage of the abortion edict were the obstetricians and gynaecologists. In many respects, these specialists were ill-prepared for the kinds of social assessments they were required by the edict to issue. To begin with, the majority of the obstetricians and gynaecologists whose opinions had been canvassed before the edict was signed had declared themselves opposed to legalization.[16] Indeed, there is evidence that some of the most prominent representatives of this specialty were caught off-guard by the actual signing of the edict in November, 1920.[17] Even more to the point, the edict was passed just as the field of obstetrics and gynaecology was emerging from a period of seven lean years (1914–21) during which time the lion's share of medical research was understandably devoted to military medicine.[18] When the field began to revive in the early 1920s, there was widespread consensus that 'uterus gynaecology' had had its day and that the female patient ought to be treated as a whole.[19] But the specialty of obstetrics and gynaecology was divided between those devotees of holism who favoured a biological approach[20] and a smaller group who favoured the sort of social approach to gynaecology that Max Hirsch was pioneering in Germany at the same time.[21]

For its part, the specialty of protection of maternity and infancy was also poised somewhat uneasily at the interstices of social and biological science. The social focus of the specialty flowed logically from its concern with such issues as child rearing, adoption, and homelessness. But the physicians who spoke on behalf of this specialty[22] insisted that child care should be categorized as a medical matter.[23] The view that the protection of maternity and infancy was part of medical science was reflected in the field's research agenda[24] and in the content of its two leading journals, *Zhurnal po izucheniiu rannego detskogo vozrasta* and *Okhrana materinstva i mladenchestva*, which devoted the majority of their space to clinical questions, reserving only a small section for social matters.[25]

How did these two groups of physicians respond to the mandate contained in the 1920 edict? This paper argues that, to a large extent, the 1920 edict medicalized not only the performance of abortion, but also the terms in which legalization was discussed by Soviet physicians. Until the last third of the 1920s, physicians opposed to legalization criticized the new policy primarily on the grounds that abortion was harmful to women's health; only at the end of the 1920s did they begin to attack that policy on the grounds that it had a negative impact on population growth. Were these terms of discourse imposed on physicians? In my view, Soviet physicians opposed to legalization not only agreed to, but welcomed, the terms of reference. Doctors critical of the new policy talked openly about the tension between the demands of medical science and the demands of social life that had been set in motion by the passage of the 1920 edict.[26] For most physicians opposed to legalization, the solution to this tension lay in confining their claims to authority to the medical aspects of abortion.

## Science Versus Social Life

The extent to which Soviet physicians in the 1920s resisted being cast as judges of the social implications of legalized abortion – e.g., its impact on the growth of population or public morality – is clear from the transcripts of the meetings of specialists in obstetrics and gynaecology and of specialists in the protection of maternity and infancy. To be sure, in the immediate aftermath of the passage of the 1920 decree, there were occasional discussions of abortion in a moral tone reminiscent of the pre-revolutionary medical debates over the legalization. For example, a 1922 meeting of the Moscow

Society of Obstetrics and Gynaecology heard a paper on the physician's responsibility toward the unborn child – an early instance of foetal rights.[27] But as they began to perform their duties under the new law, physicians increasingly confined their writing and speeches to the medical sequelae of abortion.

The earliest articles and speeches (1922–4) on the medical consequences of legalization tended to be either reports of isolated cases of rare complications after artificial abortion[28] or impressionistic accounts of the net impact of the new policy on women's health.[29] But within a short time, physicians began to conduct statistical studies of the medical consequences of abortion. In June, 1924, the VI meeting of the All-Union Society of Obstetricians and Gynaecologists heard Dr M. Karlin of the State Clinical Obstetrical/Gynaecological Institute in Leningrad report on a study of 1,362 women done over the course of the first six months of 1923.[30] Although Karlin declared that the performance of an abortion by a physician reduced the risk to women's health, his data showed that the incidence of illness resulting from abortions was substantially higher than that resulting from births. Moreover, his results suggested to Karlin that the fertility of women who had abortions and no live births was lower than the fertility of women who had no abortions (the women who had undergone only abortions averaged 1.87 conceptions apiece, whereas those women who had undergone only births averaged 2.12 conceptions). This finding was important, given the rise in artificial abortion: for every natural birth there were 2.91 artificially induced abortions.[31]

These data on differential fertility spoke directly to the issue of declining population, but significantly Karlin discussed reduced fertility from the vantage point of the individual woman rather than that of society as a whole. A somewhat different spin was put on this data by Dr Bublichenko, who had supervised Karlin's research. Bublichenko concluded that artificial abortion was a social evil 'not only in the sense of lowering the birth rate, but in the sense of harming women.'[32] In fairness, at one point Karlin did allude to the social question. Examining the pattern of births in his sample, he found that of the 44 per cent of women who had never had an abortion, 52 per cent had but one birth, 23 per cent had two births, and 25 per cent had two or more children. On the basis of these findings, Karlin concluded, somewhat prematurely, that the *Zweikindersystem* was not really widespread among Leningrad women.

To be sure, both Karlin's and Bublichenko's handling of statistics was flawed, but for this paper the statistics themselves are less significant than the polemical use to which the 'data' was put. Statistics were very much part of the argument here – much as they were in the German medical debates on abortion in the same decade.[33]

The 1924 meeting with its brief reference to the demographic implications of legalized abortion was anomalous. In the period 1921–5, public discussion by physicians of abortion was infrequent. A review of the workings of the Obstetrics/Gynaecology Society of I Moscow State University for the year 1925 recorded that of 66 reports presented at 22 meetings, only one had dealt even tangentially with the issue: this was a report on the fluctuations in the birth rate and the reasons for it.[34] At the VII All-Union Congress of Obstetricians and Gynaecologists held in Leningrad in 1926, there was no report that dealt with abortion.[35]

In the period 1925–7, Soviet physicians began to discuss abortion with increasing frequency. Both in public and in print, their discussions of the subject tended to focus on the medical sequelae of abortion.[36] Even when they linked abortions to subsequent problems of fertility, the majority of physicians wrote about the problem from the vantage point of the well-being of the individual woman rather than that of the vitality of society as a whole.[37]

When physicians began to translate their opposition into action in the second half of the decade, not surprisingly, they also justified their opposition on the medical grounds. According to one report, as early as the end of 1924, some physicians had refused to perform abortions.[38] In 1926, other physicians went further, calling for a review of the policy of legalization.[39] Speaking on behalf of the critics, Dr Ul'ianovskii explained that it was not 'bourgeois morality'[40] but science that had prompted the opposition. As he put it, 'Certainly the state decree was stronger than the authority of science. But in the depths of their souls, doctors, to whom the interests of science and its authority were dear, probably even now are opposed to the decree with all its attendant consequences.'[41]

If physicians deliberately restricted their claims to authority to medical issues, it is also true that they guarded jealously the authority they did have. A report of the annual meeting of the Leningrad Obstetrical/Gynaecological Society held on 31 January, 1925 referred to a storm of protest from physicians over a proposal to have the regional abortion commissions (*troiki*) rule on whether abortions ought to be performed for medical reasons. The doctors insisted on their right to decide the medical cases, just as strongly as they tried to distance themselves from deciding the social cases.[42]

In fairness, prior to 1927 there were isolated instances of

physicians, particularly specialists in the protection of maternity and infancy, who linked the legalization of abortion to discussions of the birth rate. For example, at the May, 1926 meeting of the Leningrad section of the Division for the Protection of Maternity and Infancy, Dr Shuster-Kadysh asserted that the extent of abortions could have an impact on the birth rate.[43] But, to an important degree, sustained discussion of the demographic implications of the legalization of abortion required a finely tuned indication of the absolute number of abortions being performed.

The data for such a portrait began to emerge after July, 1924, when women who applied to the commissions for a free abortion were required to fill out a questionnaire on their social background and on their reasons for seeking an abortion. Beginning in 1925 those questionnaires were worked through by statisticians from the Central Statistical Administration and by physicians from the Commissariat of Public Health's Division for the Protection of Maternity and Infancy.[44] At about the same time, physicians in hospitals also began to keep records on patients who came in 'having started abortions which on their own'. This body of research yielded valuable social data on the prototypical abortion patient. An important by-product was a more accurate indication of just how many abortions were being sought.

**Kiev, 1927**

After this data had been in the public domain for a little over a year, the I All-Ukrainian Congress of Obstetricians and Gynaecologists opened in Kiev in May of 1927.[45] In many ways this Congress was a landmark event. The question of abortion was the second 'programme question'; 35 reports were presented on the subject. More to the point, the significance of the distinction between legal and illegal abortions was challenged as physicians critical of the policy argued that abortion, whether performed by a licensed physician or by a back-room abortionist, was harmful to the female organism.[46]

But most important, a number of physician-delegates drew connections between the absolute rise in the number of abortions and the birth rate. For example, Dr E. F. Schinkar of Kharkov provided data showing how over a three year period, while the per centage of abortions conducted 'on the side' fell from 66.5 to 49 per cent, the absolute number of abortions rose almost 300 per cent. (Schinkar made no reference to the difficulty of measuring underground abortions!) He also showed that the ratio of abortions to live births went up, both in the cities and in the countryside.[47] In his presentation, Dr Laptev argued that the vaunted reduction of abortions performed outside medical facilities was merely relative because the absolute number of abortions had risen so dramatically after 1925/1926.[48] According to Dr Tikhandse of Tbilisi, by 1924 abortions were 50 per cent of all births in Leningrad while in the large Grauerman maternity hospital in Moscow, the figure was 43 per cent. The situation in the countryside, according to Tikhanadse, was not much better.[49] While Dr Levit of Leningrad went on record saying that the 1920 decree had no effect on the number of abortions,[50] Dr Tikhanadse insisted that legalization had raised the number of abortions. Dr Laptev took the argument one step further: the rise in the number of abortions meant that the birth rate had fallen from 18.8 per 1000 in 1924 to 15.45 in 1926 — this despite the radical rise in births per 1000.[51]

To be sure, the statistics were unreliable, confusing, and often contradictory, but the weight of opinion in Kiev on the demographic implications of legalizing abortion was clear. And yet one of the resolutions passed at the end of the Congress explicitly denied that legalization of abortion had affected the birth rate.[52]

It is interesting to note that the appearance of the demographic issue on the agenda coincided with the appearance of the moral issue. The physicians who came to Kiev in the spring of 1927 decried not only the demographic sequelae of legalizing abortion but also its moral consequences which one delegate summarized as 'sexual chaos'.[53] What occurred at Kiev, then, was a concerted outcry by physicians against the social implications of legalizing abortion.

That Kiev was the venue for the first sustained discussion of the connection between legalized abortion and the birth rate is hardly coincidental. In general, opposition to the 1920 decree was more loudly voiced outside Moscow and Leningrad. But more to the point, the Ukraine had been particularly hard hit by the population implosion that followed the War, civil war and famine of 1914–22. According to a German estimate based on official Soviet statistical sources, there was a dramatic increase in death rates in the Ukraine from the famine (75.9 for 1000; 82.4 per 1000 in the first two quarters of 1922 respectively), which in this case led to radically lower birth rates.[54] In addition, it was in Kiev that the first new research centre for demography was formed in 1919 under the leadership of M. V. Ptukha.[55] Although there was less formal contact between obstetricians/gynaecologists and demographers in the 1920s than one might imagine, demographic issues were very much 'in the air' in Kiev. Little wonder therefore that the demographic issue was raised with some force here.

The Kiev meeting put the demographic implications of legalized abortion on the medical agenda in the Soviet Union.[56] In the wake of the 1927 meeting we find one physician claiming that abortion, underground or legal, whether performed by a physician or a *babka*, had the effect of diminishing the birth rate.[57] Another from Lugansk claimed that his colleagues had been wasting their time looking at the causes of abortion, its impact on women's health and reproductive capacity; the most important question about abortion was its impact on the birth rate.[58]

And yet, the 1927 meeting did not change indelibly these physicians' long-standing habit of restricting their claims to expertise to the medical aspects of abortion. Significantly, abortion was not listed as one of the four major topics for the VIII All-Union Congress of Obstetricians and Gynaecologists held in Kiev in 1928.[59] Indeed, the main emphasis of that meeting turned out to be the relation between women's roles in the production process and their roles as mothers-to-be.[60] The lone major report in the 1927 mode was that by Dr Bronnikova who discussed the harmful effects of abortion on a woman's subsequent capacity to give birth.[61] In retrospect, the 1927 Kiev meeting turns out to have been a rather unique event in the tide of medical opposition to legalized abortion. The demographic argument, sounded with such vigour at the Kiev gathering, did not reassert itself with any force until the early 1930s.

In the last two years of the 1920s, concern for the well-being of the woman as guardian of future generations (the basis for the demographic argument) was displaced in the medical literature by concern for the health of the woman as worker.[62] Significantly, the physical welfare of the female was now discussed not only by specialists in maternity and infant care or in obstetrics and gynaecology,[63] but by industrial hygienists who considered, *inter alia,* the impact of abortion on the woman's ability to work.[64] Almost imperceptibly, the legalization of abortion began to be defended as a policy in the interests of the working woman. Thus in 1928, Vera Lebedeva, the head of the Commissariat of Public Health's Division for the Protection of Maternity and Infancy published an article in which she referred to the legalization of abortion as a policy that protected the health of the working woman.[65] In the same year, A. B. Gens contributed an article to a German journal in which he rationalized the continuing concern with abortion as a function of the increasing participation of the woman in public life.[66]

## Medical Discourse on Contraception

The near absence of the demographic argument in the discourse between the state and the physicians on the question of abortion stands out in bold relief when we examine Soviet medical discussions of contraception in the 1920s. In Russia, birth control was legalized at the end of 1923,[67] and the Central Scientific Commission for the Study of Contraceptives was established in 1925 under the aegis of the Commissariat of Public Health's Division for the Protection of Maternity and Infancy.[68]

In 1924, even before the Commission had started its work, a medical debate on the subject erupted in public. In the main, physicians who were in favour of the dissemination of contraceptive devices made their case on the grounds that birth control was the only effective counterweight to abortion and to the spread of sexual disease.[69] But there was even one argument for birth control on the grounds that it would put an end to the slavery of women – a variety of women's liberation argument that was rarely met in the Soviet medical debate over abortion.[70] Those physicians who declared themselves unqualifiedly against birth control did so on the grounds that contraception licensed a reduction in the desire to have children and thus threatened the welfare of the nation.[71]

For our purposes, there are several intriguing aspects of the debate over contraception in the period 1924–9. First, the range of the physicians' discourse differed significantly from that which characterized the discussions of abortion during the same period. Whereas until the last third of the 1920s most Soviet obstetricians and gynaecologists took care to confine their claims to authority to the medical aspects of abortion, the very same physicians did not hesitate to speak out on the social implications of legalizing contraceptive measures. For example, K. K. Skrobanskii who had deliberately avoided social issues in his argument against abortion, discussed in great detail the moral, the psychological, and the social evils involved in limiting conceptions.[72] Indeed, the issue of contraception brought out the type of wide-ranging reflection on history, on morality, and on psychology that had been characteristic of Russian discussions of abortion before the Revolution.[73] In this vein, one participant in the debate over contraception wrote a long article the main theme of which was the tension between the increased sexual desire among women and the strengthening of the maternal instinct.[74]

Second, the discussion of contraception was phrased in demographic terms. Most of the opponents of contraception argued that birth control was more dangerous to the growth of the population than was abortion. Its very effectiveness, the unlikeliness that it would harm women physically, and the fact that it would not involve women in the murder of the foetus made birth control particularly threatening to the survival of the nation.[75] To obviate the risk to the growth of population that they believed would follow, some opponents of contraception recommended limiting access to birth control devices; others entertained the idea of state involvement in maintaining high fertility.[76] (Only a few brave voices argued that what was most important was to alleviate the dire economic conditions that made women wish to terminate or prevent their pregnancies.[77]) Surprisingly, not only opponents, but also champions of birth control often argued in demographic terms, submitting that contraception could be conducive to the preservation of maternity.[78]

### Soviet Demographers and the Abortion Question

The presence of a strong demographic focus in Soviet medical debates over contraception highlights the absence of that focus in medical debates over abortion. Did Soviet physicians discussing abortion pay so little attention to the demographic argument because demographers were discussing the issue? In other words, are we dealing here with an informal division of intellectual terrain?

This question is particularly interesting because, in the 1920s, the overlap between Soviet demography and medicine was less than had been the case in the pre-1917 period. Before the Revolution, two of the leading figures in Russian demography, P. I. Kurkin[79] and S. A. Novosel'skii,[80] were trained physicians. After 1917, when new research centres of demography were being created, the importance for a demographer of medical preparation appears to have waned. In 1919, the Institute for Demography was created in the Ukrainian Academy of Sciences in Kiev. According to a reliable account, the group of demographers which began to gather there under the leadership of M. V. Ptukha[81] did not include any physicians.[82] In 1930, the Institute of Demography in the Leningrad branch of the Academy of Sciences was founded. Although V. V. Paevskii, one of the two leading figures here (along with Novosel'skii), was professor of bio-social statistics at the Leningrad Institute for the Protection of Maternity and Infancy, he had been trained as a mathematician, not a physician.[83]

To be sure, in the 1920s, the Soviet profession of demography was small. Emil Roesle, the German demographer who was consistently favourable to Russia, put it charitably when he said that a new cohort of Soviet demographers was forming slowly.[84] And yet, even in this formative stage of the discipline of demography, there is evidence that Soviet demographers shared a professional identity and a concept of the content of demography as a science.[85]

A canvass of the Soviet demographic literature produced during the 1920s reveals that demographers did not begin to deal with the question of abortion in a systematic way until the middle of the decade. In the first half decade after the revolution, they concentrated on the devastating impact of the War on the number and rate of reproduction of the population. The Commission for Research into the Sanitary Consequences of the War, 1914–20 examined such issues as the loss of fighting men in the army, the reduction in the birth rate, the increase in death rate, and the impact of the War on the dynamics of marriage rates, etc.[86] The economist Strumilin studied the impact of the war on the labour force.[87] The sanitary physician Z. G. Frenkel writing in 1923 calculated the number of children unborn during the War.[88]

As the death rate began to decrease, statisticians moved to examine the birth rate. In 1924, statisticians and demographers adduced data which showed that the birth rate in Russia, traditionally high particularly in the rural sector,[89] was returning to its pre-war level. Participants at the III Congress for the Protection of Maternity and Infancy in 1925 heard V. G. Mikhailovskii claim that the Russian birth rate was virtually at its pre-war level of 43.8 per 1000 female population.[90] According to the demographer N. A. Kuvshinnikov, the birth rate in nine *gubernii* was nearly at its pre-war level as early as 1922.[91]

Other statisticians drew attention to the rapid rise in the marriage rate. According to one view, there was a dramatic rise in the rate of marriages in Moscow as early as 1919 and in St Petersburg in 1920;[92] a more conservative estimate had marriage rates beginning to rise from mid-1922 on and rising sharply from 1923 on.[93]

Whether they were dealing with birth, death or marriage rates in post-war Russia, the perspective of the Russian statisticians was always comparative. Devastating though the effects of the War were, from all accounts Russia's recovery was more rapid than that of many other countries. Indeed, what the Russian figures underscored most strongly was the difference in the birth rate between Western and Eastern Europe.[94] To be sure, there were some authors, both Russian and non-Russian, who argued that the East-West differences were over exaggerated.[95] Whether these authors were correct that the issue of declining population growth was a constructed one cannot be assessed here. What is clear, however, is that the fear of depopulation that was so intense in Western Europe[96] played almost no role in Russia. One should add that in Russia, the fear of over-population was as remote as the fear of depopulation. As Daniel Todes has shown in his book, the enormous geographical expanse of Russia always deprived the ideas of Malthus of any significant resonance there.[97]

In the second half of the decade, the question of abortion did appear on the agenda of Soviet demographers and statisticians. In 1926 and then again in 1927, at the initiative of M. Gernet, the head of the moral statistics section of the Central Statistical Administration[98] who collaborated with physicians from the Commissariat of Public Health's Division for the Protection of Maternity and Infancy, two large-scale studies of abortion were produced. The data for these studies were the cards which women requesting free abortions from the *troiki* were required to complete from 1924 on.[99] The large-scale studies revealed that the prototypical abortion patient was not the destitute woman, but her better-off counterpart, the woman with one or more children who was either married or in a stable relationship. This finding conflicted directly with the rationale for the passage of the 1920 edict. Not surprisingly, the contradiction was never addressed directly. Instead, A. B. Gens, the official spokesman for the policy of legalization, used the findings of these studies to argue that women were not seeking an abortion with their first pregnancies and that legalization was not responsible for an up-turn in abortions. The first contention was supported by the data from the questionnaires;[100] the second was not susceptible of either verification or falsification on the basis of the data. Significantly, in these two rich studies, there was only one direct reference to the impact of abortion on the birth rate – that by the demographer V. V. Paevskii who claimed that abortions were a 'significant factor in the demography of the two capitals' – i.e., Moscow and Leningrad.[101]

The lack of sustained discussion by demographers of the abortion issue continued past 1927. If we look at one of the major statistical journals, *Statisticheskoe obozrenie*, for the years 1929–30, we find little evidence of interest by Soviet statisticians in assessing the number of abortions. Indeed, virtually until the end of the decade, Soviet demographers appeared to continue studying the natural movement of population (i.e., birth, death, marriage rates) much as they had done earlier.[102]

### Foreign Demographers and Soviet Abortion

The low level of concern among Russian physicians over the demographic consequences of legalized abortion was reinforced by the views of foreign demographers who were impressed by the advantages of Russia relative to the countries of Western Europe. In an article published in Russian in 1925/1926, the German medical demographer Emil Roesle used data collected by the Central Statistical Administration to argue that whereas the birth rate in Eastern Europe began to go up from 1923 on, in Western Europe it began to fall as of 1921.[103] In 1925 in an article printed in Germany, the same Roesle furnished data which suggested that by comparison with Germany, Russia had a huge excess of births over deaths in 1923.[104] This foreign assessment of the advantageous Russian birth rate was incorporated wholesale into Soviet discussions.[105]

There were even more direct reassurances coming from foreign demographers about the wisdom of the policy of legalization. For example, in 1926, Roesle produced what became a famous comparison of the death rates from puerperal fever in Berlin and Leningrad. On the basis of his figures, Roesle argued that in 1924 nearly four times as many women died of puerperal fever in Berlin as did in Leningrad.[106] The heightened death rate in Berlin was particularly significant because the birth rate there was 10.2 per 1000 whereas in Leningrad it was 26.6. In the same year, Roesle published a longer article fleshing out the comparison.[107] The Berlin figures were broken down into deaths from abortion and deaths from lying in, whereas those from Leningrad were not. Of the 13.14 deaths per 1000 of the population in Berlin, 80 per cent of the maternal deaths were from abortion. If those 80 per cent were eliminated, he argued, Greater Berlin would have a death rate similar to that of Leningrad (3.77 per 1000).[108] Roesle implied – even if he did not say directly – that the legalization of abortion was responsible for lowering rather than raising the death rate among women.

In Germany, Roesle was attacked by physicians for having produced an exaggerated comparison which blunted the impact of legalizing abortion on the birth rate.[109] But in Russia, the comparison was accepted without qualification. Roesle himself was described in the Soviet literature as 'a famous German statistician, one of the most important civil servants in the Ministry of Public Health and a big defender of the legalization of abortion.'[110] Roesle's comparison became embedded in the Soviet medical discussion. Leading spokesmen for the Soviet policy of legalization like A. B.

Gens used the comparison to press the point that legalization had reduced the threat to women's health – never indicating that Roesle's article had come under fire in Germany.

Initially the reassurances by Germans that by legalizing abortion the Soviets had decreased rather than increased the risk to women were taken at face value. At the end of 1927, as evidence of 'the epidemic of abortions' began to mount in Russia,[111] it seemed to many that deaths from puerperal fever were less the issue than the falling birth rate. As we saw, in the wake of the Kiev meeting, Soviet physicians began to talk more openly about the impact of abortion on the birth rate.[112]

In the Soviet setting, the question of whether the legalization of abortion was adversely affecting the birth rate was overlaid with ideology. One of the two original justifications for the decriminalization of abortion had been that legalization would reduce the number of underground abortions.[113] Reviewing the effects of the new policy after it had been in place less than four years, the Commissar of Public Health, Semashko, admitted that the total number of abortions had risen sharply since 1920, but he insisted that the increase in hospital abortions was occurring at the expense of underground terminations of pregnancy.[114]

In fact, there were two separate questions here: was abortion on the rise because it was legalized? second, did legalization reduce underground abortions? The first question, important though it was, was not susceptible of an empirical answer. All agreed that abortions had increased somewhat since 1920 and sharply increased since 1926. But was that rise attributable to legalization? Some physicians assumed that there was a more-or-less stable level of abortions (legal and illegal) in a given population; what varied from country to country was simply the ratio of one to the other.[115] Others assumed that legalizing abortion reduced the inclination of women to have children.[116]

The second question – whether legalization had succeeded in reducing underground abortions – was an empirical question, but one to which there was no clear answer. The registration cards kept by the abortion commissions covered only women who had applied for cost-free legal abortions. Judging from the number of women who arrived in hospitals or clinics bleeding from botched operations, it was plain that underground abortions were still being performed.

But how to count the underground abortions? As Soviet physicians pointed out, it was almost impossible for a doctor to distinguish between an incomplete abortion which had begun spontaneously and an incomplete abortion which had been induced artificially. At the end of the decade, in an article published in German, Dr Magid of Kiev laid out the difficulties in measurement for his foreign colleagues.[117]

That Magid published his article in German was hardly coincidental. He was responding to a pair of articles published in 1929 by Dr Sigismund Peller, the Viennese social hygienist/demographer who had recommended using the anamnestic method (the patient's case history) as the basis for counting abortions.[118] Peller suggested anamnesis not as a vehicle to differentiate legal from illegal abortions (in Vienna, except for the most clear-cut medical reasons, abortion was illegal), but rather as a device to compensate for the notorious slothfulness of midwives and insurance workers in recording abortions.

Peller's work struck almost immediate resonance in Russia. But significantly, it was not the statistician/demographers but rather the physicians in Russia who took up Peller's challenge – for their own reasons. As Dr Magid of Kiev explained in an article published in German in 1930, if one wanted to compare the number of abortions in a country where abortion was legalized against the number in a country where abortion was still a criminal offence, it was critical to use the same method of counting. Intrigued by the promise of Peller's method, Magid applied the anamnestic method to a study of abortion rates in Moscow and Leningrad. In his first publication using the anamnestic method, Magid reported that his figures for Moscow and Leningrad women in the age bracket 15–44 years corresponded roughly to those of Peller for Viennese women in the same period.[119] Magid's conclusion had a polemical bite. He underscored the similarities of the abortion figures in a society where abortion was legal and in a society where abortion was punishable by law. The implication was clear: the legalization of abortion had not reduced the total number of abortions.

Peller had a different axe to grind. In a reply to Magid published in 1931, Peller reported that his research had persuaded him that abortion had the most minimal impact on the decline of population; a much greater role was played by the planning of fertility through contraception.[120] As he put it, 'The meaning of abortion for population policy is widely overestimated in our country. From a medical standpoint, the prohibition of abortion is shameful; from the point of view of population policy, it is insignificant.'[121] He added that the Russians had become excited about the impact of abortion on the fall in population because, in contrast to Germany which had experienced a drop in population 50 years ago, Russia had just recently 'come into the waves' *(in die Welle)* of the drop in birth rate.

Magid was not willing to take these reassurances at face value. In an article published in German jointly with his Kiev colleague Dr Venkovskii in 1931, Magid compared the findings obtained using the anamnestic method against the available statistical data on abortions in Russia. The authors found that Peller's method produced a strikingly low figure. (Peller's method yielded a figure of 26,600 abortions for Moscow in the year 1927; according to Soviet statistics, the number of legal and registered incomplete abortions was 45,852.)[122] This is hardly surprising given the difficulties involved in using a patient's case history to count illegal abortions.[123] At the end of the article, Magid and Venkovskii raised the possibility that the number of illegal abortions in Russia had increased, rather than decreased with legalization.[124] Their foray into comparative research led Magid and Venkovskii to challenge the utility of the anamnestic method for Russia. Much more important, these authors effectively called into question the reassurance offered by the foreign demographers about the vitality of the Soviet birth rate.

But, by this point, demographic concerns had become more prominent in medical discourse. Those concerns, one should note, tended to be expressed in a particular form. In late 1931, a variety of medical journals began to carry articles on the rising number of abortions in the countryside.[125] For example, the author of a 1931 study of the regulation of fertility in Kolomensk region claimed that while the number of interruptions of pregnancy in the countryside relative to the number of births was less than in the city, the growth of this phenomenon in the countryside was much faster.[126]The number of first pregnancies which ended in abortion had almost doubled in the countryside between 1926 and 1930, whereas it remained virtually stable in the city. Another study examined the reasons for rural women seeking abortions.[127] To be sure, as early as 1930, there were scattered references in the demographic literature to the growing trend toward abortion among rural women.[128] But in late 1931/early 1932, the issue of rural abortion was put on the front burner by physicians.

These discussions of abortion in the rural sector reflect more than a shift of interest from the town to the countryside. For those who thought systematically about demographic issues in Russia, the countryside with its high birth rate had always been a form of safety net. Even after abortion had been legalized, the social mapping done in the mid-1920s revealed that women in the countryside were loathe to seek abortions at a rate approximating that of their urban sisters.[129] But the onset of the policy of forced collectivization in late 1929 and early 1930 coupled with the famine of 1931 may have altered that long-held reluctance. Whatever the case, by discussing the growing phenomenon of rural abortion, physicians were signalling their concern with the impact of abortion on the growth of population.

## Conclusion

The selective appearance of the demographic argument in Soviet medical debates over abortion presents us with several distinct puzzles. First, there is the virtual absence prior to 1927 of the demographic argument in the physicians' case against legalization. Our brief canvass of the medical literature on contraception showed that the reluctance to discuss the social implications of limiting fertility was specific to the issue of legalized abortion rather than to the medical specialties of obstetrics and gynaecology or maternity and infant care; indeed, physicians of both profiles discussed at great length the implications of contraception for population growth. Further, our review of the writing on population by Soviet demographers in the 1920s suggests that the terms of discourse between the state and the physicians on the abortion issue governed not only physicians but also other professional groups such as demographers. The paper showed that Soviet demographers avoided discussion of the social aspects of abortion longer than did physicians. Even the interventions of foreign demographers failed until the end of the decade to draw Soviet demographers into a discussion of the implications of legalization for the decline of population growth in Russia.

Why were physicians so reluctant to discuss the demographic issue? I have argued that confining themselves to a critique of the medical sequelae of abortion provided physicians with a certain security; given their opposition to legalization and the mandate from the state to ensure the smooth operation of the abortion system, the tension between 'science and social life' was best resolved by restricting their critique to the medical aspects of abortion over which they had been given clear jurisdiction, could claim expertise, and had day-to-day control.

The second puzzle relates to the flowering of the demographic argument against legalization in 1927. The visible increase in the number of women seeking abortions coupled with the publication of statistical data on the number of legal abortions being sought surely made the question of population growth appear more acute. But how should we understand the physicians' willingness to set aside their long-standing disinclination to discuss the demographic implications of decriminalizing abortion? This change could be considered evidence of the adroitness of the physicians as political lobbyists, responding flexibly to new information and concerns. In my view, the change in discourse was more likely a tacit admission by physicians that the objections to legalized abortion launched in the name of the health of the individual woman had been ineffective in prompting reconsideration of the policy.

Third, there is the puzzle of the virtual disappearance of the demographic argument between late 1927 and late 1930. Having articulated the demographic argument against abortion, why did physicians not continue to trumpet it? In my view, the answer lies less in the weakness of the demographic argument itself than in the strength of the particular form of medical argument which swamped it from 1927 on. In the wake of the commitment to rapid industrialization made at the XIV Party Congress of 1927, the discussion of legalized abortion – as of so many other aspects of social policy – was increasingly refracted through the lens of industrialization. In the early 1930s, the focus on the health of the woman as worker which we noted earlier became overwhelming, as the state attempted to come to grips with the trade-off between involving women in the labour force and encouraging maternity.[130]

Finally, there is the puzzle of the reappearance of the demographic argument against abortion in late 1931/1932 and its continuance, albeit in muted form, until 1935. Two alternative explanations suggest themselves. The emergence of the demographic argument may have been a response to a threat to population growth which stemmed from heightened levels of abortion in the countryside. Earlier I referred to the spate of articles published in 1931/1932 on the increasing recourse by rural women to abortion. The weakness of statistics coupled with the cleverness of rural women in hiding abortions make it difficult to know for sure whether there was really an increase in rural abortions, whether the perceived increase was an artifact of better record-keeping, or whether indeed, the issue of increased abortions was constructed in order to prepare the ground for a new policy.

The appearance in 1931 of the demographic argument against abortion could also be attributed to the Cultural Revolution (1928–31) which affected the content and personnel in so many fields of Soviet arts and science. The available evidence does not support this interpretation strongly. From all appearances, the Cultural Revolution hit the Soviet field of obstetrics and gynaecology rather late and in a comparatively mild form. Judging from the composition of the editorial boards of the two leading journals in the field, *Ginekologiia i akusherstvo* and *Zhurnal akushertsva i zhenskikh boleznei*, from the leadership of the All-Union Society for Obstetrics and Gynaecology, and from the roster of active members of the Leningrad and Moscow Obstetrics/Gynaecology Societies for the period 1928–33, there was some turnover in the top leadership in the specialty, but there was also remarkable stability in the cohort of active researchers and writers. In short, in the field of obstetrics and gynaecology one looks hard to find a major figure who was excluded from the public arena. The real turnover in personnel appears to have occurred only in early 1935. [131]

What the field of obstetrics and gynaecology did experience in the years 1931–2 was a change in the foci of attention, away from social gynaecology and toward clinical matters. This shift was formalized in a 1933 article which mandated a division of space in the premier journal: lead articles were to get three to four pages, the social gynaecology section was to be 16 pages, the clinical section 48 pages, foreign literature eight pages.[132] But in and of itself this shift would hardly explain the appearance of the demographic argument, because under the new order social concerns were given less rather than more space.

The specialty of the protection of maternity and infancy did not fare as well as obstetrics and gynaecology. At the V All-Russian Conference on the Protection of Maternity and Infancy held in April, 1931, there were references to 'class war' in the specialty.[133] There was also a change in the major journal in the field, *Okhrana materinstva i mladenchestva.* As Elizabeth Waters has noted, at the beginning of 1931, Vera Lebedeva, a physician with impeccable Bolshevik credentials, lost her position as editor-in-chief of this journal to A. P. Bogat.[134] As proof of the new broom sweeping clean, the reconstituted editorial board moved social issues to the front of the journal and medical ones to the back. For most of the 1920s, spokesmen for this specialty had insisted on their expertise in clinical matters; now clinical questions were confined to a paltry few pages. And yet the reappearance of the demographic argument cannot be attributed to the change in focus of this particular specialty because, in 1931/1932, the threats to population growth were discussed by obstetricians and gynaecologists rather than by specialists in maternity and infant care.

## Denouement: The Demographic Argument Writ Large

At the IXth All-Union Congress of Obstetricians and Gynaecologists in Moscow on 9–14 March, 1935, the question of abortion was not on the programme.[135] But, the following year, with scant warning, the issue resurfaced.[136] On 27 June, 1936, a law was passed recriminalizing abortion in Soviet Russia.[137] The text of that law reflects a strong concern with the vitality of the Soviet population. Not only the language, but the substance of the law bespeaks the preoccupation of its authors with the demographic issue. In recriminalizing abortion, the state did not make contraception more readily available or more effective; instead, it expanded the number of nurseries and increased the maternity pay for women. That this law was part of a larger pro-natalist policy is beyond question.[138] But whether that pro-natalist policy itself was motivated by a concern for future generations or by a concern for the substantial number of people that had vanished in the course of collectivization, of the famine in the Ukraine, and of the first round of the purges is a puzzle that remains to be unravelled.

## Acknowledgement

The author acknowledges with thanks the support of the Hannah Institute for the History of Medicine and the helpful comments on an earlier draft of this paper made by Professor Mark B. Adams (University of Pennsylvania), Professor Robert E. Johnson (University of Toronto), Dr Alain Blum (Institut National d'Etudes Démographiques, Paris) and Dr Jochen Richter (Forschungsstelle zur Geschichte der Sexualwissenschaft, Magnus Hirschfeld Gesellschaft, Berlin).

This article was first published in *Cahiers du Monde russe et sovietique*, xxxiii (1) (January–March, 1992), 59–82.

## Notes

1. See 'O proizvodstve abortov' in *Spravochnik po okhrane materinstva i mladenchestva* (Moscow, 1928), 78–9.
2. In November, 1919, the forensic expert Dr I. Leibovich produced a set of theses recommending the legalization of abortion. In February of 1920, the Leibovich theses were circulated by the Division of Medical Expertise of the Commissariat of Public Health to all *guberniia* health departments with instructions to solicit the opinions of the health workers, justice workers, social workers and representatives of the Women's Division of the Communist Party. See L. M. and L. A. Vasil'evskie, *Abort kak sotsial'noe iavlenie* (Moscow and Leningrad, 1924), 95.

3. See Laura Engelstein, 'Abortion and the Civic Order: The Legal and Medical Debates', in Barbara Clements Evans *et at.* (eds), *Russia's Women* (Berkeley, CA: University of California Press, 1991), 185–207.
4. A. B. Gens, *Abort v RSFSR* (Moscow, 1925), 7.
5. See Paul Weindling, 'The Medical Profession, Social Hygiene, and the Birth Rate in Germany, 1914–1918', in Richard Wall and Jay Winter (eds), *The Upheaval of War* (Cambridge: Cambridge University Press, 1988), 417–37; J. M. Winter, 'The Fear of Population Decline in Western Europe, 1870–1940', in R. W. Hiorns (ed.), *Demographic Patterns in Developed Societies* (London: Taylor and Francis, 1980), 173–95; Philip E. Ogden and Marie-Monique Huss, 'Demography and Pronatalism in France in the Nineteenth and Twentieth Centuries', *Journal of Historical Geography,* viii (July, 1982), 283–98.
6. For a close analysis of those debates, see Cornelie Usborne, 'Abortion in Weimar Germany – The Debate Amongst the Medical Profession', *Continuity and Change,* v (2) (1990), 199–224.
7. For an examination of trends in Russian fertility over the past century, see Ansley J. Coale, Barbara A. Anderson, and Erna Harm, *Human Fertility in Russia since the Nineteenth Century* (Princeton, N.J.: Princeton University Press, 1979).
8. The 1920 edict was not a strike for women's rights over their own bodies. A few months after the edict was passed, the Commissar of Public Health, N. A. Semashko, declared that only petty bourgeois anarchists could want such a thing. N. A. Semashko, 'Bol'noi vopros', *Izvestiia* 151 (11 July, 1920), 3; N. A. Semashko, 'Eshche o bol'nom voprose', *Kommunistka* 3–4 (1920), 19–21.
9 For the argument that Soviet policy makers had a consistently pro-natalist line, see Krisztyna Mänicke-Gyöngyösi, 'Geschlechterverhältnis, Modernisierung und neue Öffentlichkeit in der Sowjetunion', *Feministische Studien,* vii (1989) no. 1, 55–6.
10. V. Z. Drobizhev, *U istokov sovetskoi demografii* (Moscow, 1987), 77–8.
11. See Elizabeth Waters, 'From the Old Family to the New: Work, Marriage, and Motherhood in Urban Soviet Russia, 1917–31', Unpublished Ph.D. dissertation, University of Birmingham, (1985), 271–8.
12. *Spravochnik po okhrane materinstva,* 78–83.
13. More often than not, such certificates were issued by the consultation clinics run by the Division for the Protection of Maternity and Infancy.
14. Initially, the commissions were staffed by a physician and a member of the Women's Division of the Communist Party (*Zhenotdel*). In December, 1924, it was decreed that the commissions should include

a third member from the Commissariat of Public Health's Division for the Protection of Maternity and Infancy (Okhmatmlad). *Waters*, 'From the Old Family to the New', 272.

15. The extent of the authority granted to physicians deluded some into thinking that they had unlimited jurisdiction. For example see E. E. Rosenblum (Moscow), 'Schwangerschaft, Entbindung, Aborte, Menstruation, und ärztliche Kontrolle in der USSR' *Deutsch-Russische Medizinische Zeitschrift*, (1926) no. 10, 692–708.
16. Vasilevskie, *Abort kak sotsial'noe iavlenie*, 95.
17. The issue of legalization was on the agenda of the 3 November, 1920 meeting of the Moscow Society of Obstetricians and Gynaecologists, a meeting which was attended *inter alia* by the Commissar of Public Health, N. A. Semashko. This meeting was scheduled to continue on 17 November, but was postponed until the 25th for lack of attendance. In the interim, the abortion edict was signed. 'Otchet sekretarei B. M. T'edra i M. A. Kolosova o deiatel'nosti Moskovskogo Akushersko-ginekologicheskogo obshchestva za vremiia s 1916 po 1921 g., chitannyi v godichnom zasedanii obshchestva 16 noiabria 1921 g.', *Ginekologiia i akusherstva* (1922) no. 1, 140–1.
18. I. L. Braude, 'K reforme vysshego meditsinskogo obrazovaniia', *Ginekologiia i akusherstvo* (1922), no. 1, 100–08.
19. At the 1924 All-Union meeting of gynaecologists and obstetricians, Vera Lebedeva, the head of the Commissariat of Public Health's Division for the Protection of Maternity and Infancy complained that physicians never looked beyond the uterus to see the woman and the conditions of her life. *Trudy VI-ogo s"ezda obshchestva vsesoiuznykh akusherov i ginekologov* (hereafter Trudy VI s"ezda) (Moscow, 1925), 219.
20. G. K. Zhivatov, 'Biologicheskoe napravlenie sovremennoi ginekologii', *Ginekologiia* i akushertsvo (1928), 348.
21. M. F. Levi, 'Sotsial'naia ginekologiia i ee mesto v sisteme okhrana materinstva i mladenchestva' *Moskovskii meditsinskii zhurnal* (1927) no. 10, 61–9. For an authoritative presentation of the German approach, see Max Hirsch, 'Die Bedeutung der Sozialgynäkologie und Frauenkunde für Praxis und Unterricht', *Zentralblatt für Gynäkologie*, xliv. (1920) no. 47, 1348–50.
22. Until 1930, physicians who specialized in this area received the very same medical training as all other physicians. D. Glebov, 'O podgotovke vrachei-spetsialistov po okhrane materinstva i mladenchestva i o povyshenii ikh kvalifikatsii', *Zhurnal akusherstva i zhenskikh boleznei* (1931), 428–35. For a discussion of the training of paramedical personnel in this area, see A. I. Lagutiaeva, 'Podgotovka personala po

okhrane materinstva i mladenchestva za desiat' let oktiabr'skoi revoliutsii', *Okhrana materinstva i mladenchestva* (1927) no. 11, 55–9.

23. Waters, 'From the Old Family to the New', 210.
24. For example, the 1927 review of the activities of the prestigious Leningrad Institute for the Protection of Maternity and Infancy by its director listed research areas in the following rank order: questions of physiology, and pathology, psychology and pedagogy of early childhood; questions of physiology, diet, hygiene and pathology of the female organism in the period of sexual growth, pregnancy, birth, post-partum, and breast-feeding; and questions of eugenics(!). Last on the list were the social-legal questions; this division of the Institute had only begun its work in 1925. 'Leningradskii Institut okhrany materinstva i mladenchestva', *Sotsialisticheskoe Zdravookhranenie* (1927) no. 8–9, 35–50.
25. At the end of the decade, the journals relegated medical matters to the background and put the premium on social philosophy. Waters, 'From the Old Family to the New', 246.
26. L. V. Ul'ianovskii, 'Abort i dekret 20 noiabria 1920 goda', *Zhurnal akusherstva i zhenskikh boleznei* (1928), 179–96. Ul'ianovskii recorded that a similar tension between the demands of science and the demands of life was evident when the issue of legalizing abortion was discussed in the decade before the edict of 1920 was passed.
27. See A. P. Gubarev, 'Prava mladentsa i nauchnoe akusherstvo', *Ginekologiia i akushertsvo* (1922) no. 1, 5–18.
28. O. N. Lebedeva, 'K voprosu o nektorykh redkikh oslozhneniiakh operatsii iskusstvennogo aborta', *Moskovskii meditsinskii zhurnal* (1925) no. 2, 32–6.
29. In a 1922 speech Dr Alexandroff recorded his impression that physicians had never seen as much sepsis as they had since 1920. Reported in Serge Krassilnikian, *Russische Erfahrungen mit der Freigabe der Abtreibung – eine Lehre für Deutschland* (Berlin, 1930).
30. *Trudy VI-ogo s"ezda*, 200–04. For the long version of this research report, see M. Ia Karlin, *Abort i ego posledstvie do i posle revoliutsii* (Moscow, 1924).
31. In drawing conclusions about fertility without controlling for age or sexual activity, Karlin was on shaky ground.
32. See L. I. Bublichenko, 'Zabolevaemost' i smertnost' pri rodakh sravnitel'no s vykidyshami', *Trudy VI-ogo s"ezda*, 169–71.
33 Usborne, 'Abortion in Weimar Germany'.
34. 'Otchet o trudakh Akushersko-Ginekologicheskogo O-va pri 1-m MGU za 1925 g. (39 god sushchestvovaniia)', *Moskovskii meditsinskii zhurnal* (1926), no. 6, 85–6. The report in question

was by A. Pakhmanov, 'Rozhdaemost' i prichina ee kolebanii', *ibid.*, 88.

35. 'VII Vsesoiuznyi s'ezd ginekologov i akusherov', *Moskovskii meditsinskii zhurnal* (1926) no. 9, 97–100.
36. For example, see A. I. Lagutiaeva, 'Znachenie iskusstvennogo vykidysha dlia organizma zhenshchin', *Okhrana materinstva i mladenchestva,* (1926), no.9, 3–5; P. G. Bondarev, 'Vliianie iskusstvennogo vykidysha na zhenshchiny', *Trudy VI-ogo s"ezda,* 297–8; and L. V. Ul'ianovskii, 'K kazuistike oslozhnenii vo vremiia proizvodstva i posle operatsii iskusstvennogo vykidysha', *Zhurnal akusherstva i zhenskikh boleznei* (1926), 768–76.
37. Typical of articles in this vein was A. V. Lankovitz, 'K voprosu o vliianii iskusstvennogo aborta na rody, poslerodovoi period i plod', *Zhurnal akusherstva i zhenskikh boleznei* (1926), 41–51. The exception to this rule was an article by Shuster-Kadysh about infant mortality and birth rates. M. A. Shuster-Kadysh, 'Detskaia smertnost' i rozhdaemost' v ikh vzaimootnosheniiakh i v sviazi s sotsial'nymi faktorami s tochki zreniia okhrany materinstva', *Zhurnal akusherstva i zhenskikh boleznei* (1924), 455–81.
38. See *Zhurnal akusherstva i zhenskikh boleznei* (1924), 80.
39. In 1926, the Obstetrical-Gynaecological Section of the First All-Siberian Congress of Physicians passed a resolution calling for a reassessment of the policy of legalization. In the same year, the Third Congress of Physicians in Georgia passed a resolution arguing that one should perform abortions on medical grounds only. See V. I. Sinebriukhov, 'Abort i bor'ba s nim', *Vestnik sovremennoi meditsiny* (1929), no. 17, 908–09.
40. The charge that opponents of the legalization of abortion were slaves to 'bourgeois morality' had been levelled by Gens in his speech to the III All-Union Conference for the Protection of Maternity and Infancy in 1925. *Gens, Abort v RSFSR.*
41. Ul'ianovskii, 'Abọrt i dekret 20 noiabria'.
42. 'Protokol 1 godichnogo zasedaniia Leningradskogo Akushersko-Ginekologicheskogo Obshchestva', *Zhurnal akusherstva i zhenskikh boleznei 1927,* 131. This incident was also mentioned in Ul'ianovskii, 'Abort i dekret 20 noiabria', 183.
43. 'Otchet o deiatel'nosti nauchnogo obshchestva okhrany materinstva i mladenchestva', *Zhurnal akusherstva i zhenskikh boleznei* (1927), 123.
44. The research resulted in the publication of two large-scale studies. See *Abort v 1925 godu* (Moscow, 1926); *Abort v 1926 godu* (Moscow, 1927).
45. For the transcript of the Congress, see Dr A. Mayer, *Erfahrungen mit der Freigabe der Schwangerschaftsunterbrechung in der Sowjet-Republik*

(Stuttgart, 1933). The Congress was attended by delegates from all over the Soviet Union.

46. This argument had appeared in print earlier. See M. V. Shestopal (Kharkov), 'Legal'nyi abort i zdorov'e zhenshchiny', *Profilakticheskaia meditsina* (1927), no. 3, 76–9.
47. E. K. Schinkar, 'Der Abort vom sozialen Gesichtspunkt aus', *Erfahrungen*, 77–8.
48. M. I. Laptev, 'Abortus arteficialis', *ibid.*, 122.
49. For Tikhanadse's intervention, see *ibid.*, 229.
50. I. B. Levit, 'Einige Angaben zur Statistik der Abtreibungen vom sozialen Standpunkt aus', *ibid.*, 103. Levit had expressed the same view in Russian. I. V. Levit, 'Neskol'ko dannikh k statistike vykidysha s sotial'noi tochki zreniia', *Zhurnal akusherstva i zhenskikh boleznei* (1927), 555.
51. M. I. Laptev, 'Abortus arteficialis', *Erfahrungen*, 124.
52. According to Resolution 3, 'the increase in artificial abortions had as yet had no effect on the growth of the population in the Ukraine.' See 'Resolution des Kongresses in der Abortfrage', *ibid.*, 132.
53. B. F. Kirillov, 'Der Abort', *ibid.*, 115.
54. E. Roesle, 'Sootnoshenie mezhdu rozhdaemost'iu i smertnost'iu v ukrainskikh i inostrannykh gorodakh za gody 1922–1924', *Profilakticheskaia meditsina* (1925), no. 4, 87–9.
55. The institutional base of this group was the Demographic Institute established under the aegis of the Ukrainian Academy of Sciences. Drobizhev, *U istokov*, 26.
56. By contrast, the demographic issue was on the agenda in Germany from 1910. See Sheila Faith Weiss, 'The Race Hygiene Movement in Germany, 1904–1945', in Mark Adams (ed.), *The Wellborn Science: Eugenics in Germany, France, Brazil, and Russia* (Oxford: Oxford University Press, 1990), 8–68. In France, it was on the agenda from 1870. See William H. Schneider, 'The Eugenics Movement in France, 1840-1940', *ibid.*, 69–109.
57. V. K. Kriukov, 'Vliianie legalizatsii abortov na dvizhenii naselenie', *Gigiena i epidemiologiia* (1928) no. 8, 36–9.
58. P. I. Kordobovskii, 'Aborty i rozhdaemost', *Profilakticheskaia meditsina* (1928), no. 5, 43–5.
59. 'I Vseukrainskii s'ezd akusherov i ginekologov', *Profilakticheskaia meditsina* (1927), no. 7, 211–15.
60. Topics for this meeting included the optimum length of maternity leave; the impact of work on a woman's ability to give birth, etc. An evening session was devoted to the impact on women's reproductive life of occupational hazards.

61. 'VIII Vsesoiuznyi s"ezd akusherov i ginekologov', *Zhurnal akusherstva i zhenskikh boleznei* (1928), 531.
62. See 'Obzor nauchnykh zasedanii Moskovskogo akushersko-ginekologicheskogo obshchestva', *Ginekologiia i akusherstvo* (1929), no. 3, 404–07.
63. In 1930–1, there was a series of articles reporting the results of longitudinal studies of the harmful effects on women's health of repeated abortions. A. S. Madzhuginskii, 'Dannye patronazhnogo izucheniia vliianii iskusstvennogo vykidysha na zdorov'e zhenshchiny', *Ginekologiia i akusherstvo* (1930), no. 4–5, 501–11; Ia. A. Rusin, 'O pozdnom samoproizvol'nom aborte', *Ginekologiia i akusherstvo* (1930), no. 4–5, 563–6. See also V. N. Shaternik, 'K voprosu o perforatsii matki pri iskusstvennom aborte', *Ginekologiia i akusherstvo* (1930), no. 3, 426–33. Such articles began to fall off in late 1931. A very few physicians, notably A. S. Madzhuginskii, continued to write in this vein throughout 1932 and 1933–indeed up to 1936.
64. The best review article of this substantial literature is G. A. Batkis, R. B. Kogan and Sh. Ia. Shufir, 'Trud i proizvoditel'naia funktsiia zhenshchiny', *Sotsial'naia gigiena* (1930), no. 1–2, 17–57. Of course labour hygienists had been concerned with female workers as early as 1921. See for example, S. Kaplun, *Zhenskii trud i okhrana ego* (Moscow, 1921).
65. Wera Lebedewa, 'Neues Leben in der Sowjetunion Mutter-und Kindesschutz', *Das Neue Russland*, 5 Jahrgang (1928), Heft 2, 30.
66. A. B. Gens, 'Der Künstliche Abortus als soziale und Milieu-Erscheinung', *Archiv für soziale Hygiene und Demographie*, N.F. III Band, (1928), 555–8.
67. From the autumn of 1924 on, the Leningrad branch of the Division for the Protection of Maternity and Infancy allowed abortion commissions to take the initiative and suggest contraception as an alternative to abortion to avoid unwanted pregnancies. Waters, 'From the Old Family to the New', 294.
68. The Commission issued eight volumes of working papers (*trudy*) on the subject of birth control. See *Trudy komissii po izucheniiu protivozachatochnykh sredstv*.
69. L. G. Lichkusa, 'Rol' protivozachatochnykh sredstv v bor'be s plodoizgnaniem', *Zhurnal akusherstva i zhenskikh boleznei* (1924), 115.
70. Nik. Markov (Smolensk), 'K voprosu o vykidyshe i o znachenii protivozachatochnykh sredstv', *Russkaia klinika*, xxi (January, 1926), 71–91.
71. For example, K. K. Skrobanskii, 'Abort i protivozachatochnye sredstva', *Zhurnal akusherstva i zhenskikh boleznei* (1924), 1–13.

72. *Ibid.*
73. For the pre-1917 debates, see Engelstein, 'Abortion and the Civic Order'. One of the very few exceptions to this moralistic tone in the discussion of contraception was Zinaida Michnik who took a pragmatic approach. See Z. Michnik, 'Ogranichenie detorozhdeniia i okhrana materinstva i mladenchestva', *Zhurnal akusherstva i zhenskikh boleznei,* (1927), 337–8.
74. Markov, 'K voprosu o vykidyshe'.
75. Lichkusa, 'Rol' protivozachatochnykh sredstv'.
76. See S. A. Tomilin, 'Problema narodonaseleniia', *Vrachebnoe delo* (1927), no. 23–4, 1890, as cited in Waters, 'From the Old Family to the New', 266.
77. V. S. Gruzdeva, 'Iskusstvennyi vykidysh, kak sotsial'noe zlo, i bor'ba s etim zlom', *Kazanskii meditsinskii zhurnal* (1928), no. 1, 76–91.
78. Z. Michnik, 'Ogranichenie detorozhdeniia i okhrana materinstva i mladenchestva', *Zhurnal akusherstva i zhenskikh boleznei* (1927), 340. Michnik was interested in the preservation of maternity from the point of view of the individual woman, not that of society as a whole.
79. See brief biography of P. I. Kurkin in *Gigiena i epidemiologiia* (1927), no. 1, 142–4. The links between Kurkin and the German demographer Roesle are discussed in H. Müller-Dietz, 'Medizinische Beziehungen zwischen Deutschland und der UdSSR: E. E. Roesle und P. I. Kurkin', *Acta Congressus Internationalis XXIV Historiae Artis Medicinae* 25–31 August, 1974 (Budapestini, 1976), Tom I, 697–703.
80. For a biography of Novosel'skii, see S. A. Novosel'skii, *Demografiia i statistika* (Moscow, 1978), 7–15.
81. P. I. Pustokhod 'Institut demografii Akademii Nauk USSR', *Demografichnyi doslidzheniia,* Vyp 2 (1971), 8. For a sense of Ptukha's place in the development of Soviet demography, see Drobizhev, *U istokov*.
82. See S. A. Tomilin, 'Ob ustanovlenii sel'skikh raionov demograficheskogo izucheniia (demograficheskaia smychka s selom)', *Profilakticheskaia meditsina* (1925), no. 8, 115–16. There may have been some regional rivalry at play here. Tomilin, a trained physician, was head of the statistical section of the Ukrainian Commissariat of Public Health. At the time he wrote this article, he was based in Kharkov.
83. See the obituary for Vladimir Vladislavovich Paevskii in *Vestnik Akademii Nauk SSSR,* (1934), no. 6, 28–32. Paevskii graduated from the physico-mathematical faculty of St Petersburg University where he specialized in the application of the theory of probability to

insurance questions.

84. Roesle, 'Sootnoshenie', 99. The development of Soviet demography is described in some detail in Drobizhev, *U istokov*.
85. See the entry on 'Demografiia' in the *Bol'shaia meditsinskaia entsiklopediia* (Moscow, 1929), 8, 611–21.
86. *Trudy komissii po obsledovaniiu sanitarnykh posledstviiakh voiny 1914–1920* (Moscow/ Petersburg, 1923) cited in Drobizhev, *U istokov*, 17. Among the influential articles was 'Velikaia voina i estestvennoe dvizhenie naseleniia', *Vestnik statistiki* (1920), no. 5–8, 16–46. This was a reprint of an article by Christian Derning which had originally appeared in *Archiv für soziale Hygiene und Demographie*, BD XIII Heft 4 (1920). See also A. V. Gorbunova, 'Vlianie mirovoi voiny na dvizhenie naseleniia Evropy', *Russkii evgenicheskii zhurnal* (1922), no. 1, 39–63.
87. S. G. Strumilin, 'Trudovye poteri Rossii v voine', *Narodnoe khoziastvo* (1920), no. 18, 104–06.
88. Z. G. Frenkel, 'Griadushchie proiavleniia neotvratimykh demograficheskikh posledstvii voiny 1914–1918', *Profilakticheskaia meditsina* (1924), no. 5–6, 79–82. Frenkel estimated the number of unborn children at 10 million and predicted that the effects of the War would continue to be felt not for 4–5, but for 7–8, years.
89. See S. A. Tomilin, 'K voprosu o plodovitnosti krest'ianki i vliianii ee na detskuiu smertnost', S. A. Tomilin, *Demografiia i sotsial'naia gigiena* (Moscow, 1973), 218 –20. This article appeared originally in *Zhurnal po izucheniiu rannego detskogo vozrasta* (1929).
90. V. G. Mikhailovskii, 'O rozhdaemosti i smertnosti naselenie Soiuza SSR', as cited in P. P. Liublinskii, 'Rozhdaemost' i problema naseleniia v sovremennom obshchestve', *Russkii evgenicheskii zhurnal* (1926), no. 3–4, 155.
91. N. A. Kuvshinnikov, 'Estestvennoe dvizhenie naseleniia RSFSR v 1920–1922', *Gigiena i epidemiologiia* (1926), no. 1, 104. This article appeared originally in *Vestnik statistiki*, kn xxi (1925).
92. Gorbunova, 'Vliianie mirovoi voiny', 43.
93. Kuvshinnikov, 'Estestvennoe dvizhenie naseleniia RSFSR'.
94. Roesle, 'Sootnoshenie mezhdu rozhdaemost'iu'.
95. A Russian author claimed that the Germans over-exaggerated their low birth rate in order to justify the retention of paragraph 218-220 of the German Criminal Code which criminalized abortion. Z. A. Gurevich, 'Abort v Germanii', *Profilakticheskaia meditsina* (1928), no. 1, 62–72. In much the same way a French author claimed that the population crisis in France was constructed; the problem in post-war France was not falling birth rates but rising

death rates. Alexandre Roubakine, 'Note sur la prétendue "dépopulatio" de la France', *Bulletin de l'Academie de Médecine*, cxiii (1935), 143 ff.

96. In Germany, the concern over the declining rate of population growth intensified after the First World War when many realized that Russia might come out of the War in tact and might turn out to be the greatest biological threat to Germany. Weiss, 'The Race Hygiene Movement in Germany'. In France, there was considerable fear of being swamped by the more rapidly growing population of the new German empire. According to one source, Malthusianism held sway so long as the focus was internal matters, but when attention shifted to questions of international prestige, 'populationist' views took hold. Ogden and Huss, 'Demography and Pronatalism in France'.
97. See Daniel P. Todes, *Darwin without Malthus* (Oxford: Oxford University Press, 1990).
98. In the 1920s, the moral statistics section of the Central Statistical Administration was conducting research on a variety of 'social anomalies' – prostitution, narcotics, infanticide, suicide, to name but a few. For a collection of some of the most interesting articles from that period, see *Moral'naia statistika v 20-kh godakh. Seriia istoriia statistiki* (Moscow, 1990). It is possible that the research on abortion was conceived as part of a larger effort to map deviance.
99. *Abort v 1925 gody, Abort v 1926 godu.* There were also spin-off studies conducted using the same data. See N. Kameneva, 'Opyt sotsial'noi gruppirovki dannykh ob abortakh', *Vestnik TsSU* (1928), no. 1, 77–94; B. Sigal, 'K sotsial'noi kharakteristike sovremennogo aborta', *Zdravookhranenie* ii (4) (1929), 110–25.
100. Gens found that only 12 per cent of the women who came in for abortions were pregnant for the first time. *Abort v RSFSR,* 12.
101. *Ibid.*, 31.
102. B. Babykhin, 'Sila smertnosti v RSFSR i rost' naseleniia', *Statisticheskoe obozrenie* (1929), no. 1, 98–105; M. Kaplun, 'Brachnost' naseleniia RSFSR', *Statisticheskoe obozrenie* (1929), no. 7, 90–7; B. Iagolim, 'Rozhdaemost' po g. Moskve v sviazi s sotsial'nym sostavom naseleniia', *Statisticheskoe obozrenie* (1928), no. 10, 85–8.
103. Roesle, 'Sootnoshenie', 93.
104. E. Roesle, 'Die Bewegung der Bevölkerung in der russischen Sozialistischen Föderativen Sowjet-Republik (RSFSR) in den Jahren 1920-1923', *Archiv für soziale Hygiene und Demographie,* i (1925/1926), 202.
105. A. B. Gens, 'Geburtenüberschuss und Abtreibung in der Sowjetunion', *Neue Generation,* (1928) 24 Jr., 253–355.

106. See E. Roesle, 'Die Statistik des legalisierten Abortus', *Zeitschrift für Schulgesundheitspflege und soziale Hygiene*, xxxviii. (1925), Heft 10, 445–55.
107. E. Roesle, 'Zur Statistik des legalisierten Abortus', *Das Neue Russland* (1925), no. 9–10, 38–9.
108. Of course, in Leningrad, there were also deaths from puerperal fever after abortion.
109. See Dr Engelsmann, 'Zur Frage des legalisierten Abortus', *Zeitschrift für Gesundheitspflege und soziale Hygiene* (1926), no. 2, 49–55. Engelsmann argued that the rate of abortions was higher in Greater Berlin than anywhere else in Germany. See also Albert Niedermeyer, 'Betrachtungen zur Arbeit Roesle's "Die Statistik des legalisierten Abortus, *Zentralblatt für Gynäkologie*"' (1926), no. 19, 1267 ff. Niedermeyer charged that the figures for Berlin were broken down into deaths from abortion and deaths from lying in, whereas for Russia the data were not disaggregated.
110. Gurevich, 'Abort v Germanii', 64.
111. A physician from Volchansk recorded that in the period 1925–6, the number of abortions in the city had doubled, while in the countryside the number had tripled. As a result by 1926, the abortion commissions were no longer vetting requests for abortions; instead, using an anatomical diagram, doctors at the consultation bureaus explained to women what the operation entailed, warned about the dangers and simply handed out the permission slips. T. N. Suetin, 'K voprosu ob aborte', *Profilakticheskaia meditsina* (1927) no. 7, 85–90.
112. P. I. Kordobovskii, 'Aborty i rozhdaemost', *Profilakticheskaia meditsina* (1928), no. 5, 43–5.
113. After little more than three years of experience with the new policy, the Commissar of Public Health made it clear that it was utopian to expect that the legalization of abortion would eliminate underground abortions; it would merely reduce their number. N. A. Semashko, 'Drei Jahre Sowjetgesetzgebung in einer 'wunden Frage', *Das Neue Russland* (1924), no. 3/4, 27–9.
114. *Ibid.* This point was reiterated by the official spokesman for the policy. Gens, *Abort v RSFSR,* 17–18.
115. I. B. Levit, 'Neskol'ko dannykh k statistike vykidysha s sotial'noi tochki zreniia', *Zhurnal akusherstva i zhenskikh boleznei* (1927), 555. For the same view by a non-Soviet physician, see Sigismund Peller, 'Abortus und Geburtenruckgang', *Medizinische Klinik* (1931), 847–9.
116. For example, see S. A. Tomilin, 'Problema rozhdaemosti', in S. Tomilin, *Demografiia i sotsial'naia gigiena,* 180–5. This article was

originally published in *Profilakticheskaia meditsina* (1923).

117. Dr Magid, 'Die Statistische Terminologie und Methodologie des Aborts', *Archiv für soziale Hygiene und Demographie*, N. F. Band V (1930), 409–11.
118. Sigismund Peller, 'Studien zur Statistik des Abortus, I', *Zentralblatt für Gynäkologie*, (1929), no. 14, 861–71; II-*ibid.*, no. 35, 2216–27.
119. M. Magid, 'Zur vergleichenden Statistik des legalisierten und des nichtlegalisierten Abortus', *Zentralblatt für Gynäkologie* (1930), no. 31, 1946–7.
120. Peller, 'Abortus und Geburtenrückgang', 847. Peller had done a large study of the problem. See S. Peller, *Fehlgeburt und Bevolkerungsfrage* (Stuttgart, 1930).
121. Peller, 'Abortus', 849.
122. M. Magid and M. Venkovskii, 'Zur Statistik des illegalen Abortus', *Archiv für soziale Hygiene und Demographie*, Neue Folge Bd. vi (1931), 427.
123. I owe this point to a discussion with Robert Johnson.
124. Magid and Wenkowsky, 'Zur Statistik des illegalen Abortus', 429. Magid became preoccupied with the problem of counting illegal abortions. In an article, published in 1931, he attempted to study spontaneous abortions as a way to get at artificial illegal ones. See M. Magid, 'Über die Frequenz des spontanen Abortus und deren Bedeutung beim studium des künstlichen, speziell des illegalen Abortus', *Zentralblatt für Gynäkologie* (1931), no. 9, 531.
125. For an early article in this vein, see M. M. Tarabukhin, 'K voprosu ob aborte na sele', *Zhurnal akusherstva i zhenskikh boleznei* (1930), 540–54.
126. B. I. Burde, 'O rezul'tatakh regulirovaniia detorozhdeniia naseleniem', *Zhurnal akusherstva i zhenskikh boleznei* (1931), 840.
127. M. M. Levin, 'K kharakteristike prichin iskusstvennogo aborta', *Zhurnal akusherstva i zhenskikh boleznei* (1931), 375 ff.
128. V. Babykhin, 'Perspektivy estestvennogo dvizheniia naseleniia v RSFSR na blizhaishie gody', *Statisticheskoe obozrenie* (1930), no. 6, 121–6.
129. In 1926, Gens devoted half of his large study of abortion in Russia to the rural sector. See A. Gens, *Was lehrt die Freigabe der Abtreibung in Sowjet-Russland? Heft I: Der Abort auf dem Lande* (Wien, 1926).
130. See G. M. Agadzhanov, A. B. Gillerson, and M. F. Makarov, 'Beremennost' i proizvoditelnost' truda', *Ginekologiia i akusherstvo* (1932) no.3, 29 ff.; Ia. Zakgeim and Iu. E.Gitelson, 'Trudovaia ekspertiza v ginekologii i akusherstve', *ibid.*, no. 4, 18 ff.; E. M. Kopteva, A. D. Greibo, and E. I. Gagarinskaia, 'K voprosu ob orientirovochnykh srokakh vosstanovleniia trudosposobnosti posle operatsii isskustvennogo aborta', *ibid.*, no. 2, 9 ff. Also E. E.

Rozenblium, 'Tsentralizatsiia ili detsentralizatsiia v dele predostavleniia dekretnykh otpuskov po materinstvu', *Zhurnal akusherstva i zhenskikh boleznei* (1932), 22–7.

131. This sort of information was carried in great detail in each issue of the leading journals in the field.
132. 'Proizvodstevnnnyi plan na 1934 g', *Zhurnal akusherstva i zhenskikh boleznei* (1933), 388–9.
133. See 'V Vserossiiskoe soveshchanie po okhrane materinstva i mladenchestva (10–14 aprelia 1931g)', *Zhurnal po izucheniiu rannego detskogo vozrastva*, xi (1931), no. 9–10, especially the intervention by G. Batkis, *ibid.*, 391.
134. Waters, 'From the Old Family to the New', 245.
135. In 1935, there was a series of articles on the medical sequelae of abortion in the two large obstetrics and gynaecology journals.
136. There was no discussion preceding this law in any of the medical journals. The only harbinger of things to come was a brief set of 'spontaneous' letters to the editor of *Pravda* in June, 1936. See Alain Blum, 'La société et le politique en Union Soviétique depuis 1917– illustrations démographiques', *Rossika* (1991) (in preparation).
137. *Postanovleniia TsIK i SNK ot 27 iuniia 1936g., 34, 'O zapreshchenii abortov, uvlechenii material'noi pomoshchi rozhnitsam, ustanovlenii gosudarstvennoi pomoshchi monogosemeinym, rasshirennii seti rodil'nykh domov, detskikh iasliei, detskikh sadov, usilenii ugolovnogo nakazaniia na zaplatezh alimentov, i o nekotorykh izmeneniiakh v zakonodatel'stve o razvodakh'.*
138. See Wendy Zeva Goldman, 'Women, the Family and the New Revolutionary Order in the Soviet Union', in Sonia Kruks *et al.* (eds), *Promissory Notes. Women and the Transition to Socialism* (New York: Monthly Review Press, 1989), 59–81.

# 6

# Heinrich Zeiss, Hygiene and the Holocaust

*Paul Weindling*

While the interwar political conflicts resulted in the emergence of great dictators, the period also saw the projecting of the image of the medical researcher as an immensely powerful figure with a superhuman intellect, dictatorial powers in the emerging welfare states, and commanding mass adulation in the new media of film and radio. Contrasting images of medical research arose in antithetical social systems. Paul de Kruif's *Microbe Hunters* (of 1926) glamorized heroic personalities in accounts rich in personal foibles and idiosyncracies.[1] At the International Congress of the History of Science in London in 1932 Soviet researchers proclaimed a materialistic view of science in which great scientists were agents of social revolutions.[2] In 1936 Ludwik Fleck produced a socio-cultural account of scientific innovation focusing on Ehrlich and Wassermann (who contributed to the therapy and diagnosis of syphilis) and their relations with the Prussian state.[3] The question arises whether the heroic image of the medical researcher generated under Nazism can also be assimilated into the rising tide of relativism and of a reaction against positivism?

The legacy of these historical breakthroughs has prompted medical historians since the post-Second World War era to study the psychology and social circumstances of medical researchers. Yet the issue of a scientist's perception of research data remains crucial: here interwar Gestalt theory – demonstrating that total images were perceived on the basis of fragmentary sensory data – was vital. However, one of the first major applications of a psychological approach to the history of bacteriology and immunology has been totally overlooked. It is the maker ( and the social forces that went into the making) of this new image of scientific medicine – Heinrich Zeiss – who forms the subject of this chapter.[5]

Zeiss has been almost totally erased from the post-1945 Cold War world. For there is no Festschrift, no honorary degrees and only two brief obituary notices. This is surprising as Zeiss from 1933 was Director of the prestigious Institute of Hygiene in Berlin. Through his research and historical writings, he sought to reconcile the long-running conflict between Koch's bacteriology and Pettenkofer's environmentalism, and so merits a place in the history of German hygiene and public health. There is a curious obituary notice published in 1951 by the medical historian Diepgen in a list of historians and scientists and medical men who died within 'the German language area' since 1939 (including Isidor Fischer who died in London and Richard Koch who died in Southern Russia).[6] Diepgen knew nothing about the date, place and circumstances of Zeiss's death – which, it subsequently transpired, occurred in Vladimir in the Soviet Union on 31 March, 1949 – although the circumstances are still shrouded in mystery. Hans Harmsen, who collaborated with Zeiss in the mapping of disease and subsequently became a professor of public health noted for his eugenic activities, also published an obituary based on information provided by a returning German prisoner of war.[7] It is appropriate in Europe, at a time when its frontiers and ideological contours are being redrawn, that it is possible to evaluate the biography of an innovator in medical biography, whose career defied conventional assumptions of twentieth-century political conflicts: for Zeiss worked to support the Soviet health system in the 1920s and then Nazi expansionism in the 1930s and 1940s. Such a career was so fundamentally opposed to the Cold War era – indeed so paradoxical – that western medical history has conveniently forgotten Zeiss, and Soviet communism literally buried him (and I will show how ignominious burial was to Zeiss).

Zeiss was born on 12 July, 1888 in Frankfurt: while his father was engaged in the insurance business and the family was Calvinist, this quintessentially Weberian combination led not to modernistic rationalism but to a concern with cultural traditions. Zeiss was a typical wandering student, studying medicine at Marburg, Heidelberg, Freiburg, Berlin, Munich and then again at Freiburg. From 1909–10 Zeiss did six months' military service in Freiburg – initiating a military strand to his life, which was more broadly typical of German bacteriology as numerous professors of hygiene had begun their careers seconded as military cadets to hygiene institutes. Zeiss qualified in medicine at Freiburg in 1913 – a university which spearheaded the introduction of racial hygiene into medicine.[8] At Freiburg were youthful advocates of *Lebensraum* like Fritz Lenz, who later, as professor of racial hygiene, had the rooms once occupied by the social hygienist Grotjahn in Zeiss's Hygiene Institute. Many Freiburg professors of medicine espoused eugenics like the anatomist Eugen Fischer and the pathologist Aschoff.[9] Zeiss's medical diploma was signed by the professor of psychiatry Alfred Hoche, who was to justify compulsory killing of the incurably ill.

The career of Zeiss took on a military and tropical medical complexion. In 1913 Zeiss was assistant at Dresden when he qualified as a military doctor. From 1914 he was assistant to Martin Mayer in the bacteriological department at the Hamburg Institute for Tropical Diseases. Ironically – given Zeiss's antisemitism – Mayer, who was Jewish would be forced to emigrate to Venezuela. The Hamburg Institute, founded by Bernhard Nocht, a bacteriologist who was drafted into Hamburg public health by Koch, was a bastion of nationally-minded medical researchers who sought to establish the superiority of German medicine in the wider world.[10]

Having armed himself in the medical sciences, Zeiss did war service. From 1914–15 he saw frontline service as a military medical officer in France. His tropical qualifications meant that from 1915–16 he was adjutant to the chief military medical officer in the mission to Turkey. From 1916 he was assistant to two leading exponents of German tropical medicine: to Rodenwaldt in the Turkish 5th army, and to Viktor Schilling who was stationed in Aleppo. Here Zeiss would have been aware of the Armenian concentration camps on the fringes of the city. Zeiss thus shared in the anaesthetizing experience of death in military action, and the atrocities committed by the Turkish army hardened him to the horrors of the slaughter of civilians, so providing an ominous precedent for the Nazi Holocaust.

Zeiss returned to Germany where he worked in a malaria hospital near Dresden. Defeat, starvation and political and economic turmoil plunged Germany into crisis. For nationally - minded doctors like Zeiss it was also a moment of spiritual and intellectual crisis. Zeiss accused the allies of not only attempting to starve Germany but also of destroying his nation's scientific and cultural resources.[11] Nationally - minded doctors resolved to continue the war against the allies, especially against the loathed French who insisted on Germany's humiliation with the Treaty of Versailles.

In 1919 Zeiss returned to the bacteriological department at the Hamburg Tropical Institute, and in 1921 he became assistant port medical officer in Hamburg. Although Germany had lost its colonies, German exponents of tropical medicine were anxious to find outlets for their expertise. The Bayer pharmaceutical company had produced a new sleeping sickness drug, patriotically named *Germanin*, and Zeiss collaborated with Mühlens of the Tropical Institute on clinical trials of the new drug.

In this beleaguered situation, an opportunity came for tropical researchers to deploy their skills. The Russian author, Maxim Gorki, appealed in 1921 to the dramatist, Gerhart Hauptmann, to sponsor a call for German aid to halt the famine and disease in the Soviet Union. The Germans feared that infectious disease would sweep across Europe and eradicate the civilized races. Since the turn of the century the Germans had sought to sustain an iron curtain of quarantine and disinfection stations in Eastern Europe. Going into Russia would enable German public health officials to have an early warning system of threats of cholera, typhus and other infectious diseases. The Germans equipped a train with a bacteriological laboratory, disinfection equipment, zyklon gas (one of its first uses), an operating theatre and sanitary engineering equipment. Their aim was to support ethnic German 'colonists', whom the German authorities feared would bring infectious diseases and possibly communism back into Germany. Thus a policy of aid to prevent mass emigration was formulated. The famine was described as a holocaust with thousands of deaths and savage atrocities by populations desperate for food.[12]

Whereas the Americans sought to deal with the peripheral Soviet republics and local administrators – and were accused of undermining central Soviet government – the Germans made a point of cultivating relations with the central Soviet authorities. Zeiss established a central bacteriological laboratory in Moscow, which was praised by Trotsky. Zeiss expanded the laboratory into a clinic, experimental research institute and German cultural centre, and hoped that this could develop into a permanent German medical institute in Moscow. He argued that even greater than the hunger for food was the hunger for German culture, particularly among doctors and medical researchers among whom was a long-standing tradition of interaction with German medicine since the eighteenth century. Zeiss envisaged re-establishing German *Lebensraum* and cultural leadership. He abhored the influence of France and of the Pasteur Institute, denouncing the duplicity of Besredka (a Russian-Jewish emigré) in maintaining relations with both Czarist exiles and the communist regime. He pointed out that just as the French had encircled the Mediterranean with Pasteur Institutes, so a German outpost in Moscow was a staging post for re-establishing German influence in Afghanistan and Iran. The German Red Cross doctors cultivated links with the Southern Republics, notably with Georgia where there was a German hospital and schemes for genetic and anthropological research.

Until 1924 Zeiss's salary was paid by the state of Hamburg. He then entered Soviet employment, first at the chemotherapeutic research institute and, until December, 1930, at the Pasteur Institute for Experimental Therapy under the distinguished bacteriologist, Tarassewitsch. Throughout the period Zeiss worked in association with the German embassy in Moscow, reporting on all aspects of Soviet medicine and health conditions, and providing medical assistance for the illicitly stationed German military installations in the USSR. In 1930 the NKVD accused Zeiss of being the central figure in a spy and espionage organization initiated by the German intelligence services. His activities were so open that he was hardly a secret agent. But he was certainly in constant touch with the German embassy as an active information gatherer and transmitter. His medical qualifications gave him a privileged position, and he used his position to travel widely, and arranged material support and the sending of German books, including eugenics and racial literature, to dissident ethnic German colonists.[13]

Drawing on the concept of geo-politics promoted by expansionist German nationalists, Zeiss coined the term 'geo-medicine'.[14] With the pathologist Aschoff, Zeiss promoted studies of geographical factors in disease. From 1927 until 1932 he supported a German-Russian Institute for Medical Geography in Moscow. Zeiss also undertook serological studies of the Volga Germans establishing their origins from his own part of Germany – Hessen. He studied the interaction of constitutional and environmental factors. Zeiss opposed socialist interpretations of social hygiene linking disease to economic conditions: he argued that both German and Soviet social hygiene relied on the concept of the totality of psychological, historical and environmental influences as shaping the health of total populations. Geo-medicine was to provide a basis for preventive medicine, but beyond this he considered that eastern expansion would rejuvenate an ageing German nation.

Geo-medicine was also linked to the history of medicine. Zeiss's experiences in Turkey prompted research on the bacteriologist Otto Obermeier, who had researched on relapsing fever.[15] While in the Soviet Union Zeiss researched on Metchnikov, to whom he gave a German intellectual pedigree by highlighting contacts with Haeckel's evolutionary monism and Virchow's cellular pathology.

The biography, published in 1932, is an impressive achievement in making use of archival sources and of oral histories for which Zeiss travelled to Paris to interview Metchnikov's colleagues. He aimed to counter the narrowness of a Franco-Russian view of Metchnikov by making the fundamental point that scientific work was shaped by German-inspired philosophical preconceptions.[16] Zeiss was on the committee of the German Society of the History of Medicine and Science, and sought to establish a Metchnikov Museum as a centre of Russian medical history.

The Stalinist policies of tightening the hold of the communist party on all aspects of intellectual life and of the collectivization of agriculture undermined the basis of Zeiss's presence in the Soviet Union. The rationales of German-Soviet medical co-operation were undermined by Stalinist notions of economic and intellectual autarchy. Semashko, the Germanophile Commissar for health, was dismissed in 1930 when Zeiss's employment was also terminated by the health commissariat. Zeiss reacted against a communist avant-garde led by Bukharin in Russian intellectual circles, opposing a materialist formulation of history of science and medicine. Intellectually and politically, Zeiss became radicalized. For like the eugenicist Lenz, the medical and nationalist publisher J. F. Lehmann and numerous other German racial hygienists, Zeiss was a member of the conservative German National People's Party from 1920–8. His experience of the death and disease resulting from Soviet collectivization and the refusal of the German government to aid the evicted ethnic Germans led to Zeiss's political radicalization. He joined the Nazi Party in 1931, which was proclaiming that the ethnic Germans were being systematically exterminated. Zeiss left the Soviet Union on 23 February, 1932.

During the 1920s Zeiss steadily acquired the necessary scientific credentials becoming Privatdozent in 1924, Professor in 1925, a medical officer in 1930, and associate university professor at Hamburg in 1931. These were rewards for his nationalist activities in the Soviet Union, as were the associate professorship and directorship of the Berlin Hygiene Institute in 1933 and the full professorship of hygiene in April 1937.

During the 1930s Zeiss turned his attention westwards and indeed visited London on a number of occasions. This was partly to contact tropical researchers. With Mühlens, who was by now head of the Nocht Institute in Hamburg, he visited the Wellcome Laboratories – which they admired as the best in the world – and also the tropical researcher, Philip Manson Bahr. On return

Mühlens and Zeiss reported that British tropical researchers supported re-establishing German colonies.

Zeiss's main reason for visiting London was to rally what he called 'a consolidated army for cremation'. He was honorary member of the Cremation Society (in London), and when the International Cremation Federation was launched in 1937, Zeiss was a Vice-President. He assumed a leading role in the Nazi Gleichschaltung of the cremation movement purging it of free-thinking and liberal elements. Cremation was no eccentricity: professionally it represented the imposition of hygienic control and technologies in the management of death, ideologically it marked a rebirth of Nordic notions of fire representing everlasting life, and combined with medical expertise in disinfection, it was to be a lethal combination in the gas chambers of the Holocaust.

While in Berlin, Zeiss researched on a broad front in his Hygiene Institute and as Director of the Academy of Military Medicine. Concerned to promote positive health – particularly of the army – he researched into nutrition. He pursued preventive medicine by researching into typhus vaccines, and the efficacy of disinfectants was also a major interest. He venerated the Nazi ideologist, Erwin Liek, for holistic medicine, and he propagated notions of relations between physical and psychological health.[17]

In 1941 the NKVD circulated the accusation that the Germans had been planning a bacteriological war against the Soviet Union, and that Zeiss was masterminding these plans. This document was captured by the German army, and translated by Zeiss. In 1945 the Soviet authorities arrested Zeiss, tried him in 1947 – presumably on the basis of the earlier charges of espionage – and he died from Parkinson's disease (evident before his arrest) in the prison hospital in Vladimir.[18]

The question arises that although Zeiss was falsely accused in that the German attack on the Soviet Union did not involve actual germ warfare he was a leading Nazi medical expert with interests in the Soviet Union where the German army and SS death squads were waging a war of genocide. In what sense does Zeiss illuminate the Holocaust? Despite his involvement in typhus research, there is no evidence that he conducted medical experiments in concentration camps, or experimented on victims from concentration camps like the Berlin human geneticist Verschuer who received from Mengele heterochronic gypsy eyes. No visits to concentration camps by Zeiss are known, unlike other professors of hygiene such as Pfannenstiel, the professor at Marburg, who voyeuristically observed through a spy hole, the trial gassings with hydrocyanic acid in Belzec.

Although a member of the Nazi Party from 1931, Zeiss was not a member of the SS, and nor was he an activist in the Nazi Doctors League, and neither, unlike so many human geneticists, an adjudicator on racial ancestry. He was not (like the professors of psychiatry and mental hospital directors) involved in scanning the case histories of the mentally ill in order to decide who should be killed. Nor unlike Nauck (another sometime Red Cross doctor in the Soviet expedition and Director of the Hamburg Institute for Tropical Medicine during the 1950s), did he take the initiative in 1940 in recommending the sealing off the Polish ghettos on the basis of epidemiological evidence that Jews were carriers of typhus.

He might, like so many professors of medicine, have continued in office after the war or after a perfunctory denazification tribunal and a small fine have been rehabilitated. He might have sought the support of his old Jewish teacher Martin Mayer for a whitewashing denazification certificate or Persilschein. For as chief medical adviser in hygiene to the German army he might have pleaded patriotic duty in keeping troops free from epidemic disease. This interpretation of military medical officers heroically doing their duty under the severe conditions on the Eastern Front is one that the medical historian Kudlien has sought to defend – and so drawing a strict line between the criminal abusers of medicine, and the dutiful majority in the profession.[19]

In understanding Zeiss's function in the Nazi death machine, it is first necessary to appreciate how his diverse research projects were all geared to German conquest of the East. He related nutrition to the provision of iron rations; his researches into vaccination were to sustain the immunity of the army and German settlers from cholera and typhus; he even became interested in sauna baths as a means of maintaining the personal hygiene of soldiers; and research into disinfectants was crucial in the battle against disease in the East; finally, the issue of large-scale hygienic disposal of the dead was a motive of cremation.

The role of the German army on the Eastern Front was genocidal. Among his papers is a directive (presumably deriving from the Hygiene Department of the Waffen-SS) concerning typhus prevention: 'as all Russians and Jews are potential carriers of typhus they should be ' – using a characteristic hygienic euphemism – "cleansed"'.[20] Given that the Holocaust was in part carried out by the mobile death squads under joint military and SS command which killed millions in the Soviet Union, such an order had lethal consequences.

The activities of Zeiss provided indirect support for the notorious extermination camps in Central and Eastern Europe. The technologies of epidemic prevention – shower baths, delousing procedures, fumigation and cremation – supplied the Nazis with the means of efficiently killing train loads of Jews, gypsies and others, who had scientifically been labelled by eugenicists as degenerates. A key transition was the use of hydrocyanic acid rather than carbon monoxide used in the T4 'euthanasia' killings of psychiatric patients and crippled children. For hydrocyanic acid was easily transported in canisters, it was cheaply produced by IG Farben, and it was used to kill large numbers rapidly. Hydrocyanic acid was supplied in large quantities by the Hygiene Institute of the Waffen-SS, ostensibly for pest control, particularly as an antityphus measure. The SS trained special disinfection squads in Oranienburg and Riga (in Estonia). The use of this pesticide and training procedures in disinfection – as well as various programmes of medical experiments in concentration camps – came under the control of an ambitious SS doctor, Joachim Mrugowsky, who was a colleague of Zeiss.

Zeiss was in contact with Mrugowsky from 1936 counting him as one of the close co-workers of his Berlin Institute. He supported Mrugowsky, giving him the status of Privatdozent at the University of Berlin and undertaking joint research. Mrugowsky had a key role in authorizing and personally conducting numerous human experiments, for which he was executed in Nuremberg. There was a deep spiritual bond between the two doctors. They were interested by medical history and medical geography, and applied studies by pre-bacteriological medical authors like Murchison and of medical geographers like Hirsch to epidemiological problems. Mrugowsky advanced a holistic concept of disease as a Gestalt which he applied to the notion of typhus as a 'Gemeinschaftskrankheit' when directing preventive measures on the Eastern front. He also had a fine collection of the naturalist and geographer, Alexander von Humboldt, and he was expert on the history of medicine in the age of Goethe. His Nazi gloss to an edition of Hufeland's writings on medical ethics showed the importance of vitalist concepts of a life force and of social factors in the recasting of medical knowledge. Zeiss can be seen as endorsing such environmentalist theories of medical epistemology and historiography in contrast to racial hygienists oriented to human genetics like Fritz Lenz.[21]

Zeiss devoted effort to formulating an appropriate ideology of Sturm und Drang for medical research in the context of Blitzkrieg and genocide. This can be seen in his biography of Behring, which is an underrated classic in the history of medicine. Zeiss looked partly to Lytton Strachey for supplying a new type of biographical model highlighting psychological traits of depression and destructive personal characteristics, although the emphasis was on the superhuman transcendence of personal and social limitations. While the major intellectual in-puts into this substantial biographical project still require clarification, I would like to come back to Fleck who was at a typhus research institute under Mrugowsky in Buchenwald. Uniting the captive Fleck and the commanding figure of Zeiss was an assault on the history of medicine as an account of empirically based innovations in laboratory science. But whereas Fleck pointed to sociological dimensions of knowledge, Zeiss stressed the importance of cultural traditions. Interestingly Zeiss began work on Behring just after publication of Fleck's book. He offers a counterpart to the Nazi dramatizing of Robert Koch (in contrast to *Dr Ehrlich's Magic Bullet*, the Warner Brothers film of 1940). In a very tangible way Behring supplanted Fleck's work as the German conquerors opened a Behring Institute at Lvov (Lemberg), where Fleck had worked. Similarly Zeiss supplanted Fleck's view of medicine as a socio-cultural process. Whereas Fleck wrote about the Jewish researchers Ehrlich and Wassermann, Zeiss (who in all fairness praised Ehrlich's genius) concentrated on Germanizing the figure of Behring (who for example had a Jewish wife resulting in the embarrassment of half-Jewish children requiring a special Aryan dispensation). It is of interest to note that Diepgen sponsored further work on a biography of Robert Koch at his institute – written by the Jewish public health expert, Bruno Heymann. Here history is as paradoxical as the survival of Fleck in the typhus laboratory in Buchenwald.[22]

The importance of Behring to Nazi ideology can be illustrated by the Behring commemoration in Marburg in 1940 with its parading students in brown shirts, and the drumming up of mothers and children to salute their saviour from diphtheria.[23] The biography co-published with the Marburg virologist Bieling provides a more sophisticated picture than could the Nazi Führer ideology and notions of blood and soil. Although the original biography was planned in 1932 on the initiative of Behring's widow, with a team of authors including Alfred Goldscheider, and a publisher (the Akademie Verlag) that Zeiss later denounced as Jewish, Zeiss came to emphasize the heroic psyche of Behring as a latterday Germanic scientific warrior. In the midst of the destruction of war, Zeiss was concerned with the enduring persistence of intellectual creations, and the racial roots of science. He emphasized the interaction of cultural, psychological, philosophical and geographical influences, as with Behring's origins from modest but cultured German stock on the 'deutschen Grenzmark des Ostens', Behring having grown up as one of 12 children in an idyllic rural setting of Deutsch–Eylau.[24] Zeiss portrayed how Behring's discovery of serum therapy drew on his ability to think in terms of images and analogies, attributed to Behring's reading of Schopenhauer and Nietzsche. These provided correctives to what Zeiss viewed as the superficialities of Kantian rationalism.[25] Beneath the surface of the cool, objective scientist, there were deeper racial emotions. Zeiss focused on an entry in Behring's diary demanding personal self-sacrifice: 'Los von sich selbst – Symbolisch: Aufräumen, Verbrennen'. This placed Behring in a tradition stretching from Paracelsus to Schopenhauer – that of 'enthusiasm', so giving medical research the status of a pantheistic German ideology, emphasizing the links between national culture and scientific achievements. This also served as an antidote to Soviet historical materialism.[26] This idealistic and nationalist historical approach was opposed to Soviet dialectical materialism. The fruition of Zeiss's Germanic philosophy of medicine at the time of the German offensive in Russia and the Holocaust serves to indicate how prior contacts with the Soviet Union shaped rationales for Nazi medicine and genocide.

Zeiss offers a corrective to the traditional approach of Nazi medicine which isolates a small group of criminals. He shows the fallacy of recent interpretations of racial policy as determined by modernistic rationalizers keen to reduce disease to hereditary germs contained in the genes. Rather than any monolithic interpretation of Nazi medical research and ideology (which drawing on the Nazi prescription for meals cooked in a single pot, one might characterize as the *Eintopf* school), analysis of figures like Zeiss shows the need to establish their place within a complex and changing constellation of medical and racial theories.

Nazi medicine was pluralistic in its organizational structures and in its ideologies: for example, geneticists fought against Lamarckians, and biochemical reductionists fought holists. Zeiss illustrates that environmentalist approaches – contained in his notion of geo-medicine – interacted with inherited racial characteristics. In pursuit of the extermination of disease, the doctor was empowered to sacrifice worthless lives. Science had an affinity to authoritarian social systems, which corresponded in miniature to autocratically administered research institutes and to systems of funding and reward which cultivated elitism among researchers.

While science was hailed as providing solutions to a range of social problems, Zeiss suggests that such modernistic rationalism was not antithetical to cultural traditions and religious attitudes to nature. The forging of crucial discoveries was attributed to fiery qualities of personal greatness and of penetrating insight into nature. Discovery was not a process of rational accumulation and evaluation of data: it arose from psychological and social crises. Nazism supplied an impetus to medical science in that Germany had a special mission for a creative rejuvenation of mankind by exterminating not only Jews and communists but also sweeping away rational empiricism and supplying a new metaphysical underpinning to science.

The Holocaust was not just an episode in the history of genocide, it was very much a product of contemporary medical science. The intellectual shock waves resulting from the implementation and catastrophic destruction of human life had profound implications for the history of science. For in the vision of Zeiss the rituals of 'disinfection' and 'cremation' (to use just two of the hygienic euphemisms of the Nazis) represented the culmination of a belief in science as a simultaneously creative and destructive process that required the purging and clearance of antiquated knowledge. The sacrifice of supposedly useless and inferior lives was justified in order to ensure the advancement of science. It was in the midst of the flames of destruction that the revelation of discovery and the forging of the psychological charcteristics of a superior breed of scientific supermen would occur.

## Notes

1. I. Lowy, 'Immunology and Literature in the Early Twentieth Century: Arrowsmith and The Doctor's Dilemma', *Medical History,* xxxii. (1988), 314–32.
2. G. Werskey, *The Visible College* (London, 1978), 138–48.
3. L. Fleck, *Genesis and Development of a Scientific Fact* (Chicago and London, 1979), originally published as: *Entstehung und Entwicklung einer wissenschaftlichen Tatsache; Einführung in die Lehre vom Denkstil und Denkkollektiv* (Basel, 1935).
4. M. G. Ash, 'The Emergence of Gestalt Theory: Experimental Psychology in Germany 1890-1920', (PhD Dissertation, Harvard 1982).
5. Zeiss is a central figure in P. J. Weindling, 'German-Soviet Medical Co-operation and the Institute for Racial Research, 1927–c.1935',

*German History*, x (1992), 177–206. Biographical sources include Bundesarchiv Koblenz R 86/744 Prof Dr Heinrich Zeiss.

6. P. Diepgen, 'Verstorbene innerhalb des deutschen Sprachgebietes seit Herbst 1939', *Centaurus*, (1950–1), 81–6, 167–73.
7. H. Harmsen, 'In memoriam Prof. Dr. med. Heinz Zeiss', *Zentralblatt für Bakteriologie, Parasitenkunde, Infektionskrankheiten*, clviii. (1957), 161–4.
8. H. Zeiss, *Der diagnostische Wert der Darmcoliagglutination in der Pathologie des Sauglings*, MD Dissertation (Freiburg, 1913).
9. P. J. Weindling, *Health, Race and German Politics between National Unification and Nazism* (Cambridge, 1989), 96–101.
10. Remarkably Nocht is never mentioned in Richard Evans' voluminous study of the Hamburg cholera epidemic: R. J. Evans, *Death in Hamburg* (Oxford, 1987).
11. H. Zeiss, 'Der Kampf der Feindlichen Wissenschaft gegen Deutschland', *Suddeutsche Monatshefte* (1919), 157–62.
12. Weindling, 'German-Soviet Co-operation', W. Eckart, 'Medizin und auswartige Kulturpolitik der Republik von Weimar-Deutschland und die Sowjetunion 1920–1932', *Medizin, Gesellschaft und Geschichte*, x (1993) (in preparation).
13. Weindling, 'German-Soviet Co-operation'.
14. H. Zeiss, 'Geomedizin (geographische Medizin) oder medizinische Geographie?', *Münchener medizinische Wochenschrift* (1931), 'Die Notwendigkeit einer deutschen Geomedizin', *Zeitschrift für Geopolitik*, ix (1932) 474–84.
15. H. Zeiss, *Otto Obermeier. Die Entdeckung von fadenformigen Gebilden im Blut von Ruckfallfieberkranken* (1873) (Leipzig, 1926).
16. H. Zeiss, *Elias Metschnikow, Leben und Werk* (Jena, 1932). H. and W. Muller-Dietz, 'Bemerkungen zu der Metschnikow-Biographie von H. Zeiss', *Acta medico-historica* (Riga, 1992).
17. H. Zeiss and K. Pintschovius, *Zivilisations-Schaden am Menschen*, 2 edn (Munich and Berlin, 1944).
18. Harmsen, 'Heinz Zeiss'.
19. F. Kudlien, 'Begingen Wehrmachtsarzte im Russlandkrieg Verbrechen gegen die Menschheit; Der Wert des Menschen, Medizin im Deutschland 1918–1945, (Berlin, 1989), 333–52.
20. The papers of Zeiss are in the Humboldt University archives, Berlin.
21. J. Mrugowsky, *Das arztliche Ethos. Chr. W. Hufeslands Vermachtnis einer 50 jahrigen Erfahrung* (Munich, 1949). P. J. Weindling, 'Die weltanschauliche Hintergrund der Fleckfieberbekampfung im zweiten Weltkrieg', paper presented to 75. Jahrestagung der Deutschen Gesellschaft für Geschichte der Medizin, Naturwissenschaft und

Technike.V, 25-28 September in Jena (in preparation).

22. Weindling, 'Typhus and the Holocaust'.
23. *Behring zum Gedachtnis* (Berlin, 1942).
24. H. Zeiss and R. Bieling, *Behring, Gestalt und Werk* (Berlin, 1941).
25. Zeiss and Bieling, *Behring*, 146–7, 481–4.
26. Zeiss and Bieling, *Behring*, 13, 146–7, 481–4.

# 7

# The Sick Poor and the State: Arthur Newsholme on Poverty, Disease and Responsibility[1]

*John M. Eyler*

Between 1880 and 1920 the diseases of greatest concern to public authorities were dramatically reframed. This transformation was the product of both scientific and policy changes. On the one hand the status of such diseases as pathological entities was altered by bacteriological research. What had been known as zymotic disease processes, because of their presumed resemblance to fermentation, were reframed as infectious processes and viewed as the body's response to the growth and reproduction of specific microbes. Related research on the transmission of such specific living agents provided a biological explanation for the results of epidemiological studies which, since mid-century, had suggested that epidemic diseases were contagious and had suggested vehicles, such as food and water, for their transmission.

On the other hand, the public response to such diseases also changed. In the last quarter of the century civil authorities in Britain were much more active in trying to prevent disease and premature death. While the classic documents of the sanitary movement may date from the 1840s,[2] a comprehensive network of local health authorities was created only in 1872 with the passage of legislation that divided the nation into sanitary districts and required each sanitary authority to appoint a Medical Officer of Health (M.O.H.).[3] This legislation and the financial incentives that central government provided in the form of low cost public loans stimulated local initiative and caused the majority of local authorities to do what only a minority had previously done: construct or improve public water supplies and sewers, build public abattoirs, condemn and tear down slum housing, and appoint a corps of sanitary inspectors to visit markets and shops, common lodging houses, and private homes.[4] The reframing of epidemic and endemic disease soon redirected the local health authorities from environmental sanitation to control of infectious patients. In 1889 notification, or case-reporting, of about a dozen of the most common acute infectious diseases was made mandatory in London and a local option in the provinces, and a decade later notification was universally required.[5] Visiting homes following notification, tracing contacts and antecedent cases, isolating cases, and building isolation hospitals all followed, as persons joined things as the focus of health departments' attention. In the process local authorities began to offer treatment and other personal services to the diseased and their families in addition to the older police and regulatory functions implicit in sanitary reform. By the second decade of the new century, beginning with infants, local authorities were offering personal services to both the sick and the well in the hope of preventing future disease or disability.

Finally, and of greatest interest in the present context, is the fact that the relation of public authority to the sick poor, the most frequent recipient of these services, dramatically changed during these four decades. The clearest indicators of the altered relationship between the sick or physically helpless and the state are the new social programmes which the Liberal Party introduced between 1906 and 1914: old age pensions, national health insurance, unemployment insurance, free school meals for malnourished children, a school medical service, infant welfare services, and national systems of gratuitous treatment for tuberculosis and venereal disease.[6] These new programmes were a deliberate repudiation of the strategy of public assistance codified by the Poor Law Amendment Act of 1834. The New Poor Law established a set of deterrents and penalties intended to make the receipt of relief so unpleasant that it would be the last resort of all who applied.[7] The workhouse test, the requirement that the able-bodied receive assistance only in the workhouse, and the principle of least eligibility, the goal of seeing that the life of the pauper in the workhouse was less attractive than that of the most poorly-paid labourer on the outside, were attempts by the Poor Law reformers of the 1830s to separate the pauper from the labouring poor and to deter the latter from sliding downward into destitution and dependency. It has often been pointed out that the New Poor Law both reflected and fostered the view that destitution was a sign of personal failing and character defect.[8] To be in receipt of relief was not only to lose some of one's civil rights and sometimes one's freedom, but it meant being morally stigmatized. By contrast the new welfare initiatives of the first two decades of the twentieth century provided services as entitlements. They offered personal services on the basis of need, often without prior contribution, and without penalty or civil disability. The appearance of such programmes is ample proof that poverty as well as disease was being understood in new terms. If poverty was being reframed, then attitudes toward the sick poor might be expected to have changed as well. As we will see, among those providing the new public services, changes in conviction were less swift and conclusive than the change in policy.

We can conveniently explore this problem by considering the works of a leading British public health figure whose official career almost exactly corresponds to this 40-year period. Sir Arthur Newsholme began his public career in 1883 as part-time Medical Officer of Health (M.O.H.) to the London vestry of Clapham. In 1888 he became the first full-time M.O.H. of Brighton, and from 1908 to 1919 he served as Medical Officer of the Local Government Board, the effective head of the British public health service.[9] His public career reflects the reorientations in public health programmes necesssitated by both scientific discovery and political change. Both his prominence and his interest in the social components of disease make Newsholme's thinking revealing.

Public health activists who, like Newsholme, began their careers in the early 1880s were heirs to a well-established Victorian belief that disease was associated with poverty and destitution. At mid-century the journalist and investigator of London's poor, Henry Mayhew, noted

> Indeed, so well known are the localities of fever and disease, that London would almost admit of being mapped out pathologically, and divided into its morbid districts and deadly cantons. We might lay our fingers on the Ordnance map, and say here is the typhoid parish, and there the ward of cholera; for truly as the West-end rejoices in the title of Belgravia, might the southern shores of the Thames be christened Pestilentia. As season follows season, so does disease follow disease in the quarters that may be more literally than metaphorically styled the plague-spots of London.[10]

In such a passage Mayhew was doing little more than echoing the voices of investigators like William Farr of the General Register Office, who over the last decade, had compared the vital statistics of town and countryside, industrial town and cathedral town, working class district and middle class district to show that the urban labouring poor had much higher mortality rates, lower life expectancy, and presumably more frequent bouts of disease than other groups in the population.[11]

> The annual rate of mortality in some districts will be found to be 4 per cent., in others 2 per cent.; in other words, the people in one set of circumstances live 50 years, while in another set of circumstances ... they do not live more than 25 years. In these wretched districts, nearly 8 per cent. are constantly sick, and the energy of the whole population is withered to the roots. Their arms are weak, their bodies wasted, and their sensations embittered by privation and suffering. Half the life is passed in infancy, sickness, and dependent helplessness.... Diseases are the iron index of misery, which recedes before strength, health, and happiness, as the mortality declines.[12]

For such commentators disease and the mortality it caused were indicators of well-being, indices of civilization. The excess sickness and the premature death of the poor were evidence of social defects demanding remedy.

Even the Poor Law reformers of the 1830s who argued most forcefully for a system of deterrents in the granting of relief acknowledged that the sick poor were a special case. It was not the intention of either Edwin Chadwick or of Naussau Senior, both of whom were chief architects of the New Poor Law, that the sick poor be subject to conditions intended to force the lazy, the imprudent, or the drunken into productive labour. Both acknowledged that sickness, disability, and old age rendered some of the labouring poor unable to support themselves and their families. Such misfortune could not be blamed on the destitute themselves. These unfortunates were entitled to assistance in their own homes and should be taken into special facilities only at their own request.[13] This recognition may have been small consolation to the destitute sick who in subsequent decades, contrary to Chadwick's and Senior's intent, often found that they had no choice but to enter a general workhouse where they endured conditions which, when made public, shocked mid-Victorians, nor did it alter the fact that in the Metropolis prior to 1885 by receiving any relief, even medical relief, they were pauperized and suffered the civil penalties that the law laid on other paupers.[14] But it does show that early Victorians, even Utilitarian bureaucrats like Chadwick, were capable of recognizing a distinction between destitution caused by sickness or infirmity and that caused by the alleged character flaws which were blamed for most destitution.

Chadwick in fact recognized that sickness was a major cause of pauperism and destitution. This was a point he made repeatedly in his 1842 Report on the Sanitary Condition of the Labouring Population, where he gave several estimates of the annual loss in human life from disease as well as figures for the numbers of widows and orphans thrown on the relief rolls by the premature death of wage-earners.[15] This reading of the relationship between poverty and disease further removed the destitute sick from the stigma of pauperism. Much pauperism was due to disease which, Chadwick's medical advisers assured him, was due to environmental defects that could be prevented by sanitation. Viewing the problem in this way permitted Chadwick to broaden the appeal of public health reform and to make intervention more acceptable to an age which preferred laissez-faire economics and government retrenchment. By removing sanitary defects, defects often beyond the control of individual labouring families, one would economically prevent disease and thus reduce pauperism and the resulting burden on the rates without compromising individual responsibility or challenging personal liberty. The sanitary movement was founded on the conviction that squalor caused disease, which in turn caused destitution. Such destitution threatened the social and moral order. Viewed in these terms sanitation was the complement of the deterrent policy of the poor law. The latter would insure that the giving of relief did not undermine initiative or encourage malingering. The former would reduce the number who were thrown into destitution through no fault of their own.

Newsholme falls squarely in this tradition of viewing disease as a cause of poverty. In a paper intended for fellow Medical Officers of Health written in 1909 in response to the deliberations of a Royal Commission appointed to consider revising the poor law policy that Chadwick had helped design nearly three-quarters of a century earlier, Newsholme summarized the Commission's evidence linking together poverty and disease. A third of English paupers were sick, and half of the funds spent on their behalf went to the relief of sickness. In interpreting these results Newsholme revived the past.

> We need to learn again the lessons taught to our parents by Southwood Smith, Chadwick, and their co-workers, that one of the chief causes of poverty is disease, and that extended public health administration must continue to be a chief means of removing destitution from our midst.[16]

Pulmonary tuberculosis was a case in point. He went on to estimate that between 1907 and 1916, exclusive of lost wages from prolonged illness, fatal cases in men alone would cost the nation some £58.3

million.[17] What better investment in national efficiency could there be than preventive measures against tuberculosis? Tuberculosis was an especially important example. The disease was popularly associated with poverty, but statistics showed that mortality from this dread ailment had been falling for several decades. Was it possible that improvements in the standard of living had caused this mortality decline? In studies of the epidemiology of tuberculosis, Newsholme found a strong correlation between the decline of pauperism and the decline in the mortality from pulmonary tuberculosis in the United Kingdom.[18] He cautioned, however, that pauperism was not poverty but rather poverty relieved at state expense. He argued that closer analysis showed that a decrease in direct privation was not the crucial factor in the decline of phthisis. Using census and trade figures for various nations and capital cities, he attempted to demonstrate that the decline in the mortality from phthisis did not show a clear correlation to any of several relevant indicators of standard of living: improvements in nutrition, as measured by a fall in the price of wheat or in the total cost of a working class family's food budget; total cost of living; or improvements in housing. The most important factor in tuberculosis's decline, Newsholme argued, was institutional segregation of the sick. Poor Law records showed that as the ratio of indoor to outdoor relief increased (i.e. when the proportion of institutionalized sick paupers grew) as had occurred in England, Scotland and Wales, tuberculosis declined. But where the ratio of indoor relief to outdoor relief had fallen, as in Ireland, tuberculosis mortality, and presumably morbidity increased. These findings justified Newsholme's claim that isolation was the best preventive measure against tuberculosis, and it added plausibility to the claim that specific administrative measures rather than general social amelioration were the best solution to the health problems of the poor.

Like Chadwick and the early Victorian sanitary reformers Newsholme justified expenditures on public health programmes as community investments. Even economic calculations of the cost of sickness proved that

> by combined efforts on the part of the community the total mass of poverty and sickness can be decreased, and that such efforts are not mere unproductive expressions of altruism. They represent, in fact, the best investment that the community can make.... Health is always cheaper than disease, and without an efficient state of health progress in other social concerns is being constantly impeded.[19]

It was, of course, entirely possible to turn Chadwick's equation around and to claim that economic deprivation caused the excessive disease and premature death among the poor. This interpretation was not nearly as congenial to Victorians, suggesting as it did that intervention in the economic system would be necessary to solve the problems of both pauperism and preventable disease. While Newsholme's predecessors had considered the possibility that low income caused disease, most of them considered that low income was at best a secondary cause of ill health.[20] Newsholme's four major epidemiological studies of infant mortality reached this conclusion.[21] High infant mortality, he easily verified, was a fact of urban working-class life. But low income *per se* did not explain the distribution of infant deaths. Poor nations such as Ireland and Norway had lower infant mortality rates than Britain, and within Britain high wages did not necessarily offer protection. Jews living in great poverty in some industrial districts had remarkably low rates, while miners, who were among the best paid of the English working class, had very high infant mortality rates. If greater income reduced infant mortality, why hadn't infant mortality declined during the last 20 years of the past century when real wages had risen and the mortality for all other age groups declined? While domestic overcrowding seemed to be an important influence, it was not an invariable determinant of high infant mortality. High infant mortality was tied to the life of the urban poor, but, Newsholme concluded, some feature of the life of the industrial working classes and not low income *per se* was the major cause of preventible infant deaths.

But Newsholme was under no illusions about the hazards to health in the lives of the poor. Few middle-class observers had such regular contact with the domestic life of the poor as Medical Officers of Health. Even at the beginning of his public career he recognized that there was a barrier to the efficacy of any public health work he could undertake.

> I refer to the extreme poverty among certain sections of the population, which checkmates efforts made to prevent overcrowding and ensure cleanliness. A low rate of mortality among children is difficult to attain when they are insufficiently clad and fed, and live under conditions of poverty which by some strange fatality appear to render more rapid the multiplication of the population.[22]

Over the next few years Newsholme's thinking about poverty would respond to the more systematic social investigations of the last 20 years of the century.[23] Investigators like Charles Booth and B. Seebohm

Rowntree not only replaced Mayhew's anecdotal accounts of destitute individuals and his vivid portraits of the more colourful of London's street people with aggregate measurement of the extent and depth of destitution, but, by computing a poverty line, they showed in hard-headed terms the meagre life that even the most sober and prudent of unskilled labourers could hope to attain. Within months of the appearance of Rowntree's influential study of poverty in York, Newsholme published a careful summary of its evidence and conclusions for the medical profession.[24] He explained Rowntree's division of the town's population by social class, the meaning and use of the poverty line, a typical working-class family's odyssey above and below the poverty line as earning capacity and number of dependents changed year by year, and the fact that at the time of the survey, a period of relative prosperity, 28 per cent of York's population lived below the poverty line. He painted a sensitive picture of the plight of unskilled labourers who lived just above the poverty line. They could have no luxuries. 'The family must never spend a penny on bus or railway, or on newspapers; they must write no letters; they can join no sick club....' The calculation of the poverty line made no allowance for sickness or for pleasures like tobacco or beer. Any deepening of poverty could only be met by reducing a diet just able to sustain physical efficiency. 'To give the father sufficient food, wife and children go short.'[25] The nature and consequences of such privation were missed by more casual observers.

The growing knowledge of the life of the poor encouraged Liberal economists to discuss poverty as a problem of an economic system rather than as the personal problem of individuals. John A. Hobson, for example, attacked the complacent assumption that the poor had only themselves to blame and that education and self-help would be the primary remedies for destitution. Hobson instead taught that whatever the personal defects of some individuals among the poor, poverty was the result of economic and legal systems that denied opportunities and cheapened the value of labour.[26] In these years Medical Officers of Health, more haltingly to be sure, also began to re-examine their assumptions about the role that privation played in the health of a community. James Niven, Medical Officer of Health for Manchester, for one, regarded the casual labour system and trade cycles as major causes of both poverty and disease in industrial cities. He went on to add ignorance and irresponsibility as secondary causes.[27] While poverty *per se* need not cause disease, Niven argued, as long as the casual labourer lived a precarious hand-to-mouth existence one could fairly say poverty did cause disease. Low or irregular wages forced the poor to live in conditions which exposed them to infection and lowered their resistance.

Newsholme was also learning to view the issue in economic terms. Influenced by the investigations of the Royal Commission on the Poor Laws, he labelled the meagre outdoor relief given to widows with small children as 'extravagant parsimony'.[28] Not only would such inadequate support cause chronic malnutrition, lost 'efficiency' and disease, but the desperate efforts of such women to supplement their relief by entering the labour market at the lowest level would help depress the wages of other workers. In certain contexts Newsholme was willing to depart from the traditional Victorian position and to argue that destitution caused disease. Typically, he assigned poverty an indirect role.[29] It necessitated overcrowding in working-class dwellings. It discouraged cleanliness. And it encouraged irresponsible behaviour. But on occasion Newsholme assigned a more direct role to economic privation. In his study of the history of typhus in Ireland, for example, he concluded that extreme poverty had fostered typhus mortality by encouraging disease transmission and raising case fatality.[30] And in a context different from his writing on the epidemiology of tuberculosis which we have already considered, he could even advance a conclusion he would soon repudiate: that falling wheat prices had played a large role in the improved health of the English people and even in the decline of tuberculosis.[31]

What then was his position? Did poverty cause disease, or did disease cause poverty? He tried to explain his views with a metaphor.

> The conditions of poverty in a community exposed to typhus as to phthisis, may be compared with the dryness of timber exposed to the onset of fire. The poorer and the more over-crowded the population, the drier and the more densely aggregated the timber, the more extensive will be the epidemic or the conflagration produced by infection or flame.[32]

In a town free from fire the best measure of protection might be to fireproof buildings, but in the presence of fire, there is no time to increase the resistance of timbers to flame. The best strategy then is to protect buildings from the spread of fire. Analogously, with the exception of vaccination for smallpox, measures for increasing resistance of a population to infection work too slowly and uncertainly to be used in a crisis.

It seems then that the answer to this question was partly a matter of expediency. Poverty, Newsholme came to realize, was a complex phenomenon with economic, behavioural, and biological components. He was fond of explaining that poverty and disease, like many social evils, formed a vicious circle with each contributing to the generation of the other.[33] This fact was grounds for optimism, not for discouragement, because a circle can be broken at any point. In the present state of knowledge the most efficient means of attacking the problem of poverty was to keep people from getting sick, which in practice meant breaking the chain of contagion.[34] Knowledge of social problems, he explained in 1909, is presently in the position once occupied by the understanding of disease. Using available sociological and economic knowledge and the crude solutions they suggest, one can remove some of the symptoms of poverty. But as knowledge improves, more exact means will be available.[35] The present means of dealing with poverty, like medical treatment of the past, shows 'the mischief and the hindrance to real progress which are caused by adopting an empirical treatment of symptoms instead of a scientific treatment of disease.'[36]

That answer coming from a Medical Officer of Health was hardly surprising, and it was an answer in sympathy with the Minority Report of the Royal Commission on the Poor Laws with its insistence on attacking the causes of poverty rather than treating symptoms. Newsholme had thus reached a reasonable synthesis, one that came to terms with new understandings of poverty but which continued to justify public health work as a force for general social amelioration. But the issue here was not so simple. This question gained urgency in the first decade of the twentieth century through new political issues forced upon the nation's leaders by poverty. At home there was chronic worry, especially in the Liberal Party, about how to channel working-class aspirations and recently-acquired votes into the programmes of the traditional parties.

> By 1890 the old problem of pauperism had become a problem of poverty and the essentially economic dilemma was political and social: What, it was asked, can the governors of the nation do to prevent the poor from using their franchise to overturn a society based on capitalist wealth? As it turned out, the defence against socialism was social legislation.[37]

At the turn of the century there were more immediate racial and imperial anxieties. The nation was, in fact, facing a crisis of confidence. Foreign competition in industry, trade and agriculture, the growth of German military might, and then the disastrous showing of the British forces in the South African War shattered

Britain's complacency about its place in the world and provoked in reaction a movement for 'national efficiency' which cut across party lines and aimed at halting the nation's decline.[38] Especially troubling was the news from urban recruiting stations during the Boer War. Disease and physical defects meant that many, it seemed far too many, urban working-class males were physically unfit to help defend the Empire. This revelation gave urgency to the troubling information about the lot of the urban poor that social investigators had been collecting since the middle 1880s. Perhaps the race had grown too puny to rule a great empire. Were the British, or at least the urban working class, no longer an Imperial race? Was it possible that both poverty and disease were due to some defect or defects inherent in the poor?

Nothing reveals the strength of hereditarian thought in the Edwardian period more clearly than the use of biological arguments by the New Liberals, the economists and political philosophers on the left flank of liberalism who, at the turn of the century, provided the justification of a more active, less deterrent welfare policy. The New Liberals refashioned Liberalism to make it a political philosophy capable of dealing with the social problems of industrial society, while preserving the party's traditional commitment to individual liberty.[39] This intellectual transformation was bold and far-reaching. The New Liberals dissociated themselves from laissez-faire economics and embraced collectivism. They also moved away from their antipathy to the state and saw the state as the dominant agent for the creation of a just society. But this change of opinion depended heavily on the example provided by biology. Evolutionary biology provided assurance that the principles governing human progress were open to human understanding, and it offered encouragement to think of society as an organic entity in which collective choice, i.e. state action, was not only justified but essential.[40]

Hobson could argue mightily against the claim that the poor were responsible for their own misery.

> How shall a child of the slums, ill-fed in body and mind, brought up in the industrial and moral degradation of low city life, without a chance of learning how to use hands or head, and to acquire habits of steady industry, become an efficient workman? ... It is the bitterest portion of the lot of the poor that they are deprived of the opportunity of learning to work well. To taunt them with their incapacity, and to regard it as the cause of poverty, is nothing else than a piece of blind insolence.[41]

But even Hobson shared the common suspicion that at least some of the poor might be biologically inferior. In a passage much like the one just quoted about the disadvantages slum children face he concludes 'bad seed sown in poor earth will not grow into flourishing and fruitful plants, even if carefully watered, pruned, and protected as it grows.'[42] He could embrace eugenics in the same spirit in which he criticized the old economic system.

> Selection of the fittest, or at least, rejection of the unfittest, is essential to all progress in life and character ... To abandon the production of children to unrestricted private enterprise is the most dangerous abnegation of its functions which any Government can practice.[43]

Newsholme was also keenly interested in applying the principles of biological evolution to social problems.[44] This preoccupation is most evident in his concern for changes in human fertility patterns. He, in fact, went to greater lengths than most other observers to measure precisely the much-publicized fall in birth rates,[45] and he wondered about its economic and political consequences. Scattered throughout his writings one can find evidence of the then-common anxieties about national power, interracial competition within the Empire, and the future of Anglo-Saxon cultural dominance. Such worries were created by the realization that at home the birth rates of the middle and upper classes were falling while those of the working classes were not, and that abroad other nations and races had higher fertility rates than Britain.[46]

But Newsholme recognized much sooner than many New Liberals the dangers that lay in seeking hereditarian or eugenic solutions to social problems. His caution was first alerted in the early 1890s. It was rekindled a decade later during the investigations following the Boer War of alleged physical degeneration among the poor, and it was sustained by a lengthy disagreement with Karl Pearson and his associates who saw both pauperism and the health problems of the poor as evidence of hereditary defects and questioned the utility of preventive measures against diseases such as tuberculosis.[47]

Newsholme challenged the hereditarian assumption that current socio-economic standing reflected inherent differences in ability.[48] Success was also dependent on opportunities which were very unequally distributed.

> Even the greatest ability may fail through lack of favouring circumstances; and it is impossible to say how many mute inglorious Miltons may have failed to be discovered. The fact that the poorest are lowest in the social scale cannot be used as a

> completely satisfactory argument that – as proved by selection – they are the poorest stock.[49]

Borrowing heavily on evidence provided to the Royal Commission on Physical Training in Scotland and to the Interdepartmental Committee on Physical Deterioration he argued that although much physical debility could be found among the poor, that debility was better explained by poor nurture than by hereditary degeneration.[50] Adopting the environmentalist stance which he maintained through his entire career, Newsholme explained that the troublesome thing about difference in the birth rates between the upper and the lower classes was not that the inherently inferior were outbreeding the inherently superior classes, but that those who were least able to offer children good nurture were having the greatest number of children.[51] Newsholme also offered empirical evidence that natural selection was not working as hereditarians predicted it would. If, for example, high infant mortality served to weed out weak, inferior stock, then populations subject to high infant mortality should enjoy greater health at later ages. But in his studies on infant mortality, Newsholme showed that districts having high mortality rates in the first year of life, also had high rates at later ages.[52]

But there was yet another possibility, one that had preoccupied the early Victorians. Might not both the poverty and the disease of the poor be attributed to moral inferiority? Did the much publicized idleness, drunkenness, gambling, vice, child abuse, and congenital syphilis in the slums prove what the respectable classes had long suspected: the poor were ignorant, irresponsible, and cruel? Here early Victorian investigations of the life of the poor gave much encouragement to the view that the poorest classes were morally degraded. Both Chadwick and Mayhew, for example, confused the destitute and miserable with the filth that was alleged to cause their ill health. 'It is significant that the same words – "residuum", "refuse", "offal" – were used to denote the sewage waste that constituted the sanitary problem and the human waste that constituted the social problem.'[53] Chadwick quotes one of his witnesses as explaining:

> The bone-pickers are the dirtiest of all the inmates of our workhouse; I have seen them take a bone from a dung-heap, and gnaw it while reeking hot with the fermentation of decay. Bones, from which the meat had been cut raw and which had still thin strips of flesh adhering to them, they scraped carefully with their knives, and put the bits, no matter how befouled with dirt, into a wallet or pocket appropriated to the purpose. They have told me, that whether in broth or grilled, they were the most savoury dish

> that could be imagined. I have not observed these creatures were savage, but they were thoroughly debased. Often hardly human in appearance, they had neither human tastes or sympathies, not even human sensations, for they revelled in the filth which is grateful to dogs, and other lower animals, and which to our apprehension is redolent only of nausea and abomination.[54]

The suspicion of the moral sensitivity, if not the actual humanity, of the poor survived the discovery that poverty was an economic phenomenon. The social investigations of the last two decades of the nineteenth century left room for part of the plight of the poor to be attributed to their own behaviour. Rowntree, for example, found in York that while a total of 28 per cent of the population lived below the poverty line, 18 per cent of the town's population (almost 65 per cent of the poor) lived in what he called secondary poverty, that is, their earnings would have sufficed for their basic needs were it not for some wasteful expense including drink and gambling.[55] It was a troubling realization that those who lived near the poverty line spent, by some estimates, 25 per cent of their income on drink.[56] Certainly destitution caused by such means should be remedied by moral reform.

New Liberal economists such as Hobson demurred. He argued that temperance might be prudent behaviour for individual labourers, but it offered no solution to the problems of destitution. He predicted that if all labourers would forgo their beer the most likely result was that their wages would be reduced by just the amount they had formerly spent in the pub unless some other essential expense replaced the beer.[57] The state might have moral purposes, but, Hobson argued, moralizing was not the way to realize them. Self-help and moral reform could not be expected to civilize the poor so long as the struggle to survive absorbed all their energy.

> We cannot go to the lowest of our slum population and teach them to be clean, thrifty, industrious, steady, moral, intellectual, and religious, until we have first taught them how to secure for themselves the industrial conditions of healthy physical life .... What these people do want is better food, and more of it; warmer clothes; better and surer shelter; and greater security of permanent employment on decent wages. Until we can assist them to gratify these 'lower' desires, we shall try in vain to awaken 'higher' ones.[58]

Newsholme's differences with the New Liberals are greatest at this point. He might agree that basic problems of health and human welfare should be addressed by a broader range of state initiatives, but he did not follow those like Hobson who made little demand of individuals. By contrast Newsholme believed that some of the most difficult health problems of his age could only be adequately addressed by changes in human behaviour, moral reform in his terms. Consider the problem of alcoholism, one of those personal problems which formed vicious circles with other health and social problems. Newsholme was very troubled by the amount the working class spent on drink. As a temperance advocate he blamed the consumption of alcoholic beverages for lost national efficiency, and for crime, poverty, disease, and high infant mortality.[59] Expenditure on drink, he feared, had absorbed much of the gain in human welfare that might have resulted from higher wages.[60] But as an advocate of environmental reform Newsholme blamed the circumstances in which the poor lived for their irresponsible or destructive behaviour. Poor housing, a monotonous diet, fatigue, chronic pain, and social custom all encouraged drinking.[61] Lack of information and domestic skill made many working-class families poor managers of their small resources. The poor needed to be taught to choose and prepare nourishing foods, and to protect their health.[62]

Ignorance, of course, was not a monopoly of the poor. Newsholme had harsh words for those who would explain away the high infant mortality rates in urban working-class districts by blaming the ignorance and irresponsibility of mothers. 'It is a comfortable doctrine for the well-to-do person to adopt; and it goes far to relieve his conscience in the contemplation of excessive suffering and mortality among the poor.'[63] He explained that what makes the poor mother's ignorance or carelessness so tragic is her helplessness and economic vulnerability. Poor housing and sanitation, lack of domestic or medical help, overwork, and a pinched budget all conspire to make the consequences of her mistakes more grave than those of more prosperous mothers.[64]

But the environment could not be blamed for all the shortcomings of human behaviour. After all, in the slums one often came upon a house which was 'an oasis of cleanliness and sweetness in a desert of dirt and neglect. The structural condition of the house is not better than that of the neighbouring houses but the character of the inmates has impressed itself upon the house.'[65] Not all poor parents squandered their resources, neglected their children, or led drunken lives. Certainly part of the condition of the poor was the result of decisions made by individuals. Conquering poverty and disease would depend on more than public initiative. It would also necessitate responsible individual behaviour. Newsholme encouraged the sanitary inspector to think of himself as a 'home missionary to the poor and helpless' who by promoting 'cleanliness and self-respect' and the 'decencies of family life' made 'moral and social improvement' possible.[66] Where individual responsibility faltered public authority might have to provide added incentive. Local authorities might have to intervene to see that alcoholic parents met their responsibilities to their children even if that meant drastic measures such as the garnishing of wages.[67] Especially in his writings about alcoholism and venereal disease published after 1920, Newsholme blamed character faults, and he could be very harsh in his condemnation of individuals. Syphilis, he held, was spread almost exclusively by 'sexually immoral persons', and he argued that the disease could not be controlled until public opinion viewed 'the sexually immoral man as an enemy of society, who cannot be tolerated' and promiscuity as 'the chief enemy of the social order', a form of barbarism.[68]

Newsholme's emphasis on the reformation of character as a solution for problems of human welfare may at first seem anomalous, a late survival of his strict Methodist upbringing. It was undoubtedly that. It was also a reflection of conventional Victorian middle-class views of human sexuality, family life, and public decorum. He was offended by drunkenness, prostitution, contraception, and abortion, as well as by child abuse, and he brought to discussions of these topics an evangelical zeal that had been well-nurtured in his childhood. However, it would be wrong to pass off his prouncements so simply. Moral reform played a more reasoned part in his outlook. It provided a way for him to reconcile his politics and his science: his liberal faith in progress, amelioration, and liberty with his belief in the fundamental truth of Darwinian evolution.

Following the cue provided by Thomas Henry Huxley's Romanes Lecture, Newsholme argued that the appearance of human intelligence and co-operation sheltered humans from the brutal and blind force of the competition for survival.[69] Fitness for survival, after all, was relative, a ratio of strength of the individual to strain imposed by the environment. Hence such fitness could be increased either by increasing strength or by reducing strain. By acting collectively and with forethought humans had learned to transfer much of the pressure of the struggle for existence from the individual to the group. Newsholme held, in other words, that a process of moral evolution paralleled biological and social evolution. The self-denial that accompanied the evolution of morality created 'a new moral environment which alters very largely the results of evolution.'[70] The result was that public opinion and collective action began to protect the weak and helpless from the brutal force of competition. He held further that the progress of civilization, which recently had witnessed the abolition of slavery and the launching of campaigns to end cruelty to children and animals and to abolish the double standard of sexual conduct, reflected a grand evolutionary process in which selfishness gives way to altruism and competition to co-operation.[71] Private philanthropy, public assistance, and medical charity were all reflections of the altruism that moral evolution created. In this scheme crime, vice, and other anti-social activity were viewed as survivals of earlier and less civilized ages, and the problems of human conduct in contemporary society were reduced to the tension between coexisting human impulses: the primitive and selfish and the more evolved and altruistic.[72]

The same moral evolution had created new ethical standards which provided the fundamental reason for rejecting eugenic remedies for disease and disability. In the current moral environment a civilized nation simply could not allow a disease like tuberculosis to run unchecked.

> The logical alternative (to preventive work) is to kill off the susceptible stock or, as has been suggested, to allow them to infect their susceptible brethren and together with them perish of their disease. Such proposals have only to be stated in their crude terms in order to be apprehended and reprehended as an unsocial negation of civilization.[73]

A decade later Newsholme argued that reverting to natural selection in human affairs would destroy civilization. 'To think otherwise is the secret behind German aggression; to act otherwise is to revert to barbarism. Man has definitely replaced natural by rational selection, and will, I have no doubt, to a steadily increasing extent replace competition by co-operation.'[74]

Humans could escape the tyranny of Darwinian evolution, because they possessed the ability to act purposefully, collectively, and altruistically. In a liberal state much of the motive for right conduct had to come, he believed, from within. For this reason he found the final solution to some of the most intractable health and social problems in the reformation of human character. In this process the state could do some things. It could see that assistance did not undermine individual responsibility, and it could insist that help was dependent on responsible behaviour.[75] In some instances compulsion might be needed for 'those who do not evolve in response to the advancing tide of morality.'[76] But ultimately humans had to learn to behave responsibly. He was not unaware that he was asking a great deal of the poor, more in fact than was being asked of the more fortunate. 'Sometimes I think that those to whom a farthing is a rare coin do not realize effectively the demands on character which are made by a life in which every farthing counts.' But those oases of 'cleanliness and sweetness' in deserts of 'dirt and neglect' proved, to his satisfaction at least, that

> the necessary sacrifices can be made and made cheerfully. The constant self-denial which they entail cannot conceivably be improvised. It must result from the possession of habits both of conduct and of mind. Life without such habits in conditions which hourly call for them is not only miserable for the individual but also mischievous to the community. And yet how small a part of our national educational system is devoted to the training of character, which is, I take it, the resultant of habits of mind and conduct.[77]

On February 3, 1908, the day before he took up his duties in Whitehall as Medical Officer of the Local Government Board, Newsholme appeared as a witness before the Royal Commission on the Poor Laws.[78] The Commissioners were trying to decide whether the New Poor Law that Chadwick had helped design should remain the nation's primary response to destitution and dependency. From Newsholme's testimony it is obvious that much had changed since Chadwick's day. Newsholme condemned the Poor Law Medical services, and argued that efficient, humane care of the sick poor could only be provided by agencies completely removed from the Poor Law. His own proposals reveal not only a vastly different understanding of disease causation but the acceptance of a much expanded sphere of public initiative. Environmental sanitation was now only one routine function of many municipal health services. In addition a network of publicly-financed diagnostic and therapeutic services had evolved. Newsholme proposed to expand and unify this *ad hoc* system to create nothing less than a comprehensive municipal medical service under the supervision of the local Medical Officer of Health, which would offer gratuitous preventive, diagnostic, and therapeutic services. This municipal system would in effect take over all medical serices currently offered to the working class except those offered by the voluntary hospitals.

In other ways there are some striking resemblances between Newsholme's testimony and the views of the Poor Law reformers of the 1830s Newsholme, like Chadwick, pointed to the waste of life and money caused by preventable disease. Public health work was a good investment after all. Newsholme, more surprisingly, was also concerned with the moral effect of medical services on the recipient.

Such assistance must not undermine character. He argued that free medical care would not demoralize the recipient because co-operation and personal sacrifices would be required from the patient.

> The form in which medical aid would be given would be such as constantly to enforce on the minds of the patients their duty to the community and to themselves in matters of health. Though they would pay nothing, they would not be merely passive recipients of advice and attention. The influence of the doctor would demand from them habits of life and even sacrifices of personal taste in the interest of the health of the community, their families and themselves, which would leave them conscious of a sensible discharge of duty in return for the attention which they received. The discipline of responsibility into which the system would educate them should, in my judgment, suffice to avoid the loss of self-respect liable to arise from the merely passive receipt of gifts; and it would introduce into the national life an attitude towards matters of personal health that would have an indirect influence upon conduct, while directly restricting disease.[79]

So firm was Newsholme's commitment to the need for character reformation that it survived the scrapping of the Poor Law and the advent of the welfare state. He was most insistent on this point in discussions of infant welfare and venereal disease. Both were new additions to the public medical service in which the alternatives to voluntary changes in human behaviour were unacceptable invasions of privacy and breaches of personal liberty. But Newsholme's insistence on the necessity of high standards of personal conduct was also founded on his conviction that only ethical evolution guaranteed continued human progress. Ultimately, moral, not economic, imperatives must drive social and medical policy.

## Notes

1. The research for this piece was supported in part by NIH Grant LM03765 from the National Library of Medicine. The author gratefully acknowledges this support.
2. Edwin Chadwick, *Report on the Sanitary Condition of the Labouring Population of Gt. Britain* (1842), ed. M. W. Flinn (Edinburgh: Edinburgh University Press, 1965); & the *Report of the Metropolitan Sanitary Commission* ie Report of the Commissioners Appointed to Inquire whether any and what Special Means may be Requisite for the Improvement of the Health of the Metropolis, P.P. 1847–8, XXXII, (888, 911, 979).
3. 35 & 36 Vict., c 79, *Public Health Act*, 1872.

4. See for example Anthony S. Wohl, *Endangered Lives: Public Health in Victorian Britain* (Cambridge, Mass: Harvard University Press, 1983), 80–116 & 166–99.
5. 52 & 53 Vict., c 72, *Infectious Disease (Notification) Act, 1889*; & and 62 & 63 Vict., c 8, *Infectious Disease (Notification) Extension Act, 1899*.
6. For descriptions of the new welfare services see Bentley B. Gilbert, *The Evolution of National Insurance in Great Britain: The Origins of the Welfare State* (London: Michael Joseph, 1966); & Deborah Dwork, *War is Good for Babies and Other Young Children: A History of the Infant and Child Welfare Movement in England 1898–1918* (London & New York: Tavistock, 1987).
7. Perhaps the best introduction to Victorian attitudes toward poverty and pauperism is Gertrude Himmelfarb, *The Idea of Poverty: England in the Early Industrial Age* (New York: Alfred A Knopf, 1984).
8. Gilbert, *Evolution of National Insurance*, 21.
9. There is no biography of Newsholme. He did leave two accounts of public health work which are autobiographical in character: Arthur Newsholme, *Fifty Years in Public Health: A Personal Narrative with Comments* (London: George Allen & Unwin, Ltd., 1935); & Arthur Newsholme, *The Last Thirty Years in Public Health: Recollections and Reflections on my Official and Post-Official Life* (London: George Allen & Unwin, Ltd., 1936). See also the following for the more useful obituaries *B.M.J.* (1943), i 680–1; *Lancet* (1943), i 696; & *Nature*, 151 (1943): 635–6.
10. Henry Mayhew, 'A Visit to the Cholera Districts of Bermondsey', *Morning Chronicle*, 24 Sept,. 1849, cited in Himmelfarb, *The Idea of Poverty*, 315.
11. For a brief discussion of Farr's studies of urban mortality see John M. Eyler, *Victorian Social Medicine: The Ideas and Methods of William Farr* (Baltimore: Johns Hopkins University Press, 1979), 123–54.
12. William Farr, 'Letter to the Registrar-General', *Annual Report of the Registrar-General of Births, Deaths, and Marriages in England*, i (1838), 88–9.
13. Himmelfarb, *The Idea of Poverty*, 158, 160–1, 164.
14. For a brief description of the 1866 investigations of the condition of the sick poor in Metropolitan workhouses see Brian Abel-Smith, *The Hospitals 1800–1948: A Study in Social Administration in England and Wales* (Cambridge, Mass.: Harvard University Press, 1964), 50–64. See also *ibid.*, 124–7 for the ending of pauperization of patients in the Metropolitan Asylums Board.
15. Chadwick, *Sanitary Condition*, 76–9, 254–76. See also S. E. Finer,

*The Life and Times of Sir Edwin Chadwick* (London: Methuen, 1952), 147–9, 154–63, 209–29.

16. Arthur Newsholme, 'Some Conditions of Social Efficiency in Relation to Local Public Administration', *Public Health*, xxii (1909–10), 404–5.
17. *Ibid.*, 408.
18. For the following comments see Arthur Newsholme, 'The Relative Importance of the Constituent Factors involved in the Control of Pulmonary Tuberculosis', *Trans. Epidemiological Soc. Lond.*, ns xxv (1905–6), 49–65; Arthur Newsholme, 'An Inquiry into the Principal Causes of the Reduction in the Death-Rate from Phthisis during the Last Forty Years, with Special Reference to the Segregation of Phthisical Patients in General Institutions', *J. Hygiene*, vi (1906), 324–50; Arthur Newsholme, *The Prevention of Tuberculosis* (New York: E. P. Dutton & Co., 1908), 224–51; & Arthur Newsholme, 'The Causes of the Past Decline in Tuberculosis', *Charities*, xxi (1908–09), 217–22.
19. Newsholme, 'Conditions of Social Efficiency', 408.
20. For Farr's consideration of this problem see Eyler, *Victorian Social Medicine*, 125–6.
21. Arthur Newsholme, *Report on Infant and Child Mortality. Supplement to the Thirty-ninth Annual Report of the Medical Officer of the Local Government Board* (London: His Majesty's Stationery Office, 1910), 54–6, 60–3, 68–9; Arthur Newsholme, *Second Report on Infant and Child Mortality. Supplement to the Forty-second Annual Report of the Medical Officer of the Local Government Board* (London: His Majesty's Stationery Office, 1913), 73–8; Arthur Newsholme, 'Preliminary Report by the Medical Officer', in *Third Report on Infant Mortality dealing with Infant Mortality in Lancashire. Supplement to the Forty-third Annual Report of the Local Government Board* (London: His Majesty's Stationery Office, 1914), 14, 21; & Arthur Newsholme, *Report on Child Mortality at Ages 0-5 in England and Wales. Supplement to the Forty-fifth Annual Report of the Local Government Board, 1915–16* (London: His Majesty's Stationery Office, 1916), 68–71.
22. Arthur Newsholme, *Report of the Medical Officer of Health for the Third Quarter of 1889* (Brighton, 1889), 1.
23. For a brief discussion of the variety of investigations and the proposals for scientific social reform to which they were tied see Gilbert, *Evolution of National Insurance*, 40-58.
24. Arthur Newsholme, 'Poverty in Town Life', *Practitioner*, lxix. (1902), 682–94.

25. *Ibid.*, 690.
26. J. A. Hobson, *The Crisis of Liberalism: New Issues of Democracy* (London: P. S. King & Sons, 1909), 159–75 & John A. Hobson, *Problems of Poverty: An Inquiry into the Industrial Condition of the Poor*, 8th ed. (London: Methuen & Co. Ltd., 1913), 171–82).
27. James Niven, 'Poverty and Disease', *Proc. Roy. Soc. Med.*, Pt. 2, Epidemiological Section, iii (1910), 4–11.
28. Newsholme, 'Conditions of Social Efficiency', 406.
29. Arthur Newsholme, 'A Discussion on the Co-ordination of the Public Medical Services', *B.M.J.* (1907), ii 656–7.
30. Arthur Newsholme, 'Poverty and Disease, as illustrated by the Course of Typhus Fever and Phthisis in Ireland', *Proc. Roy. Soc. Med.*, Pt. 1, Edidemiological Section, i (1908), 2–3 & 10–14.
31. Arthur Newsholme, 'Alleged Physical Degeneration in Towns', *Public-Health*, xvii (1904–05), 299.
32 Newsholme, 'Poverty and Disease', 4.
33. Newsholme, 'Conditions of Social Efficiency', 406; Newsholme, 'Causes of the Past Decline', 222; & Arthur Newsholme, *Public-Health and Insurance: American Addresses* (Baltimore: The Johns Hopkins University Press, 1920), 148.
34. Newsholme, 'Co-ordination of the Public Medical Services', 657.
35. Newsholme, 'Conditions of Social Efficiency', 409.
36. Newsholme, 'An Address on Social Evolution and Public-Health', *Lancet*, 1904, ii 1334.
37. Gilbert, *Evolution of National Insurance*, 19.
38. For good discussions of the political response to the post-war crisis see G. R. Searle, *The Quest for National Efficiency: A Study in British Politics and Political Thought, 1899-1914* (Oxford: Basil Blackwell, 1971); Gilbert, *Evolution of National Insurance*, 59-101; & Bernard Semmel, *Imperialism and Social Reform: English Social-Imperial Thought 1895-1914* (Cambridge, Mass.: Harvard Univ. Pr., 1960), 53-82.
39. For an excellent study of this problem see Freeden, *New Liberalism.*
40. *Ibid.*, 76-116.
41. Hobson, *Problems of Poverty*, 177.
42. Hobson, *Crisis of Liberalism*, 165.
43. J. A. Hobson, *The Social Problem* (London, 1901), 214 in Freeden, *New Liberalism*, 178.
44. Arthur Newsholme, 'The Influence of Civilization upon the Survival of the Fittest', *Annual Report of the Brighton and Sussex Natural History Society, 1893-54*, 5–12; & Arthur Newsholme, 'Some Aspects of Heredity', *ibid.*, 1894–5, 6–8.
45. Arthur Newsholme & T. H. C. Stevenson, 'The Decline of Human

Fertility in the United Kingdom and Other Countries as Shown by Corrected Birth-Rates', *J. Roy. Statist. Soc.*, 69 (1906), 34–87; & Arthur Newsholme, *The Declining Birth Rate. Its National and International Significance* (London, New York, etc.: Cassell & Co. Ltd., 1911).

46. See, for example Newsholme, 'Influence of Civilization', 10–12; Newsholme, *Declining Birth Rate*, 57–8; Arthur Newsholme, 'The Control of Conception', in *Sexual Problems of To-Day*, Mary Scharlieb (ed.), (London: Williams and Norgate, Ltd., 1924), 152 & 153; & Arthur Newsholme, 'Some Public Health Aspects of "Birth Control"', in *Medical Views on Birth Control*, James Marchant (ed.), (London: Martin Hopkinson & Co., Ltd, 1926), 132.
47. Newsholme, *Prevention of Tuberculosis*, 187; Karl Pearson, *The Fight against Tuberculosis and the Death-rate from Phthisis* (London: Dulau & Co., 1911); Karl Pearson, *Tuberculosis, Hereditary and Environment* (London: Dulau & Co., Ltd., 1912); Newsholme, *Second Report on Infant Mortality*, 46–8; & Karl Pearson, 'The Check to the Fall in the Phthisis Death-rate since the Discovery of the Tuberculosis and the Adoption of Modern Treatment', *Biometrika*, 12 (1918–19), 374–6.
48. Newsholme, *Declining Birth Rate*, 44 & 49–52; & Newsholme, 'Public Health Aspects of "Birth Control"', 145–6.
49. Newsholme, *Declining Birth Rate*, 51–2.
50. Newsholme, 'Alleged Physical Degeneration', 293–4; Arthur Newsholme, 'Physical Inspection', *J. Roy. Sanitary Institute*, xxvi (1905), 67; & Newsholme, *Declining Birth Rate*, 49–50.
51. Newsholme, 'Control of Conception', 154.
52. Newsholme, *Report on Infant & Child Mortality*, 9–18, 78–82; & Newsholme, *Second Report on Infant and Child Mortality*, 43–53.
53. Himmelfarb, *Idea of Poverty*, 358.
54. Chadwick, *Sanitary Condition*, 164–5. This passage is reproduced and discussed in Himmelfarb, *Idea of Poverty*, 358–9.
55. Newsholme, 'Poverty in Town Life', 685 & 688.
56. Newsholme, 'Social Evolution', 1336.
57. Hobson, *Problems of Poverty*, 178–9.
58. *Ibid.*, 175.
59. Newsholme, 'Alleged Physical Degeneration', 300; Arthur Newsholme, 'Alcohol and Public–Health', in *The Drink Problem in its Medico-Sociological Aspects*, T. N. Kelynack (ed.), (London: Methuen & Co., 1907), 122–51; Newsholme, *Public Health and Insurance*, 123–4; Newsholme, *Second Report on Infant and Child Mortality*, 78–82.
60. Newsholme, 'Alleged Physical Degeneration', 300.

61. Newsholme, 'Conditions of Social Efficiency', 406; & Newsholme, *Public Health and Insurance*, 149–50.
62. Newsholme, 'Social Evolution', 1333; Arthur Newsholme, 'On the Study of Hygiene in Elementary Schools', *Public Health*, 3 (1890-91), 134–6.
63. Newsholme, *Report on Child Mortality*, 64.
64. Newsholme, *Report on Infant and Child Mortality*, 70–4; & Newsholme, *Report on Child Mortality*, 64–6.
65. Newsholme, 'Social Evolution', 1333.
66. Arthur Newsholme, 'The Duties and Difficulties of Sanitary Inspectors', *Sanitary Record*, ns x (1888–9), 412.
67. Newsholme, 'Social Evolution', 1336; & Newsholme, 'Conditions of Social Efficiency', 405.
68. Arthur Newsholme, *Health Problems in Organized Society. Studies in the Social Aspects of Public Health* (London: P. S. King & Son, Ltd., 1927), 107, 177–9, 188.
69. Newsholme, 'Influence of Civilization', 6–8; Newsholme, 'Social Evolution', 1331 & 1332. See also Thomas Henry Huxley, 'Evolution and Ethics', (The Romanes Lecture, 1893) in *Evolution and Ethics and Other Essays* (New York: D. Appleton & Co., 1899), 46–86.
70. Newsholme, 'Influence of Civilization', 7.
71. Newsholme, *Health Problems*, 98–9, 118–19.
72. *Ibid.*, 118–19, 182–3.
73. Newsholme, *Prevention of Tuberculosis*, 189.
74. Newsholme, *Public Health and Insurance*, 165.
75. Newsholme, 'Social Evolution', 1334–5.
76. Newsholme, *Health Problems*, 119.
77. Newsholme, 'Social Evolution', 1333.
78. For Newsholme's testimony see *Report of the Royal Commission on the Poor Laws and Relief of Distress*, Appdx. Vol 9, P.P., 1910, XLIX. (Cd. 5068), 155-82.
79. *Ibid.*, 164–5.

# 8

## The Metamorphosis of Dawson of Penn

*Charles Webster*

Bertrand Edward Dawson, Viscount Dawson of Penn (1864–1945), is one of the legendary figures of British medicine in the twentieth century. His celebrated report of 1920 is justly regarded as a classic of medical planning, and it is looked back upon as one of the cornerstones of the National Health Service. Dawson therefore figures prominently in accounts of the genesis of the National Health Service, but it is noticeable that comment relates almost exclusively to the narrow period from 1918 to 1920. Only Dawson's biographer has surveyed the long formative period before 1918, and his long career after 1920.[1] Dawson is conventionally applauded as the respected elder statesman of British medicine. He served as President of the Royal College of Physicians during the 1930s, at the time when the government was forced into taking the first tentative steps towards integrated medical planning. He was President of the British Medical Association (BMA) during the Second World War, when the first concerted attempt was made to evolve a medical scheme fitting into the government's plans for post-war reconstruction. Dawson not only occupied influential medico-political offices, but he was also the main spokesman for the medical profession in the House of Lords, and his position as a court physician gave him useful connections in the highest social circles. His *B.M.J.* obituary was headed 'Physician to Kings', while the list of major honours awarded to him fills a whole page at the opening of his biography.[2] Consequently, by virtue of numerous channels of influence Dawson was the medical leader best placed to intervene in medical planning throughout the long formative period leading up to the National Health Service, and the Dawson Report granted him an authority which all others lacked. It is therefore helpful briefly to review

Dawson's place in medical planning from 1918 until his death in 1945, and this paper will be devoted to that purpose. This will help to resolve some of the obscurity surrounding Dawson and correct errors on points of detail which commonly occur in accounts of medical planning. The general lack of real familiarity with Dawson is indicated by the frequency with which his first name is given erroneously, even in widely known sources.[3]

The background of Dawson was unremarkable. He came from the comfortable suburban middle class, younger son of an architect. His scientific and medical education was obtained at University College London and the London Hospital. He rose smoothly through the ranks at the London Hospital to become one of the most respected Honorary Physicians. Basic to his success was engagement of the confidence of Sydney Holland, Viscount Knutsford, Chairman of Governors. It was also advantageous to be married to the daughter of Alfred Yarrow, Clyde shipbuilder and one of the London Hospital benefactors. Dawson was well-educated, but he possessed only a minor scientific reputation. Even a friendly source admitted that his 'contribution was respectable rather than remarkable'.[4] Unlike Yarrow, he was not elected a Fellow of the Royal Society.

The reputation of Dawson was founded on his sagacity as a physician and energy as a member of professional organizations. There was little remarkable about his intellectual position, although he developed an interest in questions of social hygiene, and joined in the clamour for eugenics, in which capacity he was in the vanguard movement for birth control.

In 1914 Dawson enlisted in RAMC and rose to rank of Major-General. Rapidly, Dawson established himself as a respected and dominant thinker in the army medical establishment. The war in France, and the vast scale of casualties, provided an important object lesson in the co-ordination and development of medical services. Dawson showed himself to be an intelligent planner and open to new ideas, many of which were applicable in the civilian sphere.[5]

Even before the end of the War, Dawson began reflecting about the reorganization of civilian medical services. A diary entry, perhaps from the latter half of 1917 recorded:

> I want some time now for thinking over the big difficulties, for people are beginning to ask me how to solve them. I cannot yet see how the Insurance Act is to be linked with Health Service and yet it has to be.[6]

This diary entry also recorded that 'this medical reconstruction is catching on, and the men over here want me to address them so that conferences and discussions may follow'. It is therefore clear that Dawson was at least in part responding to the increasingly popular wave of support for post-war reconstruction, a phenomenon which was repeated with much greater vehemence in the forces during the Second World War. The diary entry also indicates that interested laymen were lacking in guidance, and that Dawson was recognizing a responsibility to turn his attention to this question of acute public concern. Although the introduction of National Health Insurance in 1911 (NHI) was proclaimed as a great reform, as Dawson noticed, it had produced an entirely separate health administration, lacking any co-ordination with the existing local government machinery responsible for most of the remaining publicly-funded health services. Equally serious, the voluntary hospitals lacked any meaningful relationship with the central and local government health services. Towards the end of the First World War, when reconstruction was achieving its maximum political profile, Dawson set about evolving a scheme which would reproduce in the civilian services something like the harmonization established in the emergency military situation.

Dawson made a sudden leap into public prominence when he announced his ideas in 1918. He was then aged 54, with no previous reputation for activism in the planning of civilian health services. This represented a splendid piece of opportunism. It was not occasioned so much by Dawson's high stature, but the low stature of those around him. There was a surprising lack of leadership within the medical elite concerning the future direction of the British health services. The most likely source of inspiration on planning matters was likely to emanate from the public health specialism, but this had failed to generate any figure of anything like the stature of Sir John Simon, who had died in 1904. As pressure for action on reconstruction mounted there was an urgent requirement on the political right for ideas to counteract the schemes emanating from the left. Into this vacuum stepped the middle-aged physician from the London Hospital.

An opportunity for the comprehensive exposition of Dawson's ideas came in 1918, when he was invited to give the Cavendish Lectures at the West London Medico-Chirurgical Society. These two lectures entitled 'The Nation's Welfare: The Future of the Medical Profession' were delivered on 4 and 11 July, 1918. This was not a particularly auspicious platform, but the lectures were obviously well-attended and they were widely publicised in the

*B.M.J.* and *The Lancet*, as well as attracting substantial newspaper coverage. The lectures were also published in pamphlet form in September, 1918.[7] Dawson's effort should be seen as part of a race for the high ground of medical planning. Dawson immediately gained recognition as the apostle for the medical profession, espousing ideas congenial to the political centre and right. Working in parallel were Sir Robert Morant and advocates of reform of the machinery of government, and the Labour Party, advised by the Webbs and the State Medical Services Association.

The latter represented a small rump of mainly public health doctors subscribing to the idea of more advanced state involvement in health services than was acceptable to the majority of the medical profession.[8] Dawson's wartime experience placed him at an advantage to his competitors. He was one of the few military medical leaders capable of translating the hard-won experiences of war into the language of peacetime reconstruction.

Although it is doubtful whether Dawson was acquainted with the debate about welfare among political theorists, he was intuitively in line with New Liberal thinking in reaching towards a more positive conception of the role of the state in health maintenance. He appreciated that it was no longer realistic for the state to confine its role to the residuum of the poor, or to limit its intervention according to standards representing the minimum to protect life:

> A growing appreciation of the fact by the profession and the public that much disease is preventable; a growing sense that health is of supreme interest alike to the state and the individual; that the best means for preserving health and curing disease should be available for every citizen, irrespective of his position, and by right and not by favour.[9]

The definition of objectives for the health services was repeated in the Dawson Report, and with little modification it was taken over by the Beveridge Report in 1942, the 1944 White Paper, and the 1946 National Health Service legislation.

As suggested by the original title of his lectures, Dawson was as much concerned with the interests of the medical profession as with the rationalization and extension of health services. Reconstruction was recognized as an invaluable opportunity to enhance the power and prestige of the medical profession. Dawson insisted: 'The initiation, execution and fulfilment of any policy of Health must in large measure be the work of doctors (and those skilled in the sciences allied to Medicine), for they alone possess the requisite knowledge'.[10] Basic to the realization of this objective was a Medical Advisory Council which Dawson insisted should be part of the permanent organization of a new Ministry of Health.

Dawson's proposals drew heavily on military and educational models of hierarchical organization. He sought to devise a comprehensive health service which would not entail dominance of public health doctors or moves towards a state medical service of the kind favoured in Labour and public health circles. Whole-time salaried service was denounced as 'a machine without a soul or hope of salvation'.[11] Dawson recognized an urgent need to reinvigorate general practice. He was clearly not convinced that National Health Insurance had resolved the crisis faced by this large segment of the medical profession, the fortunes of which were adversely affected by incursions from both hospital specialisms and by the rapid expansion of public health medicine.

Dawson was confident that the tide could be turned. By exploiting efficient teamwork, recognizing the potentialities of preventive medicine, and gaining access to modern diagnostic facilities, the general practitioner might establish himself with renewed authority as 'father of his people':

> ... the fact that growth of knowledge makes measures for preventing and curing disease more complex; that these measures are no longer within the power of individual effort; that they need combination of effort – in short, team work; that for such work equipment and apparatus are needed, and these in turn need organization and involve increased cost.
>
> If you admit that these organized measures are to be within the reach of all members of the community, two things follow – namely, that efficient service cannot be self supporting; that its provision implies not only men but equipment and that both must be distributed according to the needs of the community.[12]

Dawson warned that there was no future in traditional bedside medicine. He was somewhat ahead of his contemporaries in appreciating the revolutionary potentialities of medical intervention, calling for a high level of public investment in high technology medicine, with the aim of building up a comprehensive spectrum of specialized services organized in a co-ordinated hierarchy of institutions. However, future curative services were not to be developed at the expense of preventive medicine. Building on his experience with rehabilitation of soldiers, Dawson evolved extravagant plans for convalescence homes, spas, swimming baths and sportsfields, which he made integral to his plan.

At the time of delivering his lectures Dawson had evolved no settled terminology for the various elements in his organizational hierarchy. He applied such terms as 'clinic', 'health organization' or 'settlement' to the local centres of primary care. The term 'health centre' was inserted in the pamphlet-form of the Cavendish Lectures, being at that stage restricted to the explanatory note and folding plan of a 'Model Health Centre' produced by Major Biddulph-Pinchard of the RAF. Dawson's recognition of the appropriateness of this term is undoubtedly indicated by the attention drawn to the folding plan in the extended title of his pamphlet.[13]

The Cavendish Lectures confirm that in the space of little more than a year since the beginning of his deliberations Dawson had elaborated a comprehensive blueprint for the future of the civilian health services. Generous acknowledgements confirm that he was drawing extensively on specialist advice. In particular his plan represented a distillation of ideas drawn from military informants. *The Nation's Health* showed a further advance in his ideas. The Dawson Report essentially reiterated the principles of *The Nation's Health.* Indeed it is arguable that most of Dawson's later contributions represented a recombination of elements derived from the developed version of the Cavendish Lectures.

The Cavendish Lectures placed Dawson ahead of the field. A Labour Party committee began work on its proposals for a state medical service in April, 1918, but publication of this plan was delayed until 1919.[14] Dawson's ideas were attractive to both Dr Christopher Addison and Sir Robert Morant, who were appointed respectively the first Minister of Health, and first Permanent Secretary of the new Ministry of Health. Both were confident that Dawson could be converted to the realities of public administration and medical politics. With this influential backing Dawson was introduced to Lloyd George and having made a favourable impression he was appointed first Chairman of the newly-created Consultative Council on Medical and Allied Services, which represented a realization of the Medical Advisory Council advocated by Dawson in *The Nation's Welfare.*

Indicative of Dawson's stature, he seriously considered taking up the Regius Chair of Medicine at Oxford upon the death of the famous Sir William Osler. Osler's predecessor was Burdon Sanderson and his successor Archibald Garrod, both figures of incomparably greater intellectual distinction than Dawson. However, Dawson elected to concentrate on public affairs and he was given an additional platform when he was raised to the peerage, the first doctor chosen specifically to represent the interests of medicine in the House of Lords.[15]

The Consultative Council began work in October, 1919. Its Interim Report was published in May, 1920.[16] Such expedition was possible because of the compelling authority Dawson held over the inexperienced, incohesive and mainly undistinguished Consultative Council.

On main principles as well as many points of detail the Dawson Report followed the Cavendish Lectures. The most obvious related to terminology. In order to underline his preventive and promotive philosophy, Dawson adopted the term health centre for institutions at the local and district levels of health service organization.[17] To describe these tiers he imported the 'primary' and 'secondary' terminology from educational administration. The primary health centre was expected to fulfil Dawson's aim to revive general practice and establish the general practitioner as the central pillar of any scheme of reconstruction, whereas the secondary health centre was the forerunner of the modern district general hospital.[18]

The organization of health centres was discussed in detail, and sample architectural plans were included. The report also gave an account of the Gloucestershire experiment in co-ordination, which Dawson identified as having many objectives in common with his own scheme. His report avoided commitment on the crucial question of local administration of the expanded health service, apart from insisting as in the Cavendish Lectures that the 'Health Authorities' of the future should be subject to strong medical guidance.[19]

Failure to relate his plan to the existing system of local administration severely reduced the impact of the Dawson Report. Sir Edward Forber of the Ministry of Health dismissed Dawson's plan as a 'compound of theoretical symmetry, BMA aspirations and of an actual plan prepared by the county MOH of Gloucestershire.'[20] Dawson faced much sceptical comment, most of it pointing to the unrealistic or utopian qualities of his thinking. He paid the penalty for having taken little account of his critics, and having made too little attempt to come to terms with dominant political or bureaucratic forces. It is therefore not surprising that the Dawson Report, although greeted with acclaim, failed to make any lasting impression. Furthermore, Addison quickly lost credibility at the Ministry of Health as his ambitious plans for housing and health fell to pieces. His preface to the Dawson Report was lukewarm. In April, 1921 he was removed from his office. Even more disastrous for Dawson, Morant died of influenza in 1920 and he was replaced by the conventional Sir Arthur Robinson. Sir George Newman, the first Chief Medical Officer to the Ministry of Health, enjoyed a good reputation, but he was recruited from local government and was committed to the slow, incremental build-up of services administered by Medical Officers of Health and staffed by whole-time, salaried public health doctors. Newman therefore represented precisely the trend in policy which Dawson sought to circumvent.

Notwithstanding its later reputation as a classic in medical planning, the Dawson Report was largely forgotten during the inter-war period. The Consultative Council was allowed to lapse, and in public affairs the influence of Dawson was drastically reduced. Despite Dawson's activism in the BMA, and his selection as President in 1932, its centenary year, there was no reference to the Dawson Report in *A General Medical Service for the Nation*, the planning document issued by the BMA in 1930 and in a revised form in 1938. The latter contained copious references to other official reports on the health services, including the report of the Scottish Consultative Council, which paralleled Dawson's own Council. Sir George Newman's *The Building of a Nation's Health* (1939), made only passing reference to Dawson and made no mention of his report, which contrasts with the lavish praise accorded to Morant. In retrospect Dawson blamed the Ministry of Health, and by implication Newman, for his difficulties. He castigated the Ministry for having 'cold-shouldered or opposed' suggestions like the ones emanating from his report, during 'many years of obscurantism' throughout the inter-war period.[21]

Notwithstanding his disappointment concerning the official reaction to his report, Dawson continued to lecture on the future development of the health services. Increasingly he became preoccupied with the evils of a state medical service, which he now identified with the threat posed by communism. He realized that unwittingly his advocacy of collectivism was playing into the hands of socialists and Bolsheviks. This prompted a radical qualification of his previous arguments. Collectivism in medicine was made conditional on protection of the traditional liberties of the medical profession and by implication the traditional values of capitalist society.

In an address to the Brussels Congress of the Royal Institute of Public Health in 1920, Dawson warned against the creation of a 'state medical service by instalments, almost by stealth', stressing the dangers consequent on the loss of free choice of doctor or sacrifice of the 'stimulating force of rivalry'.[22]

In 1922 he wrote more philosophically about the dangers of

state systems undermining the 'charmed inner circle' of the individual personality. Communism was dangerous because it replaced 'freedom and initiative' by the 'tyranny of uniformity'.[23]

In 1924 he spoke of the difficulty of reconciling organization with freedom and flexibility. It seemed that anything undertaken by the state would be accompanied by state regulation. He warned that the medical profession was highly susceptible to damage by such control. Accordingly he increasingly looked to the development of national health insurance for workers, hospital savings schemes, and provision of private insurance plans to provide comprehensiveness within the system. He became a Director of the Guardian Assurance Company, one of the major beneficiaries of the NHI scheme.[24]

Consistent with the promotive ethos of his report, Dawson became the figure-head of the campaign for national fitness. During the inter-war period Dawson's interventions on specific issues were often more productive than his involvement on the national scene. For instance he established a reputation for drawing the Royal College of Physicians into greater prominence in medical affairs.[25] As a firm advocate of imperial responsibility, he was active in the establishment of the British Post-Graduate Medical School.[26] However, not all of his encounters produced happy results. For instance his invitation to join the Medical Research Council in 1931 led to an ignominious controversy between clinician and bio-medical science interests.[27] This exercise in co-operation proved counter-productive, serving to worsen relations between the Royal College of Physicians and the Medical Research Council, and the dispute extended over a broad front, leading to a power struggle over the control of medical research and the direction of major charities engaged in medical research. Dawson's intervention over the Local Government Bill was also a failure. In the House of Lords he led the attempt to protect the interests of the voluntary hospitals by preventing the unrestricted development of a municipal hospital service. Clause 13, which became familiarly known as the Dawson clause, survived into the Local Government Act 1929, but in a watered-down form, merely requiring a degree of consultation over proposals for the extension of local government hospital services.[28] Dawson's pleas for co-operation largely fell on deaf ears. Co-ordination in any form took place in only isolated local circumstances. Failure to develop a co-ordinated health service of the kind envisaged in the Dawson Report contributed to a financial crisis within the voluntary hospitals, among the worst afflicted being the major teaching hospitals in London. These hospitals were increasingly threatened by the policy of expansion energetically followed by the

London County Council (LCC). At a meeting convened by the Ministry of Health to discuss this problem, Dawson made one of his characteristic calls for harmonization:

> What I care most about really, having worked in both sets of hospitals and being convinced that the hospital service is going to play an increasing part through larger strata of the community, and it is going to assert itself not only for curing of illness but for the creation of health, and I am one of those who believes that the two should not be separated in idea, nor should they be separated in education, they all ought to be brought together into one consolidated effort...and achieve the efficiency of a hospital service harmoniously working and economically carried through ... the time has come to end what has been a perfectly ridiculous thing to have in a great City like this, two sets of hospitals working side by side instead of co-operating together, for the common end.[29]

Considering the importance attached by Dawson to a central advisory body, it is surprizing that he was not more active in promoting this objective. He seems to have accepted passively the demise of the Consultative Council. He joined a successor Medical Advisory Committee in 1929, and this small, informal group met occasionally, but its remit was limited to technical issues. This committee was strengthened at the request of the Minister of Health in 1936, and Dawson was invited to take the lead, but this expanded advisory committee was as inconsequential as its predecessor. Although this committee stumbled on through the Second World War, it made no effective intervention on major policy questions.[30] Dawson's further involvement over the future of the health service took place through his status as an elder statesman directly representing the interests of the medical profession and the voluntary hospitals.

Between 1920 and 1940 Dawson experienced a complete role reversal. In 1920 in medical circles he was regarded as an agent of the central bureaucracy, and was accused of over-zealous response to the post-war fervour for reconstruction, thereby making too many concessions to the conception of a state medical service. This reputation for radicalism may well have prompted George V to query his elevation to the House of Lords.[31] The Dawson Report represented an attempt to balance collectivist and individualist interests. Thereafter he rapidly lost confidence in state collectivism, and deflected his energies into promotion of organized effort in medicine through 'collaboration', 'co-operation' and 'partnership' between existing agencies. By the time of the renewed fervour for reconstruction at the beginning of the Second World War Dawson's metamorphosis was complete. Now, as a veteran medical politician and spokesman for voluntary hospital and professional lobbies, he sought to obstruct any significant extension in state intervention, even if this entailed sacrificing some of the objectives which had been central to his thinking in 1918.

At the outset of the Second World War, now in his mid-70s, Dawson was swept back into prominence. Suddenly his Report was unearthed and his influence was invoked as an indispensable part of the propaganda campaign of the BMA and the medical establishment. On the one hand it was as necessary for the BMA and its allies to concede the inevitability of reorganization of the medical services. On the other hand it was imperative to mobilize these reforms for protecting the financial interests and ideological position of the profession. Dawson provided the philosophical underpinning for this exercise. He was trusted because he was more distrustful of collectivism than other leading figures of hospital medicine such as Buzzard, Cohen, Morant or Ryle. On account of his age and remoteness, he was more trustworthy than Horder or Webb-Johnson.

Dawson is credited with an influential role in the reconstruction initiatives of both the medical profession and the voluntary hospitals. He was involved with the BMA operation to set up the Medical Planning Commission (MPC) in May, 1940 to act as the forum for the profession as a whole. He also played a leading part in committees of the London voluntary hospitals concerned with preparations for the post-war situation, and he was a guiding hand in policy statements produced by the King's Fund.[32]

Dawson reiterated the line of defence for the voluntary hospitals that he had developed during the inter-war hospital crisis. Essentially repeating his intervention at the meeting with the LCC, he insisted:

> The voluntary and municipal hospitals, though both of them necessary for the needs of modern life, must maintain their individual life to develop along their own lines with complete freedom, but with an ever-increasing co-operation so that they may produce between them a united and ordered policy.[33]

The main difference in the post-war situation would be the greater element of public subsidy needed by the voluntary hospitals. In order to extricate these hospitals from increasing dependence on local authority subsidies Dawson proposed that payment for public services would be handled through a Central Hospitals Board. By this means voluntary hospitals might enjoy the benefit of extensive public subsidy, without risking the loss of their traditional independence.

Dawson's idea of a dual system was pursued by the voluntary hospitals, and it was nominally adhered to by the policy makers until the election of the Labour government in 1945. However, as early as 1941 officials in the Ministry of Health were convinced that the voluntary hospitals were approaching their demise, and their plans increasingly assumed that a unitary system involving public ownership of all hospitals was the only feasible option. Dawson completely misjudged the scale of the dangers confronting the voluntary hospitals. He frequently assured his audiences that these institutions of charity were sacrosanct parts of the national heritage. He believed that any politician daring to confront the voluntary hospitals would be indulging in an act of madness.[34] However, the greater folly lay in Dawson's failure to realize the strength of administrative and constitutional objections to the system he was advocating.

The case of the MPC demonstrated that it was not always easy for conservative voices within the profession to control events. Given its omnibus character, there was a real risk that the MPC would fail to replicate the voluntary hospitals' unanimity of opposition to state medicine. As a pre-emptive move, the surgeon Henry Souttar, the chairman of BMA Council, was proposed as chairman of MPC at the suggestion of Dawson, seconded by Webb-Johnson. Notwithstanding such careful preparations the draft interim report of the MPC produced in 1942 was regarded as a frighteningly radical document, too favourable to state (now 'socialized') medicine.[35] The interim report was the first major planning document since the Dawson Report to attach central importance to health centres, but there was no acknowledgement of Dawson, and the report as a whole was more inclined to consider the possibility of whole-time salaried service of general practitioners than Dawson was ever willing to contemplate. Dawson suffered the indignity of seeing his health centre idea appropriated without acknowledgement and for alien purposes.

Faced with this disharmony within the profession, Dawson unearthed his 20 - year - old arguments against state medicine, essentially unchanged. At the opening meeting he reminded the MPC of the work of his Consultative Council. He then urged them to accept the 'inevitability of gradualness', perhaps forgetting that critics had used precisely this argument against the Dawson Report.[36] The first problem to be addressed in Dawson's view was that of regional coordination. He argued that schemes for regionalization offered the soundest basis for action. Indeed he claimed that 'the movement of 1920–1 has been reborn and extended under the name of regionalization'.[37] The revival of regionalization was the work of the newly-established Nuffield Provincial Hospitals Trust, an organization with which Dawson was not involved. Dawson's own regional activities had been limited to his involvement with the King's Fund of London, with only inconsequential results, as underlined by the rapid development of regionalization under Nuffield auspices in the provinces in the months before the outbreak of War.

Dawson anticipated that the reorganization of health services would take place incrementally, and that the same incremental approach would be followed by the MPC, which he advised to divide into sub-committees, which would produce a series of specialized reports, beginning with hospital regionalization. This perhaps explains the paradox that his opening address to the MPC contained no reference to health centres. This subject was clearly regarded as a subsidiary topic for later consideration. This gradualist approach had not been adopted by his Consultative Council, and Dawson's advice was disregarded by the MPC.

Dawson's address 'Medicine and the Public Welfare' in May, 1942, was published one week before the interim report of the MPC. Dawson now found himself attempting to stem the tide of enthusiasm for health centres. He accepted that in principle a 'system of health centres was necessary as a system of schools'. However, they should not rush to develop medical services on the model of education. Doctors could not be treated like teachers. They must allow the system of medical practice to evolve slowly, building on existing traditions to form a system congenial 'to the habits of thought of our people'. He repeated customary warnings about the evils of state intervention. The new health service required 'collectivism for its fabric and individualism for human relationships. And individualism will not flourish easily within the rigid boundaries of a State service, but needs the freer atmosphere which belongs to the voluntary hospitals' tradition'. Dawson was altogether uncertain how to realize this objective in practice. His preferred option is somewhat surprising, given the circumstances of the time, but it was essentially consistent with his earlier views. He advocated a technocratic system in which authority was delegated to the medical profession. He freely admitted that this represented a novel conclusion, but one which would represent 'an advance of political science'. Dawson frankly admitted that his model was derived from totalitarian regimes. Such 'autocracies avail themselves of that knowledge with greater readiness because the dictator sets up the appropriate technical body and without delay adopts or refuses its advice, whereas democracies dilly-dally because so many departments that do not understand the technical problems must have a say'.[38] Perhaps more than any other speech, 'Medicine and the Public Welfare' demonstrates the basic inconsistency of Dawson's approach. He was willing to countenance rapid movement towards an integrated medical service when authority was vested in *ad hoc* health authorities under medical control, whereas the same goals became objectionable and only to be countenanced as a gradual, evolutionary process, subject to stringent limitations, when taken up by the agencies of democratically elected governments.

Dawson's mood of caution and suspicion towards central government and local authorities reflected the predominant mood within the BMA. He was therefore a natural choice for selection as President during the negotiations with the coalition government over the establishment of a national health service. Dawson had already served as President during the centenary year, 1932. The exceptional opportunity for a second term of office came about owing to the unexpected death of the gynaecologist, Sir Beckwith Whitehouse.

Whitehouse, who served as President in 1942, was an uncompromising defender of tradition. His presidential address had contained a sustained and vitriolic attack on socialized medicine, in the course of which he deferred to Dawson and recommended that the latter's 'Medicine and the Public Welfare' should be 'read and reread by all who have the conservation of the national health and the welfare of the medical profession in their keeping'.[39] Dawson was therefore the ideal choice of President to guide the BMA during one of the most sensitive periods in its history.

Dawson's involvement in the complex negotiations between the government and the medical profession was limited. His health was deteriorating. However, he continued to make public pronouncements, the most notable being his presidential address to the BMA, two interventions in the House of Lords, on the Beveridge Report and on the NHS White Paper. In circumspect and statesmanlike terms, Dawson warned that the government's proposals for immediate establishment of a universal and comprehensive service, involving whole-time salaried service for doctors, would destroy the finest traditions of British medicine and provoke a head-long confrontation with the medical profession. He insisted on gradualism. The proposed machinery of administration was not acceptable. Local government, which represented the 'unguarded control of uninstructed people', could not be entrusted with administration of the health service. Ideally he wished to see the health service administered by Health Councils dominated by the medical profession. As a compromise elected bodies might take their instructions from powerful medical advisory bodies. He was not satisfied that the new scheme gave sufficient guarantees for the survival of voluntary hospitals, warning that 'closing down of the voluntary hospitals would result in chaos'. Even health centres were not to be adopted before being subjected to a prolonged experimental trial. The idea of whole-time salaried service for doctors was described as 'sheer madness'. Dawson aroused the suspicion that even experiments with health centres were dangerous, because they were likely to become 'foci of infection', which would end in compulsory whole-time salaried service.[40] Thus Dawson drifted into condemning the institution of which he was the virtual founder. This retraction indicates the degree to which the figure who was acclaimed as an audacious reformer in 1920 had retreated from his earlier positions. It is therefore important that the conventional view that Dawson was an early architect of the NHS should be suitably modified to take into account his record during the Second World War as the leader of opposition to the government's reform proposals. This case history also suggests that serious qualifications must be applied to the prevalent notion that the period 1918–1945 marked the emergence of consensus about health policy.

## Notes

1. Francis Watson, *Dawson of Penn* (London: Chatto and Windus, 1950). It has not been possible to trace the majority of the Dawson manuscripts available to Watson. The family and relevant libraries hope that some light will emerge on the fate of these important documents. The present author thanks members of the family and the many librarians who have assisted in the search for Dawson's papers. See also obituary notices, *The Times*, 8 March, 1945, 7. *B.M.J.* (1945), i 389–92. *The Lancet* (1945), i 353–6. *Dictionary of National Biography* (by Lady Sybil Eccles, eldest daughter).
2. *Dawson of Penn*, vi
3. The worst error occurs in V. Navarro, *Class Struggle, The State and Medicine* (Oxford: Robertson, 1978), 18, where Dawson is designated as the first Minister of Health.
4. *The Lancet* (1945), i 353.
5. Sir W. G. Macpherson (ed.), *History of the Great War Medical Services. General History*, vol. 2 (London: HMSO, 1922). *Dawson of Penn*, 111–47.
6. Quoted from *Dawson of Penn*, 142.
7. *B.M.J.* (1918), ii 23–6, 56–9; *The Lancet* (1918), ii 51–2, 83–5, the latter being included in a special issue of 20 July, 1918, 'Future of the Medical Profession'. *The Nation's Welfare. The Future of the*

*Medical Profession ... with Introduction and a Folding Plan of a Model Health Centre* (London: Cassell, 1918).

8. For the SMSA, see F. Honigsbaum, *The Division in British Medicine* (London: Kogan Page, 1979), 54–5, 80–7, 106–7.
9. *The Nation's Welfare*, 13. See also *Dawson Report*, para. 3.
10. *The Nation's Welfare*, 3.
11. *The Nation's Welfare*, 22.
12. *The Nation's Welfare*, 13, 17.
13. I have suggested elsewhere that Dawson adopted the term health centre from Labour Party sources, C. Webster, 'Conflict and Consensus: Explaining the British National Health Service', *Twentieth Century British History*, i (1990), 115–51, 136–7.
14. Labour Party, Advisory Committee on Public Health, *The Organisation of the Preventive and Curative Medical Services* (London: Labour Party, 1919).
15. *Dawson of Penn*, 148–65.
16. Consultative Council on Medical and Allied Services, *Interim Report on the Future Provision of Medical and Allied Services*, Cmd. 693 (London: HMSO, 1920). (Hereafter *Dawson Report*). For a recent sound evaluation of the Dawson Report, F. K. Prochaska, *Philanthropy and the Hospitals of London. The King's Fund 1897–1990* (Oxford: Clarendon Press, 1992). See also Honigsbaum, *Division in British Medicine*, for full discussion of the medico-political situation.
17. *Dawson Report*, paras. 9–12.
18. Elsewhere I have suggested that Morant provided Dawson with the primary-secondary terminology, Webster, 'Conflict and Consensus', 122. See *The Nation's Health*, 16 for the status of the general practitioner.
19. *Dawson Report*, paras. 94–104.
20. Sir E. Forber, 'Regional Organisation of Hospital Service', 23 November, 1939, PRO, MH80/24. For an account of the demise of the Consultative Council and failure of subsequent advisory committees, 24 December, 1943, PRO, MH80/26.
21. Dawson, 'Medical Service and Social Change: Some Reflections and Convictions', *B.M.J.* (1943), ii 429–30, 2 October, 1943.
22. Dawson, 'Medicine and the State', *B.M.J.* (1920), i 739–43; *Medical Officer*, xxiii (1920), 223–4.
23. Dawson, 'An Address on Professional Secrecy', *The Lancet* (1922), i 619.
24. Dawson, 'Address to the London Insurance Institute', *The Times*, 18 November, 1924.
25. A. M. Cooke, *History of the Royal College of Physicians*, vol. 3 (Oxford: Oxford University Press, 1964), 1060–7.
26. G. Rivett, *The Development of the London Hospital System 1832–1982*

(London: King's Fund, 1986), 211–14.

27. J. Austoker, *A History of the Imperial Cancer Research Fund 1902–1986* (Oxford: Oxford University Press, 1988), 85, 150–1, 158, 171; J. Austoker & L. Bryder (eds), *Historical Perspectives on the Role of the MRC* (Oxford: Oxford University Press, 1989), 30–2, 193–6.
28. W. A. Robson, *The Development of Local Government* (London: Allen & Unwin, 1931), 317. Prochaska, *Philanthropy and the Hospitals*, 111–13.
29. Meeting of Voluntary hospital representatives, the LCC and Ministry of Health, 27 January, 1939, PRO, MH 79/513. Rivett, *London Hospital System*, 222–5.
30. See especially, PRO, MH 71/50. For Dawson's interventions on eugenics, see G. Jones, *Social Hygiene in Twentieth Century Britain* (London: Croom Helm, 1986), 56, 124.
31. Prochaska, *Philanthropy and the Hospitals*, 90.
32. Prochaska, 145–8. The relevant documents are: *National Health Service. Draft Statement of Principles* (April, 1944), *National Health Service. Statement of Principles* (July, 1944), and *Memorandum on the National Health Service* (July, 1944), PRO, MH77/100 and MH80/34. For a report on the views of Dawson and the King's Fund, 10 April, 1943, PRO, MH80/25.
33. Dawson, Address to King's Fund General Council, 1939, quoted from F. Long, *King Edward's Hospital Fund for London. The Story of its Foundation and Achievements, 1897–1942* (London: King's Fund, 1942), 87.
34. Dawson, 27 January, 1939 (see above n. 29) 'I have never heard anybody with a sense of responsibility express the desire to displace either of them. It would be sheer madness to make any attempt to do so.'
35. *Draft Interim Report of the Medical Planning Commission* (London: BMA, 1942), and *B.M.J.* (1942), i 743–54.
36. Dawson, 'Scope of the Commission', *B.M.J.* (1941), i 60.
37. Dawson, 'Medicine and the Public Welfare', *B.M.J.* (1942), i 573–5, 573.
38. *Ibid.*
39. Sir Beckwith Whitehouse, 'The British Tradition and the New Outlook', *B.M.J.* (1942), i 457–9, 458.
40. Dawson, 'Medical Service and Social Change: Some Reflections and Convictions', *B.M.J.* (1943), ii 429–30. *House of Lords Debates*, vol. 126, cols. 256–63, 25 February, 1943; vol. 131, cols. 101–10, 16 March, 1944. See also 'First Reflections on the White Paper', February, 1944, in *Dawson of Penn*, 327–36.

# 9

# Christopher Addison: a Realist in Pursuit of Dreams

*Frank Honigsbaum*

## Summary

Addison was the only politician present at the start and end of the legislative process that produced the National Health Service. Having established a national reputation as an anatomist at the age of 41, he abandoned medicine for politics, entering Parliament in 1910 as a Liberal, moving to Labour in 1923, accepting a peerage in 1937, and ending as Leader of the Lords from 1945–1951. His life in politics was as long as the one before it – 41 years – with all but 11 as a member of one House or the other. He served in three Cabinets, holding eight offices while in the lower House and four in the upper. Lacking debating skill or a charismatic personality, he owed his advancement to his industrious character and the regard with which he was held by two prime ministers, David Lloyd George and Clement Attlee. Though doubts were raised about his administrative ability, no one ever questioned his courage, diligence, perseverance or ability to adapt to whatever task he undertook. He pursued radical goals throughout his long life but always with regard to the realities of politics. His most important contribution, certainly in the field of public health, lay in the part he played in the creation of the panel system and the Ministry of Health.

## Introduction

Only one politician participated in the legislative process that produced the National Health Service when it started in 1911 and ended in 1948. His name was Christopher Addison and not only was he a doctor but he became Britain's first Minister of Health in 1919. Having established a national reputation as an anatomist at the age of 41, Addison entered Parliament as a Liberal in 1910 in time to help one Welshman, David Lloyd George, implement a National Insurance Act that offered GP care to the working population. Then, after having moved to the Labour Party in 1923 and been elevated to a peerage in 1937, he lived long enough to help another Welshman, Aneurin Bevan, expand that restricted insurance system into a comprehensive service that covered the nation as a whole. In the process, he displayed a combination of qualities rarely seen in British government. Not only did he make his mark as a courageous social reformer but he knew when that idealism had to be tempered by the realities of politics. Principle, purpose and pragmatism were the hallmarks of his life.

His sterling character was moulded by a rural heritage. Born in 1869 the son of a Lincolnshire tenant farmer, he learned the discipline of agricultural life. A capacity for long hours of hard work, common sense, a practical approach to problems, ability to withstand adversity and a simplicity of outlook with little regard for the superficial formalities of urban society were characteristics he never lost. He was and remained a no-nonsense countryman throughout his long life.

But his politics took a different direction. Though his father came from a rural Conservative background, Addison early displayed radical tendencies that held firm throughout his life. Nor did he become a farmer like his brothers; his parents gave him the benefit of a costly medical education which he did not take long to justify or repay. By the age of 30 he had become a professor of anatomy at Sheffield University and soon made his mark in medical history as the developer of 'Addison's plane', a major contribution to understanding the abdominal organs and the progress of surgery.

Still, medicine did not satisfy him. His thoughts turned more and more in a political direction and they were reinforced by marriage in 1902 to Isobel Mackinnon Gray, the daughter of a wealthy shipping owner who had also strayed from her Conservative roots to become a Christian socialist. Her politics, indeed, were more radical than her husband's and remained so throughout their long and happy marriage. It was her wealth that probably made Addison's political career possible for he entered Parliament one year before payment of MPs began.

## Role in National Insurance

Adopted in 1907 as the Liberal candidate for the Hoxton division of Shoreditch, Addison won both elections in 1910 and became a leading medical MP when Lloyd George introduced his National Insurance Bill in May, 1911. In his memoirs, Addison claims he did not meet Lloyd George until after the Bill was presented to

Parliament and thereby implies that he had no part in its preparation.[1] But Lloyd George once gave him credit for having been 'mainly responsible' or 'almost mainly responsible'[2] for the clause in the Bill which devoted funds to medical research and paved the way for the later emergence of the Medical Research Council. To the biographer of the renowned Canadian physician, Sir William Osler, actively involved in the promotion of medical research in Britain during the Edwardian era, there was no doubt: Addison *was* the instigator.[3] As early as March, 1910, Addison showed his concern for the subject by criticizing in Parliament the small sum spent on research into tropical disease.[4] Though he never claimed authorship of the Insurance clause, the biographers who have made the closest study of his life found it to be 'highly possible that he was the originator'.[5]

Addison also played a part in the admission of dividing societies to the Insurance Act long before the Bill was presented to Parliament. His constituency, Hoxton, was the home of the leader of the dividing societies, Percy Rockliff, who had close ties with the solicitor acting on behalf of the industrial assurance offices, Kingsley Wood. From 1908, Lloyd George had led the friendly societies to believe that only they would be admitted to the Act as approved societies but Rockliff, working in conjunction with Addison and Wood, planned otherwise. According to Rockliff's journal, as early as July, 1910, Lloyd George promised Addison and Rockliff that neither dividing nor deposit societies would be barred[6] and his claim is supported by *Hansard*, for in response to a Parliamentary question raised by Addison on 16 June, 1910, Lloyd George gave the same reply.[7]

In January, 1911, Rockliff told Lloyd George how dividing societies could be admitted by permitting them to form separate sections which met the tests set for approved societies, and this paved the way for the assurance offices to participate as well.[8] With Addison later taking action on behalf of the doctors, the stage was set for the demise of friendly society power and that may have contributed to his appointment in 1929 as a trustee of one of the leading offices in the assurance world, the Liverpool Victoria.[9]

All of this suggests that Addison may have played a greater part in the planning of the Bill than he dared to reveal. There is no doubt that the account in his memoirs of his first contact with Lloyd George is suspect. He claims this occurred after the Bill was introduced and that it was he who first warned Lloyd George of medical hostility to friendly society rule.[10] But Lloyd George did not need Addison to tell him; it was a point of recurrent publicity during the Edwardian era. Not only had the doctors raised a public clamour since the 'battle of the clubs' began in 1895 but Lloyd George had two medical friends in his North Wales constituency (Drs Robert Parry of Carnarvon and Emyr Owen Price of Bangor) who had long been active in British Medical Association (BMA) affairs and the fight against the friendly societies.[11] A month before the Bill was presented to Parliament, Lloyd George made his own feelings clear to the Cabinet, calling for the eventual removal of medical benefit from friendly society control.[12]

Once the Bill was presented to Parliament, Addison took the lead in sponsoring amendments designed to free the doctors from society rule and developing a panel system that would secure their support. But Lloyd George could not go as far as the profession desired; the friendly societies had too much influence for that. A medical revolt arose in 1912 and Addison devised the means to meet it – a mobile corps of 2,000 doctors willing to practise anywhere.[13] The panel system began in January, 1913, with more than enough practitioners willing to accept the terms the government offered.

**Partnership with Lloyd George**

Addison's role in the Insurance dispute is crucial for understanding his political life, for, without it, it was doubtful whether he would have attained ministerial office. He was not a good speaker, he did not perform well in Parliament until late in life; he was not good at backslapping, his pugilistic manner aroused hostility and, unlike Lloyd George, he had no taste for massaging the media. Sir Robert Morant, the civil servant who worked closely with him in developing health provision, once described Addison as 'a queer chaotically minded person with no belief in clear organization'.[14] From the way he performed in at least one office, this seems too harsh a judgement and no one can deny that Addison displayed an amazing facility to adapt to the variety of tasks he undertook. But Sir Percy Barter, his private secretary in three ministries, also found his administrative skill lacking[15] and Addison certainly did not have the personality or tactical skills needed for advancement.

What enabled him to rise was his relationship with Lloyd George. The Welshman had staked his political career on the Insurance Act for it aroused opposition not only from the doctors but from the public and even within the Cabinet itself.

There had been no popular demand for the Bill and its call for compulsory contributions stirred hostility from all sides of the political spectrum much as the poll tax did in 1990. If the doctors had managed to destroy the Act as they tried to do, Lloyd George's political career might have ended.

More than anyone, Addison saved him and thereafter Lloyd George did much to advance the doctor's career. In 1914 Addison became Parliamentary Secretary to the Board of Education and in the following year, when Lloyd George took charge of the new Ministry of Munitions, Addison went with him in the same capacity. Throughout this period, they worked closely together and there is no doubt that it was the happiest of Addison's life. With a shared belief in social reform, they were intent on adding to the welfare edifice erected by the pre-war Liberal government. As Addison so colourfully put it: 'We encourage each other to dream dreams but to base them on existing realities.'[16]

Addison hesitated before accepting the move to the Ministry of Munitions because he did not like the thought of having to exchange 'curing for killing'.[17] But thereafter he could take pride in his performance. Lloyd George had no liking for detail and let Addison organize production. Contrary to Morant's judgement, Addison at Munitions showed a keen sense of administration and not only vastly increased output but saved the country millions of pounds.

Lloyd George had further reason to prize his colleague for it was Addison who paved the way for the 'palace revolution' that put the Welshman in power in December, 1915, at the head of a coalition government. As early as May of that year, Addison drew up a list of Liberal backbenchers willing to support Lloyd George and thereafter worked tirelessly to make him Prime Minister in place of Herbert Asquith.

## Addison as Minister

Addison's reward was to become Minister of Munitions but the first sign of a deteriorating relationship came in May. Addison was confronted with a serious labour dispute which he managed to settle but, briefed by the Prime Minister's publicity officer, William Sutherland, the press gave Lloyd George the credit. Addison's reputation was badly damaged and, though the Welshman tried to make amends, in the months that followed he repeatedly sought to move Addison from Munitions, finally succeeding in July by giving him the chance, as Minister of Reconstruction, to plan the reforms they had dreamed before the war.

How well did Addison perform at Reconstruction? Many dismissed the post as an irrelevance, simply a way 'to build fairy castles for some dim and distant future'.[18] Addison was given only a small staff and Lloyd George, who was preoccupied with the War, did not provide the necessary support. But the American historian who has made a careful study of the department concluded that its pre-armistice planning was 'very extensive, courageous and far-sighted'[19]; only in its implementation did things go wrong and that was largely due to events beyond Addison's control.

One reform was realized – the creation of the Ministry of Health in 1919, bringing together under one department all, or nearly all, the health duties that had been scattered throughout Whitehall. With Addison himself as Minister, it was possible for the first time to give central direction to health policy though it took many years before major reforms were realized.

Nevertheless, the creation of the Department was no mean feat; it had been sought by reformers and the medical profession for years. Within the coalition government, Addison faced the same opposition from Conservative politicians who had resisted the Insurance Act in 1912 – Walter Long and William Hayes Fisher (later Lord Downham). They wished to leave the Poor Law and municipal health duties under the control of the crusty old department where they had long been lodged – the Local Government Board (LGB), then under the direction of Hayes Fisher.

Addison's own account of the struggle is woefully incomplete and suggests that he failed to understand the forces against him. Not until late in the day did he become aware of Long's machinations, seeing him first as a friend rather than a foe.[20] Even more serious, he lost touch with his main ally, the medical profession, and did not even contact its leader, Sir Bertrand (later Lord) Dawson, until Lloyd George suggested it.[21] His account also leaves out the legislative danger posed by Hayes Fisher who, in a desperate move to preserve the LGB, secured the passage in 1918 of what Morant described as a 'villainous maternity bill'.[22] As this incident suggests, it was Morant who recognized the tactics of their opponents and without his aid, it was doubtful whether Addison could have created a new department.

## Failure of Health Policy

In setting the health policy of the Ministry, Addison had the aid of two civil servants with whom he had worked closely – Morant, who became one of the two Permanent Secretaries, and Sir George Newman, who was appointed Chief Medical Officer. All three had long held the view that all publicly provided health services should be brought under local authority control and they regretted that the panel system, as well as Poor Law provision, had remained outside it.[23]

From the moment Addison entered Parliament in 1910, he had supported the move to bring Poor Law medical services under municipal control through the Minority Report prepared by Beatrice and Sidney Webb for the Royal Commission on the Poor Laws.[24] He had also shown a strong interest in the preventive services provided by the municipal world, introducing Bills for the feeding of infants and the hygiene education of schoolchildren.[25] Together with Newman, he was instrumental in committing the Government to the medical treatment of schoolchildren.[26] In 1914 Addison had gone so far as to declare that too high a value had been placed on treatment and he welcomed the way the excessive costs of the cash sickness benefits provided by the Insurance Act had stirred public concern for prevention.[27]

But Addison was still fully aware of the need to extend public provision for treatment beyond the limited range prevailing in 1919.[28] The panel system covered only insured persons, not their dependants, and it offered only GP care, not hospital or specialist services. Yet it provided the best hope for extension because it was acceptable to the profession as well as the public. Not only did it avoid the hated stigma of the Poor Law but it offered doctors a form of state employment free from their aversion to salaried payment. Though Addison, like Morant and Newman, would have preferred a salaried service under municipal direction, he knew there was no chance of securing medical acquiescence. The profession could only be weaned slowly in that direction.

Addison therefore set his sights on an extension of the panel system with the hope that it would supplant the Poor Law and be linked in some way with municipal provision. In the face of the high infant and maternal mortality rates then being revealed, the greatest need was to give dependants access to the GP care they had been denied before the War. Hospital treatment for the whole population could come later; extension, in Addison's view, had to start with community care.

How were these aims to be realized? The four consultative councils provided by the Ministry of Health Act offered the way. The one created for the doctors would set the ideal scheme towards which the Department should work and Addison hoped it would not only call for the extension of the panel system to dependants but accept some form of municipal administration. Then, the council formed for patients would bring pressure to bear for extended provision while the details of local unification were worked out by the council established for local authorities. Hopefully, all of this would prove acceptable to the council on which the approved societies (the bodies responsible for paying the cash benefits under the Insurance Act) were represented.

As it turned out, only the first part of this process progressed very far and it did not turn out the way the Department desired.[29] The medical council under Dawson's direction was too preoccupied with the threat of salary to make the recommendations Addison wanted. In place of the dependant coverage which they feared might add enough patients to the panel to justify a salaried service, the doctors wanted institutional provision to come first. The Dawson Report which they issued set forth an interlocking network of hospitals and health centres which, among other benefits, gave GPs as well as consultants access to beds. Nor did the doctors think this service should necessarily be free; all they declared was that it should be 'available'. They were even less helpful where local unification was concerned and it took a plea from Morant to persuade them to leave the question open.

Addison hoped the patient's council would have an offsetting effect and, indeed, it did prepare reports which called not only for maternity care but for a comprehensive service under municipal control that would cover the population as a whole, thereby uprooting Poor Law provision and anticipating the action which Aneurin Bevan took 26 years later. But the whole effort collapsed in the face of an economy campaign, led by defenders of the Poor Law and others opposed to any increase in public expenditure. The reports of the patients' council were never published and Addison failed, through the guise of a Miscellaneous Provisions Bill, even to put Poor Law infirmaries under municipal control. In the end all he could do was make minor changes in the panel system and these, by including provision for the periodic inspection of the medical records kept by panel doctors, exposed the Department to a vitriolic press campaign charging it with a violation of medical secrecy and a 'new inquisition'.[30]

## Conflicts within the Ministry of Health

Within the Department no one showed any enthusiasm for the Dawson Report. Morant died before it appeared but he knew what was coming and left no record of support. Newman, however, was swift to criticize the Report. As Chief Medical Officer, he felt threatened by the creation of a medical advisory council[31] and he not only called attention to the doctors' failure to consider the 'financial implications' of their programme but dismissed their Report as a 'somewhat disappointing document from the point of view of practical suggestion and official administration'.[32]

For this, however, Addison himself was responsible for he asked the medical council to produce only an ideal scheme.[33] If the document showed signs of hasty preparation, that also was Addison's fault for, fearful of the loss of the reform fever generated by the War, he had pressed Dawson to produce an interim report and no final one ever appeared.[34] The Minister was hopeful that the scheme would be accepted before the many doctors who had entered the armed forces returned home and settled back into practice.[35]

Newman had other reasons for disliking the Dawson Report; in particular, he showed no interest in its call for primary health centres that would provide hospital beds for GPs. Like his colleague in the BMA, Dr (later Sir) Henry Brackenbury, Newman saw the GP mainly as an instrument of social reform and wanted him to spend most of his time in or near the homes of patients, teaching them how to live healthier and saner lives.[36]

Addison no doubt shared this view but he was too pragmatic to let any opportunity for an extended service slip by. As late as March, 1921, only just before he left the Department, he was hopeful that at least 'common centres' would be built by local authorities 'even if Insurance companies were against it' (by which he meant the approved societies).[37] He also looked forward to the day – perhaps a decade away – when everyone would be covered by insurance and treatment would be free.

But Addison faced opposition not only from the Treasury but from his own Permanent Secretary, Sir Arthur Robinson, who had been appointed a year earlier following Morant's untimely death. Robinson did not share Morant's passion for health; he not only urged Addison to reject the reports of the patients' council but called for the disbandment of the body itself.[38] Now, when considering the proposal for 'common centres', he doubted whether it was desirable to encourage local authorities in a scheme which was not a business proposition.[39]

Addison left office before further action could be taken. No health centres on the Dawson model, not even a few experimental ones, were ever built.

### Housing and the Break with Lloyd George

Health, however, was not the issue that brought Addison down. He suffered a more serious defeat in the field of housing, a duty he inherited as a result of the absorption of the LGB within the Ministry of Health. Throughout the nineteenth century, public health had been seen mainly as an environmental matter, with attention centred on sewers and sanitation rather than personal care. It seemed natural then to have it attached to a department concerned with local government, housing and the Poor Law.

The doctors had long wanted a Ministry of Health confined to health issues alone and the approved societies – particularly the friendly societies who had striven throughout their history to provide protection against means tests – abhorred any connection with the Poor Law. But when the new Department was created, it was not possible for political reasons to absorb only the health side of the LGB. Nor was it desirable if the plan of a complete health service under local authority control was ever to be realized. Moreover, environmental duties were then inextricably interwoven with personal heath considerations – then much more than now. How, for example, could the problems of tuberculosis and infant and maternal mortality be separated from that of slum housing? Only later, as new drugs developed, did clinical medicine breed a life of its own.[40] Indeed, it was not until 1951 that housing and local government duties were removed from the Ministry of Health.[41]

In 1919, therefore, Addison had to deal with housing and great expectations had been aroused during the 'coupon' election which returned the coalition government to power. Lloyd George had made a 'land fit for heroes' the slogan of his campaign, holding out above all the promise of better housing for demobilized soldiers than they had enjoyed before the War. Hayes Fisher, as President of the LGB, had been responsible for making the plans and when Addison took charge prior to the department's absorption in the Ministry of Health, he was shocked to find that little had been done.[42] With fears of a social revolution stirring the Cabinet, he had to act quickly to fill the huge gap in housing, some 500,000 houses estimated as the number that was needed.

However, neither the Treasury nor Addison's Cabinet colleagues were willing to provide the funds or powers needed to meet this target. In their haste to return to a free market economy, they removed controls over prices and building materials as soon as the War ended, leaving Addison to cope with impossible conditions. Spurred by a severe labour and materials shortage, costs rose sharply and by the time Addison was removed from the Ministry in March, 1921, only 25,000 houses had been built and at twice the price expected in 1918.[43]

When Addison first took charge of housing affairs, Lloyd George had been quick to support him. In March, 1919, he warned the Cabinet of the need to implement the promised reforms in the face of the Bolshevik danger: 'Even if it cost a hundred million pounds, what was that compared to the stability of the state.'[44] But as the threat of revolution receded with the collapse of trade union power and the onset of the long depression in 1921, the Prime Minister found he could no longer keep his Conservative colleagues at bay. An anti-waste campaign, launched by the Northcliffe and Rothermere press, began with the aim of unseating him and making Addison the target of attack. Lloyd George, who as early as 1918 seemed more concerned to placate his enemies than to defend his friends, turned on the staunchest ally he had. Addison was made a Minister without Portfolio in March, 1921, and then forced to resign in July after a brutal blow in Parliament delivered by the Prime Minister he had worked so hard to put in power.

In doing so, Lloyd George won only a temporary reprieve; 15 months later, he himself was toppled, destined never to hold office again. Why did the Welshman betray his best friend? He apparently thought Addison had mismanaged housing and there may have been cause for this belief. As noted earlier, even the civil servants closest to Addison thought he was a poor administrator and he lost the most valuable members of his staff in 1920. Morant died in March and Sir John Anderson, the other permanent secretary at the Ministry of Health, was moved to the Board of Inland Revenue. Addison, who had appointed Anderson only as the result of Morant's persistent urging,[45] did not carefully select replacements. There were able juniors on the Ministry's staff but instead of seeking their promotion, Addison accepted the services of Sir Arthur Robinson, a civil servant in the more traditional mould.[46] Morant certainly would not have let Addison make the mistake of uniting the opposition by combining health and housing in a single Miscellaneous Provisions Bill which the Lords threw out in December, 1920. To give local authorities power to build general hospitals, Morant had suggested only a short enabling measure.[47] Addison thus not only failed to secure relief on housing but lost hope of reforming the Poor Law. Eight years had to pass before health care was removed from board of guardian control and placed in the hands of local authorities.

Nevertheless, whatever his weaknesses, they were not the main reason for failure. Addison was overwhelmed by economic conditions and political forces that no minister could have resisted. If it did nothing else, his 1919 Housing Act at least established housing as a social service.[48] There was no cause for Lloyd George to have treated him as brutally as he did. Addison had a genius for making friends of political opponents and Lord Carson, an Ulsterite who resisted Addison's attempts to promote Home Rule for Ireland, rose strongly to his defence.

Addison never fully recovered from the blow Lloyd George delivered; two decades later he still agonized over it. For 12 years he had worked closely with the Welshman and enjoyed access to the summits of power. Though his political life was far from over, he never again felt the exhilaration of those early years. The tie with Lloyd George meant so much to him that after a decade of hostile exchanges, he was ready to restore relations in the 1930s.

**Addison joins Labour**

This also marked a watershed in Addison's political career. Freed from the need to compromise with coalition Conservatives, he gave full bent to his radical views, moving left as he aged rather than right in the customary fashion. Though he fought and lost the 1922 election as an Independent Liberal, he stood for Labour in 1924, losing to Sir William Bull in Hammersmith. There was much irony in this contest since Bull, perhaps unknown to Addison, financed the medical revolt against the Insurance Act in 1912 and was closely linked with Long and Hayes Fisher throughout the struggle for a Ministry of Health.[49]

No sooner was that election over than Addison moved even further left, joining the Independent Labour Party and publishing in 1926 two volumes for the Labour Party on 'Practical Socialism'. This drew on his experience at the Ministry of Munitions and was intended to show how state control of production in war could be applied to a peacetime economy.

Surprisingly, health care was no longer his main concern; though he supported the Socialist Medical Association when it was formed in the 1930s, he took no part in the many efforts made between the wars to extend the panel system or municipal service. Instead, returning to his rural roots, he concentrated on agriculture. This was a wise choice since, aside from Noel Buxton, the Labour Party had few farming experts while it had many who specialised in health and social services.

Following his victory at Swindon in the 1929 election, Addison was appointed to the Ministry of Agriculture, first as Parliamentary Secretary, then as Minister in 1930 when Buxton, who had held the post, became a peer. Though Addison's stay in office was cut short by the economic crisis of 1931, he did manage to establish the principle of marketing boards for basic foodstuffs, thereby saving farmers from destructive price competition during the depression. The policy was so badly needed that it was followed by the Conservative, Walter Elliot, when he took over the department under the National Government in 1932. Elliot, himself a doctor and destined to become the only other medical Minister of Health between the wars, had supported Addison's health and housing reforms in the post-war years, retaining so much respect for his predecessor that he made use of Addison's expertise during his stay at Agriculture. No matter what duty he undertook Addison tried to rise above party politics and nowhere did he succeed more than in farming affairs.

However, once Addison joined the Labour Party, he held fast to socialist principles. He had no interest in following the Labour Prime Minister, Ramsay Macdonald, when he formed a National Government in alliance with Conservative and Liberals in 1931. Indeed, Addison was the only middle class member of the Cabinet who voted against the 10 per cent cut in unemployment benefit that destroyed the Labour Government. His wife, radical as ever, wrote to *The Times* denouncing Macdonald and Philip Snowden, Chancellor of the Exchequer, for having ignored socialism during their two years in office.

**Addison in the House of Lords**

Addison lost the 1931 election and returned to the Commons for only one more year following a by-election victory in October, 1934. When he failed to repeat the performance in the general election of 1935, he found it hard to face the fact that at the age of 66, he was not likely to win again. But his political career was far from over. Clement Attlee, with whom Addison had established close ties, became leader of the Labour Party in 1935 and persuaded Addison to accept a peerage to defend Labour interests in the House of Lords. Addison relented only after much soul-searching since he had campaigned for abolition of the upper house in 1910. Had his first wife not died in 1934, his resistance might have stiffened but he was duly appointed in July, 1937, and four months later, took as his second wife, Dorothy Low, daughter of a Conservative party agent. Addison's cross-party ties now extended to family affairs; both his sons, Christopher (who died in 1976) and Michael, took the Tory whip when they inherited their father's peerage.

When Churchill formed his coalition government in 1940, he did not offer Addison a place despite the long record of relations between them. Churchill had not been happy with what he found when he succeeded Addison at the Ministry of Munitions in 1917 and may have had no faith in the doctor's administrative ability. But the more likely reason lay in the ambivalent stand Addison took on foreign policy during the 1930s. With Churchill he attacked appeasement in 1937, but he also displayed pacifist tendencies somewhat like those shown by Lloyd George. Indeed, in the summer of 1939, Addison was cited as one of several public figures who might arrange talks between Hitler and the British government.

Addison's failure to impress Churchill did not prevent him from playing an active role in the House of Lords, raising the stature of the body and showing the same facility for cross-party ties as he had displayed in the First World War. When Labour came to power in 1945, he was the natural choice for Leader of the Lords, holding office also as Dominions Secretary until 1947 when he succeeded Arthur Greenwood as Lord Privy Seal. By now 76 years old, Addison not only had a seat in his third Cabinet but had the ear of the Prime Minister, his good friend Clement Attlee. With Addison's Buckinghamshire home close to the Prime Minister's retreat at Chequers, they met frequently at weekends. In this way, Addison established a relationship not unlike the one he had with Lloyd George 30 years earlier.

As Leader of the Lords and a member of many Cabinet committees Addison's influence extended across a broad front, but he took great satisfaction in piloting Aneurin Bevan's National Health Service Bill through the upper House. Though he seems to have played no part in planning the programme, he supported Bevan's controversial decision to nationalize the hospitals and made sure the leader of the Commons, Herbert Morrison, who strongly opposed the move, did not sabotage it in the timing of legislation.[50] For Addison, Bevan's Bill was the realization of the dream he had only dimly perceived in 1920.

Nor was his contribution to medical science forgotten: in 1948 Addison became Chairman of the Medical Research Council he created in 1919. Two years later, when Labour returned to power with a majority reduced from 100 to 6, he retained his dual position in the Lords and served on the Cabinet committee created in 1950 to review Health Service administration. When Bevan threatened to resign over denture and spectacle charges in April, 1951, Addison, pragmatic as ever, implored him not to do so, stressing the precedent that had been set with the proposed charge for prescriptions. But Bevan refused to listen. The following year, Addison's long political career came to an end with the Conservative victory in the October election, but by then, he had only two months to live, dying at the age of 82 in December.

## A Retrospective View

Addison was nothing if not a survivor in British politics. He entered Parliament in 1910 and left it for only six years in the 1920s and five years in the 1930s, serving in one House or the other until his death in 1951. Among his achievements, four stand out: his aid in starting National Health Insurance, the enormous increase in production he achieved at the Ministry of Munitions, the creation of the Ministry of Health, and the establishment of marketing boards for foodstuffs. Though he held no office at the time, the first was probably his greatest contribution, since the start of the panel system in 1913 set Britain firmly on the road to wider public provision. It took Lloyd George's charm and negotiating skill to push the Insurance Bill through Parliament but the Welshman might not have won the doctors over without Addison's assistance.

## References

A complete record of Addison's life was published by Kenneth and Jane Morgan in 1980, superseding the less adequate biography by R. J. Minney in 1958. These works, together with Addison's own accounts of his political life until 1919, were the main sources for the material in this paper. References for these books are as follows:

Kenneth and Jane Morgan, *Portrait of a Progressive, the Political Career of Christopher, Viscount Addison* (Oxford: Clarendon Press, 1980).

R. J. Minney, *Viscount Addison: Leader of the Lords* (London, Odhams, 1958).

Christopher Addison, *Politics from Within 1911–1918*, 2 vols. (London: Herbert Jenkins, 1924).

Christopher Addison, *Four and a half years, a personal diary from June 1914 to January* 1919, 2 vols. (London: Hutchinson, 1934).

Page references to these books have been included in the numbered notes below wherever specific citation was needed. Addison's private papers, also cited in the notes below, are held in the Bodleian Library, University of Oxford. Newman's papers are held in the Hereford County Record Office.

## Notes

1. Addison, *Politics from Within*, vol. 1, 20.
2. Lloyd George made this revelation at a dinner honouring Addison in February, 1914. Reports appeared in the national press on 7 February and in the medical press later. The reports in *The Times* and *The Lancet* (18 February, 483) contain the words 'mainly

responsible' while those in the *Morning Post* and the *Daily Telegraph,* among others, added the qualification 'almost mainly responsible'.

3. Harvey Cushing, *The Life of Sir William Osler* (London: Oxford University Press, 1940) 1151, note 1.
4. *House of Commons Debates,* vol. 14, cols. 1051–2, 3 March, 1910
5. Morgan, *Portrait of a Progressive,* 24.
6. *Thrift,* June, 1911, 10, 13.
7. House of Commons Debates, vol. 17, cols. 1469–70, 16 June, 1910.
8. In his history of negotiations over the Insurance Bill, Bentley Gilbert did not attach any importance to Rockliff's role but the assurance industry certainly did. For Gilbert's dismissive remarks, see his *The Evolution of National Insurance in Great Britain* (London: Michael Joseph, 1966) footnote on p. 378. For the assurance industry tribute to Rockliff, see *Insurance Mail,* 4 November, 1911, 692–3.
9. *Liverpool-Victoria Review,* December, 1951, 74. See also Addison's introduction to the publication honouring the Society's 100th anniversary, *Centenary Celebration, 1843–1943* (London: Liverpool Victoria, 1943).
10. Addison, *Politics from Within,* 1, 20.
11. For a profile of Parry, see the obituary notices in the *North Wales Observer,* 14 October, 1926, and the *B.M.J.* (1926), 2, 812. For a profile of Price, see the obituary notices in the *North Wales Chronicle,* 14 February, 1919, and the *B.M.J.* (1919), 1, 234.
12. Sir Henry N. Bunbury (ed.), *Lloyd George's Ambulance Wagon, being the memoirs of William J. Braithwaite 1911–1912* (London: Methuen, 1957) 141–2.
13. Minney, Viscount, *Addison,* 130. Lloyd George paid tribute to Addison for this aid at a conference celebrating the 25th anniversary of National Health Insurance. *National Insurance Gazette,* 1933, 337–8.
14. Paul Barton Johnson, *Land Fit for Heroes, the Planning of British Reconstruction 1916–1919,* (Chicago and London, University of Chicago Press, 1968) 354.
15. Johnson, *Land Fit for Heroes,* 70.
16. Addison, *Four and a Half Years,* vol. 1, 22.
17. Addison, *Four and a Half Years,* 1, 416.
18. Addison, *Four and a Half Years,* 1, 416.
19. Johnson, *Land Fit for Heroes,* 505.
20. Addison, *Four and a Half Years,* vol. 2, 435, 553.
21. Addison, *Four and a Half Years,* 2, 563.
22. Frank Honigsbaum, *The Struggle for the Ministry of Health 1914–1919,* Occasional Papers on Social Administration no. 37

(London: G. Bell & Sons, 1970), 43.
23. Honigsbaum, *Struggle for Ministry of Health,* 16–19.
24. *House of Commons Debates,* vol. 14, col. 434, 24 Feb,. (1910). See also *B.M.J.* (1910), 2, 158; (1910), 2, Supp., 244–5.
25. *B.M.J.* (1910), 2, 2034; (1911), 1, 958–9; 1912, 1, Supp., 547–51.
26. *Daily News,* 8 Feb., 1912; *Daily Telegraph,* 7 Feb., 1914; *B.M.J.* (1914), 1, 379–82.
27. *B.M.J.* (1914), 1, 379–82.
28. *B.M.J.* 1, 729–80; 1914,1, Supp., 191–2. Addison Papers, box 12, letter from Addison to Lloyd George, 10 April, 1914.
29. For the failure of Addison's reform plans, see Frank Honigsbaum, *The Division in British Medicine, a history of the separation of general practice from hospital care, 1911–1968,* (London, Kogan Page, 1979) 73–8.
30. Honigsbaum, *Division in British Medicine,* 93–9.
31. Honigsbaum, *Division in British Medicine,* 62–3. At one point Newman even felt threatened by his close colleague, Morant, who, he feared, wanted to head the medical as well as the lay administrative side of the Department. Morant showed great concern for Newman's feelings by telling Addison he was ready to leave the Ministry if it would help. 'As you remember, I always said I was willing if you wished it to see him on top and for me to vanish.' Newman papers, folder with notes for autobiography, entry for 3 and 4 July, 1919. Addison Papers, box 53, folder 505, letter from Morant to Addison, 28 August, 1919.
32. Honigsbaum, *Division in British Medicine,* 100.
33. Honigsbaum, *Division in British Medicine,* 64.
34. Honigsbaum, *Division in British Medicine,* 93.
35. *The Times,* 26 May, 1919.
36. Honigsbaum, *Division in British Medicine,* 122.
37. Addison Papers, box 73, folder 42, Poor Law Reform, third conference, 2 March, 1921.
38. Honigsbaum, *Division in British Medicine,* 77
39. Addison Papers, box 73, folder 42, Poor Law Reform, third conference, 2 March, 1921
40. Honigsbaum, *Struggle for Ministry of Health,* 26.
41. Hugh Dalton, *High Tide and After, Memoirs 1945–1960* (London: Frederick Muller, 1962) 349–56.
42. Addison Papers, box 12, letter with memorandum from Addison to Prime Minister, 8 July, 1919.
43. Mark Swenarton, *Homes Fit for Heroes, the Politics and Architecture of Early State Housing in Britain,* (London: Heinemann, 1981), 122.
44. Johnson, *Land Fit for Heroes,* 345–6, 370–1.

45. Johnson, *Land Fit for Heroes*, 354.
46. Addison Papers, box 53, folder 543, bundle of letters dealing with Addison's offer of First Secretary to Robinson, 9 April, 1920. See also the leader in *Local Government Chronicle*, 9 April, 1921.
47. Addison Papers, box 73, folder titled *The Hospital Problem*, introduction with minute by L. G. Brock to Minister, 26 March, 1920.
48. A. J. P.Taylor, *English History 1914–1945* (Oxford: Clarendon Press, 1965), 147–8.
49. Honigsbaum, *Struggle for Ministry of Health*, 42–3.
50. Frank Honigsbaum, *Health, Happiness and Security, the Creation of the National Health Service* (London: Routledge, 1989), 177–8.

# 10

## John Ryle: Doctor of Revolution?

*Dorothy Porter*

### Introduction

John Alfred Ryle was a man who found a mission. As Regius Professor of Physic at Cambridge University between 1935 and 42, he expressed serious doubts about current trends in modern medicine. He believed that modern medicine had greatly benefited from technical advances but had become less surely attuned to human needs. Major social changes had taken place which had brought about an epidemiologic transition. But he claimed 'We are still, as a profession, thinking more about curing than preventing, more about medical care and its huge costs than about the economies which could be effected by attacking the basic causes of disease.'[1] Ryle's answer to the clinical dilemmas of the twentieth century was to re-create medicine as a humanistic science, governed by what he called 'social conscience as well as scientific intent'.[2] He devoted the last decade of his career, and indeed his life, to fulfilling this aim. But it was a goal which linked an epistemological revolution in medicine to broader changes in society as a whole.

My aim in this essay is to locate Ryle's beliefs about changing both clinical and preventive medicine within debates about science and society in the twentieth century. Let me begin with some essential background to this study. In 1971 the historian Paul Forman put forward his now famous, provocative thesis that a culture of anti-causality in physics in Weimar Germany was produced by a surge of anti-rationalist ideology in national consciousness.[3] Defeated after the First World War Germany sought cultural solace in a neo-Romanticization of the past. The *Lebensphilosophie* of the pre-war literary, artistic and musical expressionism became transformed by the defeat of war and the German and Russian revolutions into a dominant cultural force. Insecure in the present Germany looked to the glory of the

Romanticism of Goethe and Schiller and rejected the utilitarian values of its victors. Symbolic of this milieu was Oswald Spengler's book *The Decline of the West* in which causality, conceptual analysis and physics were equated and held accountable for the destructive force of Western materialism. Mechanistic causality, the science of Newton and the epistemology of Descartes, was spurned in favour of a new intuitist and holistic model of knowledge and human thought. The rejection of Anglo-French positivism in favour of holism was expressed in neo-vitalist biology, Gestalt psychology, Weyl's famous intuitist attack on mathematics and in the phenomenology of Husserl. It also, according to Forman, nurtured the internal critique within German physics which produced the search to embrace an acausal quantum mechanics.[4]

The most provocative feature of Forman's thesis was his sociological analysis of the historical force of broad cultural values upon the internal development of scientific knowledge. He stimulated a powerful debate within the history of science which has yet to be resolved.[5] Other historians of science have pursued many of the issues which Forman problematized. Most recently, for example, Anne Harrington has explored the relationship between anti-mechanistic epistemology in the development of holistic neurobiology in Germany in the 1920s and 1930s.[6] The central question that Forman raised, however, was the spectre of anti-science within the scientific community itself. In examining the career of John Ryle in the development of social medicine I wish to discuss the rise of an anti-scientific philosophy within medicine.

A number of themes explored by Forman are directly relevant to the study of social medicine in Britain. Holistic philosophy was central to social medicine along with the political role of science in the construction of society. But Forman's crucial theme was the critique of scientific epistemology by elite scientists. In analyzing the rise of social medicine I wish to explore why a critique of scientific, technologically advanced medicine should occur from within the highest echelons of the British academic medical profession itself. Why should an elite medical intellectual like John Ryle turn against the bioscientific model of medicine? And why should he look to social science for the salvation of what he believed was the true Hippocratic spirit of the medical art?

Ryle believed a renaissance in medicine could be achieved by clinicians forming 'new partnerships in our science and practice'.[7] Like a number of his academic contemporaries the partnership he had in mind was what one of his colleagues, the biometrician and geneticist Francis Crew, described as 'the almost virgin territory which lay between the provinces of the medical and social sciences'.[8] From 1943, Crew, Ryle and a small group of leading British medical academics, attempted to pursue this partnership by creating a new medical discipline called social medicine.

Ryle and Crew thought that social science would provide an heuristic device for making a critical assault upon the dominance of the biomedical model of disease, sickness and health. In this way they were not the first, in Britain, either to question the role of biomedical science in the clinical art or to turn to the social sciences for a critical theory. David Armstrong, for example, has cited the expansion of the dispensary in the early twentieth century. Armstrong suggests that Robert Philip initiated a primitive form of health survey with his famous 'walk-past' dispensary inspections of healthy and sick children in search of undiagnosed tuberculosis.[9]

But Ryle perceived a political role for social science in medicine. He made a connection between changing medicine through social science and changing social values through scientific humanism as a political force. Did this make Ryle a revolutionary? I shall explore this question through a discussion of Ryle's politics of epistemology and how it was linked to the politics of scientific humanism as a new secular ethic for governing a rational society. Then I wish to locate this within the politics of science and society which characterized Ryle's intellectual epoch. How did Ryle, and his politics of epistemology, science and society, fit in to what Gary Werskey once called the *Visible College* of mid-twentieth-century socialist scientists?[10] And what are the implications of this story for the politics of scientific epistemology in this era in Europe?

## Epistemological Revolution

Elsewhere I have discussed the personal and professional biography of Ryle and the career path which led him to the first chair of social medicine in Britain.[11] Here I wish to concentrate on Ryle's critique of experimental science in medicine and his vision of an alliance with the social sciences.

From the early 1930s Ryle deplored the increasing influence of experimental over observational methods in modern medicine.[12] The laboratory, he claimed, had narrowed the study of the aetiology of disease.[13] According to Ryle the true Hippocratic function of the physician was to observe the entire biology of disease which included the analysis of its soil as much as its seed. This involved the holistic study of the 'conflict between man (or animal) and the noxious agencies in his environment'.[14] The physician should be a naturalist of disease and, like an ornithologist, observe the entire ecology of his species.[15] According to Ryle, the physician should study the diathetical tendencies in the constitution of each individual; his/her age; physical and social environment; psychological history; and exposure to various pathogens. Equally Ryle stressed that a holistic ecology understood the experience of disease from the patient's point of view[16] as much as that of the experimental pathologist, biochemist, physiologist, or neurologist etc. A duodenal ulcer was not simply a circular lesion situated just distally to the pyloric sphincter destroying one or more coats of the intestinal wall. It was also a type of severe hunger pain experienced periodically, occurring more frequently in men than in women, which has a tendency naturally to heal but will be perpetuated by stress. According to Ryle the experimental model of clinical science pursued detailed knowledge of the particular at the expense of 'universality' concentrating on atoms and neglecting 'wholes'. Regrettably, Ryle claimed, this had eliminated the 'sick man' from the clinical view.[17]

By the late 1930s Ryle's mission was to capture the medical curriculum and restructure the methodological and epistemological basis of medicine. Ryle claimed that the new dilemmas facing clinical medicine in the mid-twentieth century necessitated such major reforms. The demographic and epidemiological changes which had taken place in western societies produced an increasingly large proportion of the elderly suffering from chronic disease. Ryle thought that reliance on the laboratory had proved disastrous for tackling chronic illness. The unilinear logic of the experimental bio-medical sciences had eliminated a broader, environmental approach to explaining causation.[18]

By the early 1940s Ryle's holistic approach to aetiology ultimately led him out of the clinical ward into society itself. Amid the human ecology of disease, Ryle increasingly identified the most salient factors to be social and economic.[19] Coronary disease and duodenal ulcer were diseases of affluence, he asserted, just as surely as tuberculosis and rheumatic heart diseases were diseases of poverty. They were due to 'a complexity of causes which vary with time and place and social change and which can, by appropriate methods be unravelled'.[20]

By the time Ryle arrived at Oxford he identified the 'appropriate method' to be the science of social pathology.[21] His conception of it had something in common with the first science of social pathology outlined by the late-nineteenth-century social hygienist, Alfred Grotjahn.[22] Ryle differed from Grotjahn, however, in emphasizing the relationship between medicine and social science. 'Much that is truly aetiology', he emphasized, 'extends beyond the relatively confined province of pathology and invades the broader territory of social science'.[23] The science of social pathology would shift the boundaries of aetiology out of the laboratory of the microscope into the laboratory of the 'living community'; out of the hands of the biochemist and under the eye of the social scientist.[24] The new methods of social pathology would examine the morbid processes at work amongst human groups and populations, in the same way as clinical pathology examined the morbid processes within the body of the individual. As the clinical pathologist used a scalpel to complete his post-mortem, so the social pathologist used the tools of statistics, sociology and epidemiology.[25]

The most important tool in the social post-mortem was the 'social survey'. The social survey had been the mainstay of British empirical social science in the work of Chadwick, Farr, Rowntree and Booth. Later Patrick Geddes had adopted the survey methods of Le Play in the development of what he called 'civics' to produce historical analyses of settlements and their social development.[26] Ryle depreciated purely descriptive surveys of 'down-town' populations and their family relations. He believed that the information contained in them would be better provided by a novelist.[27] He believed instead that sociomedical inquiry required rigorous biostatistical surveys of health conditions that could be completed only by multidisciplinary teams which included clinicians, medical social workers, statisticians and sociologists.[28] Ryle's precise conception of social science remains obscure. While he used the term sociology in articles from the 1930s he refers only to the contribution of social workers rather than 'sociologists' in the multidisciplinary team work of social pathology. Ryle did believe, however, that social science was a moral enterprise, in which theory-building was inherently linked to social improvement:[29]

> A social science differs from a natural science in that it has other motives besides the advancement of knowledge. Its objectives are also humanistic or utilitarian. Social hygieology and pathology seek not only to increase our understanding of human health and disease and their causes, but also to furnish indications for the improvement of the former and the prevention of the latter. An additional purpose of these sciences should be to balance the emotional with the rational components of a developing social conscience.

The model of science underlying social medicine rejected experimentalism and narrow specialization in favour of observation and multidisciplinary teamwork. It was an ecological field study rather than a laboratory science. Equally it included both the natural history of disease and the sociobiology of health. Thus, it focused not only upon on the issue of disease reduction but aimed instead at the construction of positive health, and human wholeness. Social medicine was a study of the relationship of heredity and environment on human biology and happiness. For Ryle the marriage of social science and medicine would turn medicine into a humanistic enterprise and allow it to participate in the political agenda of scientific humanism.

## The Sociology of Positive Health and the Science of Biological Betterment

Ryle described social medicine as a third epoch of prevention. The first was the sanitary era of public health in the mid-nineteenth century. The second began to attack chronic diseases such as tuberculosis and venereal disease. The time had now come, however, to identify the *social* causes of *health* and to construct it through sociomedical reforms.[30] As he stated in *Changing Disciplines* in 1948, the science of social pathology was inherently linked to the science of what he called 'hygiology' – the study of health in order to identify the normal and measure deviations from it.[31] Ryle's concept of health was grounded in the relationship between the individual organism and harmony with its environment. The term healthy, Ryle pointed out, came from the term 'hale', meaning whole. Healthiness was wholeness.[32]

In his classic study of the *Social Function of Science*, J. D. Bernal, the communist crystallographer whose career at Cambridge overlapped with Ryle's, has a section on health.[33] Bernal insists that the task of modern medicine should be the improvement of health rather than the treatment of disease, and for this reason medicine needed to become 'in all its branches a public service in which research and practice are developed side by side'. Bernal suggested that the best root to follow would be the study of sickness through the observation of health.[34] This was at the heart of Ryle's concept of social medicine. He referred to Bernal's book in his lecture notes.[35] Sickness could not be assessed socially, and pathology could not be determined clinically without an understanding of what constituted health.

According to Ryle health and disease knew no sharp boundary – there was no normal and abnormal there were only the extremes and the normal of the range of variability determined by environmental conditions.[36] The object of the science of health, Ryle argued, was to define the normal range of human biological variability and identify deviations accurately. The clinician confronted with the extremities of the range of natural variability had to be able to identify 'at what point is normality passed and should we account the organ, structure, or function as diseased?' Ryle claimed that only through the study of health was it possible to measure normality in order to derive an accurate practical discrimination between 'the healthy, the unhealthy, and the borderline'.[37]

Normal variability, Ryle contended, consisted both of temporal variation within one individual as he adapts to a changing environment and species variation, i.e. variation between man and man upon which 'communal equilibrium' and 'adaptability' depended. Without species variation there would be 'no maintenance of a stock by the emergence of types better fitted for survival in a changing and exacting world or submergence of those less fitted; no natural distribution of functions within the group; no slow adaptations to the environmental changes of climate, time and place, changing occupations and social systems. In brief, alike in the individual and the community, there could be no adaptability without variability'. Ryle considered that 'Physiological and biological constants are both unthinkable.'[38]

For Ryle, biological normality was the quantifiable range of physiological variability which resulted from adaptation necessary for survival in a given environment. Good adaptability was an expression of health but he emphasized that this should always be qualified in terms of particular environmental conditions. Thus, when talking about adaptability or fitness it was necessary always clarify as to 'fitness for what'. Successful physiological harmony with the conditions which pertain to life in an office would be inappropriate to meet the hazards of life of a paratrooper.[39] Study of variability would help to explain innate resistances and predispositions to disease – i.e. help deepen an understanding of diathesis.[40]

Within his biologically evolutionary concept of health Ryle believed that it was caused by the interrelations of ancestry and environment.[41] For example, nutritionally deficient mothers produced constitutionally weak babies. Nutritionally deficient children grew into adults who then produced weak babies. Thus heredity was inextricably linked to both physical and social-economic environmental conditions. For Ryle, the study of health was the social biology of the normal range of variability and adaptability of man in modern societies.[42] It investigated the processes underlying human biological evolution and was equally a science of human biological betterment.[43]

As a science of human biological betterment Ryle viewed the study of health to be linked to Francis Galton's original agenda of eugenics as 'the study of agencies under social control that may improve or impair the racial qualities of future generations either physically or mentally'.[44] Equally Ryle's science of health bore remarkable similarities to Julian Huxley's agenda for eugenics and society in the 1930s.[45] In 1936 Huxley who, like Ryle, was a fellow of the Eugenics Society, conceived of eugenism as a social science of human betterment through the biological improvement of man by environmental equalization and genetic progress.[46] Ryle's understanding of the relationship of the social environment to evolutionary development of human variability paralleled Huxley's conception.[47]

Ryle shared Huxley's view that knowledge was also control.[48] The physical sciences had taught man how to control nature.[49] The way to control health – and thereby the range of variability – was, Ryle believed, through the marriage of medicine, eugenics and sociology. As early as 1938, Ryle wanted a sort of new 'preventive medical research council' to be set up which would orchestrate medical, eugenic and sociological studies into the social reorganization necessary for health. Health must be studied but also *taught.* Ryle pointed out that the literal meaning of the word doctor was teacher – the medical profession must therefore become health instructors to individuals, society, and its leaders about race, in the sense of human race, betterment. In the clinical situation doctors had many opportunities for communicating eugenic advice to their patients. As health instructors to government, the medical profession must emphasize the environmental determinants of health on the one hand and on the other stress the importance of encouraging the creation of an optimum quality and quantity of population stock.[50]

Social medicine focused not only on disease reduction but was also aimed at the construction of positive health, and human wholeness. The study of the human ecology of health, required a marriage of medicine with the social sciences and team partnership. Social medicine was a study of the effect of heredity and environment on human biology and happiness. Its object was human social and biological evolutionary progress and thus it possessed an educational imperative for community action. Social medicine was educative and directional as much as it was investigative.

## From Epistemological to Political Revolution

How then should the science of health fulfil its function in the rational planning of human biological betterment? And how did

Ryle perceive this function to be part of the role of social medicine in the promotion of scientific humanism?

From his twenties Ryle believed passionately in science serving humanitarian principles. In 1917, when he was on active service in Belgium, he wrote to Miriam, his wife, that he planned to write an essay 'on science and the influence of War'.[51] The moral that he wanted to stress was that science had hitherto been applied to 'the processes of destruction and death' but that after the War 'the great revolution that peace must bring will be the prompt turning of all existing sciences into the opposite direction – of maintaining, preserving and encouraging life'. 'Here', he believed, 'medical science especially will have an opportunity of a great renaissance, and all its branches, whether as physiology or public health or any other sister study must find a new inspiration, and must become in the fullest sense *applied* sciences to the great science of humanity.'[52]

By the 1940s Ryle had become demonstrably political. He used his position on the Medical Planning Committees of both the government and the Royal College of Physicians to promote his proposals for the nationalization of medicine – a cause he had always believed in.[53] He despised the commercial principle of private practice and supported the salaried employment of physicians. After publishing his views in the *British Medical Journal* in 1942[54] he corresponded with an irate 'X' – but I believe it was Lord Horder whom Ryle described as an old friend – that the commercial stress of private practice meant that doctors 'have not the freedom to think properly, to get any post-graduate education, to get adequate rest or holiday to keep fit for their work, to examine their patients thoroughly, to see their patients as often as is sometimes necessary, because of the financial relationship'. 'Equally', Ryle argued, 'their patients too only have a limited freedom unless they are rich.' Sadly, he concluded, in medicine on a commercial basis 'The business idea has conflicted with the service idea.'[55] Ryle believed that 'social and individual medicine will find a better opportunity under a reorganized, co-operative and comprehensive medical and health service'.[56]

In his professional life he never made any secret of his political principles. 'My positions are well known', Ryle wrote to his wife when he accepted the Oxford Chair in November, 1942, 'and I don't intend to alter them.' Upon his wife's advice he had never joined a political party. 'It was *you* who advised me strongly not to join the Party' he reminded her on one occasion, 'and you have *often* made me cut bits from my papers and lectures.' But Ryle acknowledged the need for discretion: 'The same caution', he told

Miriam 'requires the department – if it is to achieve the best for the future – must do so by being a good department *and* by its *teaching and research* help to create the absolute necessity for reforms which we can simultaneously work for in many ways'. At Oxford he told Miriam, 'I want us to have as many contacts as possible with the young and the left.' Wilson Jameson had told Ryle that unlike Cambridge, 'there are far more socialists who want to get things done'. Ryle believed that Oxford would give them both a chance to 'work together with our science and our humanism'.[57]

He acknowledged that compulsory institution of health was incompatible with a democratic system. Although there were instances when he regretted this to be the case, 'Such is our respect for the liberty of the individual', he argued, 'and, I might add, our disrespect for the race – that we cannot yet control, by segregation or sterilization, the excessive fertility of village half-wits who perpetuate their kind with multiple illegitimate births. We cannot at present even do much towards encouraging the general fertility of the fit and discouraging the general fertility of the unfit.'[58] Ryle believed that before the Second World War the only successful planning model for health was the Soviet system as described by the Webbs, Henry Sigerist and Arthur Newsholme.[59] Although imperfect, Ryle believed that the USSR offered the greatest hope for the future. 'My own belief', he told his father-in-law in 1941 'is that the new civilization will come from there [USSR] too. The old world has had its day and its disorder must give place to planning and abolition of the profit motive, the gradual emergence of a classless society, and the elimination of superstitions and religious irrationality in favour of sanity and science. It is possible.'[60] But for Ryle party politics and policy-making were secondary to the real issue of changing social values through science.

For Ryle the 'social conscience and scientific intent' of social medicine would help to establish scientific humanism as a new secular ethic governing social, economic and political behaviour. Ryle was convinced that 'science without humanism may work with atoms but it will not work with men', [61] and he stressed that 'the ideas and tasks of social medicine may be justly regarded as essential contributions (perhaps the most essential and practical of any at present within our range) to the developing philosophy of scientific humanism.'[62]

In a book on the 'new humanism' called *Fears May Be Liars*, in 1941, Ryle agreed with Julian Huxley that history hitherto had been dominated by the physical sciences which had built the technologies of mass warfare but that the biological and social sciences would, between them, build the technologies for peace and social harmony.[63] Ryle shared Huxley's view of 'the new humanism', as the rational control of society and biology through the social and biological sciences which mirrored the rational control the natural-physical world by the physical sciences.[64]

Both Ryle and Huxley emphasized that scientific humanism entailed the sacrifice of egotism, selfishness and individualism for altruism and mutual aid. I cannot judge whether Ryle would have agreed with Huxley that Karl Marx was the 'John the Baptist' of social science[65] but Ryle was convinced that Peter Kropotkin was right in believing that evolutionary progress was based upon the psychological faculty of altruism and the sociological effects of mutual aid in nature.[66] For Ryle, as for Huxley, scientific humanism was a secular religion which replaced individual salvation with social salvation. It consisted of abandoning fantasies of other-worldly gains for the planning of evolutionary progress. Ryle's sympathy with Huxley's vision is especially revealed through the citation at the beginning of *Changing Disciplines* from *The Uniqueness of Man*: 'What are the aims before humanism? One phrase, to my mind, really contains them all: to have life and to have it more abundantly ... A humanism that is also scientific sees man endowed with infinite powers of control should he care to exercise them.'[67]

Ryle contended that as the study of the social biology of health part of the agenda of social medicine was 'the direction of legislation on behalf of national health and efficiency', and it placed the physician in a position where, as Ryle quoted Henry Sigerist having pointed out, the physician 'must assume leadership in the struggle for the improvement of conditions'.[68] This function, Ryle insisted, did not constitute either medical or any other form of politics. It was instead, the foundation upon which political decision-making could be based.

As the medical consultant of the EMS to the Ministry of Health Ryle's influence may have been substantial on NHS planning. His hopes for sustaining general medicine were realized in the subsequent structure of the NHS which secured a major role for general practitioners.[69] Ryle believed that 'social and individual medicine will find a better opportunity under a reorganized, co-operative and comprehensive medical and health service in which the uneconomic and often inequitable separations into 'voluntary and municipal', 'private and panel', and 'preventive and remedial' services will no longer obtain'.[70] He did not feel, however, that it was the job of social medicine to advocate these changes but it would provide the means for 'the people, as voting citizens, and their municipal or parliamentary representatives to know and act'.[71] Apart from academic departments of social medicine, Ryle believed that the pre-war health centres had done pioneering work in the field of health promotion and had integrated it into the practice of both preventive and remedial medicine. He was greatly disturbed by the absence of provision for their establishment under the new National Health Service in 1948.

For Ryle, however, the 'social conscience and scientific intent' of social medicine went beyond the arena of parliamentary politics. It placed the physician at the centre of the movement to establish scientific humanism as a new secular ethic governing social, economic and political behaviour. Even in the midst of war, Ryle retained an optimistic hope of the imminent advent of 'new and possible worlds' in which 'the profession and the sciences which have the most intimate concern with man himself' will provide a 'rational and humane enrichment'.[72] Designing an 'equality of opportunity for health' was one task of social medicine as scientific humanism. Assisting the establishment of a religion of rationalism in a new social order was another. Ryle envisaged medicine becoming a leading force in scientific humanism through the incorporation of social sciences.

## Medicine and Zeitgeist

To what extent did these philosophical and political battles within medicine reflect broader movements within the politics of science and social responsibility in mid-twentieth-century Britain? To what extent did the values expressed by Ryle identify him as an intellectual of his epoch? Although Forman's original analysis dealt with the rise of quantum mechanics, he pointed to similar relationships between neo-Romantic irrationalism and anti-positivism in the biological sciences. Anne Harrington has extended Forman's account into a study of holistic models of the brain in Germany in the 1920s.[74] Harrington argues that a reaction against the 'mechanistic' model of the brain and associationist psychology in Germany was a feature of the cultural response to military defeat and social insecurity. In the late-nineteenth-century German brain scientists embraced the Lockean theory of empirical knowledge acquired through sensation and the theory of associationist psychology. Filtered through the work of Hughlings Jackson, the mechanical brain appealed to positivists such as Ernst Weber, Gustav Fechner and Wilhelm Wundt.[75] Ultimately it led Carl

Wernicke to adopt a basically reflex loop model of a brain full of messages being passed up and down telegraph wires.[76]

By the 1920s, however, this highly successful model of the brain was perceived to be grounded in 'dust and facts' empiricism supported by a rigid, positivist epistemology. Neurobiologists and psychologists such as Kurt Goldstein, Constantin von Monakow and Jakob von Uexkull rejected positivist epistemology along with mechanistic modernity. The mechanistic philosophy, of Newton, Descartes and Darwin, underlay, they believed, the soullessness of automated society filled with atomistic automat. They looked for an alternative in biological vitalism and above all in the philosophy of holism. This found vivid expression in Gestalt psychology which posited that organisms were not merely collections of organs and that humans were not merely physics and physiology but possessed an essence or essential personality. The original Berlin school of Gestalt psychology was criticized by other holistic psychologists for not sufficiently grasping the irrationalist, intuitist spirit of the true Goethean Gestalt tradition. But at the Leipzig school of holistic psychology Felix Krueger, during the Hitler years, committed Gestalt to epistemological irrationalism, the primacy of immediate nonverbalized experience, and to grasping the ultimate psychological meaning of social events.[77]

In Britain the politics of epistemology was also linked to broader cultural politics by various scientists working in the biotheoretical sciences. Gary Werskey, for example, has described a *Visible College* of socialist scientists who believed that the time had come for science to fulfil its true destiny of controlling society in the way that it controlled nature.[78] Amidst this group science *was* socialism and the critique of epistemology was crucial.[79]

As in Harrington's story of German neurobiologists and psychologists, the question of holism versus mechanism was seminal. John Burdon Sanderson Haldane, the eminent mathematical biochemist, grounded his science and his Marxism in the philosophy of holism.[80] Indeed his father, John Scott Haldane had been one of the few remaining British thinkers still admired by the Germans for his philosophical neurobiology.[81] Holism ran just as deeply with J. B. S. Haldane and he expounded it in his scientific cosmology as much as in his Marxist politics.[82] Haldane's holism, however, did not involve the repudiation of Darwinism. Early in his career Haldane attempted a mathematicization of the Darwinian theory of natural selection. Later his work in population genetics was central in the formation of what Peter Bowler has analysed as the twentieth-century 'evolutionary synthesis', in which the work of Haldane's friend, Julian Huxley, was equally influential.[83]

The biology of Huxley and Haldane was not, however, reductionist and remained imbued with a vitalist aura.[84] They were both able to give vent to the metaphysics of Darwinism in their support for eugenics.[85] Haldane ultimately became one the most outspoken and damaging critics of eugenics but both his and Huxley's holistic synthetic biology contrasted sharply with the highly positivistic sociobiology of their contemporary socialist Lancelot Hogben.[86] All three, together with Francis Crew, were founding members of the Society for Experimental Biology in 1932 and shared an interest in the interface between social and biological organization.[87] Hogben was, like Haldane, a mathematical human geneticist as well as a biochemist. He was heavily criticized for his rigid positivism, however, by a contemporary socialist biologist Joseph Needham. Needham, also an associate of both Huxley and Haldane, accused Hogben of being a reductionist mechanical philosopher especially with regard to his theory of consciousness. Hogben pioneered support for behaviourist psychology in Britain and relentlessly preferred the concept of 'conditioned behavioural responses' to the concept of 'mind'.[88]

Hogben fiercely defended epistemological positivism and ferociously attacked theories such as eugenics which he believed was based on crass prejudice and irrational values. He thought that values could be divided into private bigotry and what he called 'publicist' objectivity. Publicism was the world of social knowledge where objective values were communicable, verifiable and consensual. Such was the nature of scientific values. Needham eventually recommended that Hogben's 'publicism' should ultimately replace dialectical materialism as the theory of knowledge supporting socialism.[89]

Hogben attacked 'holism' with equal ferocity. He believed that holism constituted a theistic idealism which had invaded science and he lambasted Arthur Eddington, Alfred North Whitehead and J. B. S. Haldane for adopting it.[90] He decried their infusion with the ideas of the South African philosopher of holism General Jan Smuts who had studied at Cambridge before the First World War and returned to South Africa eventually becoming the Prime Minister.[91] Hogben claimed that the holists attacked mechanistic and materialist epistemology because the latter did not provide supernatural sanction for privilege. He persisted with his fight against fashionable philosophical idealism because he believed it could flourish only 'among those with leisure enough to study when their privileges are not compromised by unrest'.[92] For Hogben only empirical science offered a universal emancipation from the constrictions of metaphysical religion and inegalitarian social or intellectual privilege.

While these radicals differed in their epistemological politics, divided into mechanists and holists, all were united in believing science to be the means to discovering universal truths. Equally they all looked to science for the rational governance of social organization. In this they were united with another radical, J. D. Bernal, who believed that science was in fact communism. While only some of the group became card-carrying communists they all believed that socialism meant the rational organization of society by scientific principles. And all believed that rational scientific thought could become the new ethic, or glue, which held society together.[93] Huxley expressed this as science replacing mysticism – such as medieval Christianity – as the belief system which fulfilled the religious impulse of society.[94] Bernal described it as the *Social Function of Science* and its historical destiny. All were waiting for science to bring in a new order, take its hour upon the stage of history and replace doctrinaire morality with rational ethics.[95]

John Ryle was clearly a participant in the radical debates between science and politics which reverberated throughout the pre-war European scientific community. Like the German holistic neurobiologists he attacked the rigidity of the positivist epistemology of experimental science. Ryle rejected the reductionism of the mechanical philosophy.[96] But, like Huxley and Haldane he remained wedded to Darwinism and was greatly influenced by the philosophy of Smuts. Smuts had written a book on *Holism and Evolution* in 1925.[97] In it he argued that although mechanism and holism appeared to be opposed they were in fact synthetically united in the process of evolution. Life, claimed Smuts, had been proved to be a structure or structure-like.[98] Mechanism was a primitive form of structure which was succeeded by a superior form of structure, holism. 'Mechanism ... is a phase, an earlier immature phase of Holism; just as life is an intermediate phase, and mind is a later phase ... Holism is a mediating concept; it is the reality which underlies all the phases. And in the self-fulfillment of Holism, one phase passes into another.' Smuts believed that all thought was 'structural' because it was 'relational', and 'Hence I have adopted the imagery of the structures, ever more complex structures embracing the same material as the earlier structures.' Furthermore he suggested that 'in its interpretation of the physical world thought has already adopted the imagery of structures. I have therefore represented Holism as structural at all its known phases, and have distinguished the phases as differences of, and advances in, structure.' [99] Smuts reconciled holism and mechanism within an evolutionary framework and concluded that Darwinism was the greatest expression of holism. 'From the holistic point of view ... the grandeur of the Darwinian vision ... stands out in even greater fullness.'[100] Smuts acknowledged that Darwinism had been 'tacitly considered a victory for the mechanical view'.[101] But, he suggested, if the principle of natural selection was considered to be subordinate to that of variation, then Darwinian theory was in reality an expression of ecological holism. Smuts' view of evolution appears to have been an odd mixture of Darwinism with Lamarckian theories of adaptation but it relies upon privileging the principle of variation as the motor force of development. Ultimately, Smuts claimed that his holistic interpretation 'brought us back to the great Darwinian vision of universal adaptation'.[102] He went on to suggest, 'Holism has done more; it has enabled us to realize the pervasive creative unity which makes all the diverse elements of existence the co-operative members and inhabitants of an essentially friendly universe'.[103] Echoing the theories of Kropotkin, Smuts believed that the universe possessed a pre-established harmony based not upon alien destructiveness but upon 'mutual adaptation and adjustment'.[104] The mechanisms of adaptation and variation must, he claimed, be studied by biology within the unifying holistic factor. 'Above all, biological science must ever keep before itself the standpoint of the whole, without and apart from which all the details ... are meaningless.'[105]

Smuts's influence on Ryle is clear. A holistic conception of Darwinian evolution gave priority to the principle of adaptive variation based upon a co-operative, altruistic view of nature.[106] Both Huxley and Haldane, as I mentioned also influenced by Smuts, subscribed to holism while, like Ryle, retaining a fervent enthusiasm for Darwinism. Like them, Ryle incorporated his theories into the modern evolutionary synthesis. Yet like the mechanist, Lancelot Hogben, Ryle also believed in the necessity for a marriage of the biological and social sciences.[107] Hogben became active in social medicine founding the *British Journal of Preventive and Social Medicine* with Francis Crew. Above all Ryle's socialism was essentially an expression of J. D. Bernal's belief in the realization of the social function of science. Ryle's intellectual construction of social medicine, therefore, embodied not a few of the many contradictions which pervaded both the politics of epistemology in twentieth-century science and the politics of science as the new social ethic of rational society.

### Revolutionary Humanism or Panoptical Surveillance?

Social medicine was born of politics, the pre-war radical politics of epistemology, science and society. For Ryle social medicine was revolutionary in the sense of being a renaissance, a revolution of ideas. It was a re-evaluation, a revival of values of classical medicine in order to fuel a radical agenda for the future. The radical politics of one era, however, have appeared as the essence of authoritarianism to another. By the 1960s visionary 'scientific socialism' was accused by Hegelian Marxists of justifying an Orwellian nightmare of technological totalitarianism leading *Toward a Rational Society* inhabited by *One Dimensional Man.*[108] Since then the authoritarian agenda of social medicine itself has been singled out not by a Marxist but by a Foucault-informed critique. The historian and sociologist, David Armstrong, has suggested that the effect of social medicine in Britain has been to create a *Political Anatomy of the Body.*[109] In particular he believes that the marriage of medicine and the social sciences enhanced the social power of medical knowledge to achieve a panoptical form of surveillance.[110] Physiological medicine focused upon the organs and tissues of objectified patients' bodies. Social medicine, Armstrong claims, has extended the medical gaze to the social spaces which surrounds individuals. Ryle believed holistic philosophy could emancipate medicine from dead mechanistic reductionism. Armstrong argues alternatively that holistic medicine adds a totalitarian force to the social power of medical knowledge.[111]

Armstrong contends that the social survey was central to the extension of the panoptical medical gaze. The social survey facilitated the study of the normal in order to identify the sick. The medicine of the social believed that everyone was ill because the borderline with health was simply a matter of variation. The social survey identified the population of the hospital as the tip of a clinical iceberg and created new clinical foci such as the life and health of the school child or mass neurosis within the community. Armstrong claims that the social survey of the normal facilitated the development of placebo therapeutics and enhanced the methodology of the clinical trial by using control groups to show the natural course of the disease, correcting the common clinical fallacy of *post hoc propter hoc*. Armstrong argues, therefore, that the social survey constituted medical surveillance by mass observation.[112]

Armstrong also believes that social medicine significantly changed the doctor-patient relationship. A central aim of Ryle's programme was, in his own words, to 're-instate the sick-man' into medicine. In a seminal article in 1976 the sociologist, Nicholas Jewson, described how the sick man had disappeared from medicine since the eighteenth century. At one time medicine had relied heavily upon the patient's own narrative to provide a key to diagnosis. With the birth of the clinic this was replaced with the clinical observation of symptoms and morbid anatomy of organs. In turn the hospital was substituted by the laboratory as the ultimate diagnostic medium.[113] Already, however, in the 1930s John Ryle had been well aware of these historical developments which had divided the patient up into his organs and microbiological processes. Ryle wanted to re-unite the organism of the patient and place the whole person at the centre of medical practice. But whole-person medicine, according to Armstrong, turned the patient from a passive object into an active subject. Not only was the patient's narrative of his own disease important but his entire personal, social and psychological history.

Armstrong suggests that subjective medicine changed the role of the patient. Beginning with the problem of the defaulter in venereal disease treatment, the examination of patient motives and intentions became more significant in the clinical encounter.[114] The importance of the subjectivity of the patient was most elaborately expressed in the work of Michael Balint. In the 1950s Balint identified the psychoanalytic functions of general medical practice. He suggested that the psycho-dynamic of the doctor-patient relationship was central to the analysis of disease, diagnosis and treatment. The doctor himself, Balint claimed, was the drug which the patient was really seeking. Thus the doctor's personality was crucial to the process of recovery. For Armstrong this type of holistic medicine expanded medical policing by designating the entire subjective experience of the patient as a legitimate area of inquiry. So that the move from the patient as a passive object to an active subject expanded medical surveillance from organs, tissues and cells to patients' entire lives and experiences.[115]

Armstrong has a 'strong' programme of interpretation of the effects of social medicine upon medical practice in Britain. It is a species of argument produced by another association of medicine with social science after the Second World War, i.e. medical sociology. Initially Ryle and his contemporaries envisaged the role of social science as that of a handmaiden to medicine. And indeed many autobiographical accounts by sociologists confirm this view.

But as Strauss pointed out in 1957, the function of sociology *in medicine* (contrasted to that of the sociology of medicine)[116] was achieved, Raymond Illsely has suggested, when sociology was promoted to 'observer status'.[117] Subsequently the self-proclaimed function of medical sociology has been critically to appraise medicine as simply another species of social behaviour and interaction. Historically, medical sociology has always presented itself as a radical underdog nipping at the heels and toes of the vastly privileged establishment of medicine as a system of social organization and mobilization of power.[118] The accuracy of medical sociology's own image of its function awaits historical deconstruction, but Armstrong's critique of social medicine is a classic representation of it. It is also one of the finest and most superbly insightful pieces of historical medical sociology of recent times.

Aspects of Armstrong's interpretation of social medicine are correct. He is correct to point to the heightened importance of the social survey in medicine since the Second World War. The adoption of more heavily based sociological techniques has been crucial in enhancing the status of epidemiology in British medical research, the most powerful example perhaps are the studies done by Bradford Hill and Richard Doll, published in 1950, on the correlation of smoking and lung cancer.[119] Armstrong is also right to highlight the important changes brought about by placing the whole-person patient at the centre of medical practice. However, it is not clear that these developments constitute a metamorphosis of medical power. The social sources of medical power are multifarious in modern society. But the simple analytical models proposed either by Foucault, upon whom Armstrong relies heavily or, another mentor, Ivan Illich are limited.[120]

Social medicine as an academic discipline failed as an institutional enterprise. Despite the extraneous efforts and enormous enthusiasm of the standard-bearers of social medicine in the 1940s they failed to convince either medical schools or the public health profession that they had sufficiently defined a new epistemological constituency.[121] By the 1950s social medicine had already turned into something resembling an expanded concept of epidemiology. When Francis Crew and Lancelot Hogben founded the *British Journal of Social Medicine* in 1947 it was primarily epidemiological rather than sociological or interdisciplinary. The difficulties of defining the disciplinary constituency of social medicine ultimately led Jerry Morris to invent a new concept of 'community medicine' in the late 1960s, which focused largely on the systematic study of long-range health planning.[122]

While the grand evolutionary pursuits of social medicine were lost it succeeded, however, in remaining a powerful intellectual force within academic medical research and in the theory of medical practice. It remained a powerful force amongst the intellectual medical elite in Britain who were committed to a liberal ideal of medicine which was antagonistic to the constraints of technological medicine. Social medicine also became a powerful ideological justification for changing the role of the general practitioner into that of a social investigator and social worker. GPs served as the gate-keepers on the use of medical services under the NHS. They also served as monitors of morbidity within the community and new listening banks for the expression of alienation in twentieth-century society. But few, if any GPs actually transformed themselves into Balintian psychotherapeutic counsellors or into Ryle's ideal doctor-demographer, William Pickles.[123] The influence of social medicine took generations to become significant amongst ordinary medical practitioners, and even then only in a highly pragmatic and dispersed way. Similarly, although sociomedical surveys became central tools of epidemiological research, epidemiology itself remained a poor relation to the ever-expanding empire of laboratory science. The latter continued massively to accelerate the process of medical specialization and technical practice. The formal successor of social medicine, Jerry Morris's 'Community Medicine', was a damp squib which never exceeded the disparaged status of the old public health.

The panoptical medical gaze remains a Foucaultian abstraction rather than a material reality in post-war British medicine. The advocates of social medicine continue to be dissident voices in a world of high-tech medicine. Medical interest in the value of social science is confined to a narrow intellectual elite. But the influence of social medicine beyond the confines of the seminar room and scholarly article remains tenuous. The goal of transforming modern medicine into Ryle's vision of a humanistic science remains only distantly attainable. Perhaps the dismissed radical politics of the past may yet still offer lessons for the agenda of science in society.

## Notes

1. J. A. Ryle, *Changing Disciplines* (London: Oxford Medical Publications, 1948), vi.
2. J. A. Ryle, 'Social medicine', *B. M. J.*, i (1942), 801.
3. Paul Forman, 'Weimar Culture, Causality, and Quantum Theory, 1918–27: Adaptation by German Physicists and Mathematicians to a Hostile Intellectual Environment', *Historical Studies in the Physical*

*Sciences*, iii (1971), 1–115.
4. *Ibid.*
5. See, for example, John Hendry, 'Weimar Culture and Quantum Causality', *History of Science*, xviii (1980), 155–180; W. Laqueur, *Weimar, a Cultural History 1918–33* (London: Weidenfeld & Nicolson, 1974).
6. Anne Harrington, 'Other "Ways of Knowing": The Politics of Knowledge in Interwar German Brain Science', in *idem* (ed.), *So Human a Brain. Knowledge and Values in the Neurosciences* (Boston: Birkhäuser, 1991), 229–44.
7. Ryle, *op. cit.* (ref. 1), vi.
8. F. A. E. Crew, 'Social Medicine as an Academic Discipline', in Arthur Massey (ed.), *Modern Trends in Public Health* (London: Butterworth, 1949), 46–69, 66.
9. David Armstrong, *Political Anatomy of the Body. Medical Knowledge in Britain in Twentieth Century* (Cambridge: Cambridge University Press, 1983), 7–18.
10. Gary Werskey, *The Visible College* (London: Allen Lane, 1978).
11. Dorothy Porter, 'Changing Disciplines: John Ryle and the Making of Social Medicine in Britain in the 1940s', *History of Science*, xxx (1992), 137–64.
12. J. A. Ryle, 'The Hippocratic Ideal', *Lancet*, ii (1934), 1263–68, 1264.
13. J. A. Ryle, 'Aetiology: A Plea for Wider Concepts and New Study', *Lancet*, ii (1942), 29–30; *idem*, 'Medicine 1910–1935', *Lancet*, i (1935), 1049–51, 1050.
14. J. A. Ryle, 'The Physician as Naturalist', *Guy's Hospital Reports*, lxxxi (1931), 278–96, 290, reproduced in J. A. Ryle, *The Natural History of Disease* (1st edition, 1936; 2nd edition, 1946; reprinted London: The Keynes Press, 1988), 1–19, 12.
15. *Ibid.* 10.
16. J. A. Ryle, 'Social Medicine and Hospital Practice', *B. M. J.*, ii (1947), 628.
17. Ryle, *op. cit.* (ref. 12), 1264, Ryle, *op. cit.* (ref. 14), 16–17. For discussion of the importance of natural history and field science amongst British intellectuals, David E. Allen, *The Naturalist in Britain. A Social History* (London: Allen Lane, 1976).
18. Ryle, *op. cit.* (ref. 1), 85–100.
19. Ryle, *op. cit.* (ref. 13), 30.
20. J. A. Ryle, 'Coronary disease', *Lancet*, ii (1946), 692–3, 693.
21. See Editorial, 'Social Pathology', *Lancet*, i (1947), 413.
22. Ryle had this pointed out to him directly by Major Greenwood, 'Social Medicine', *B. M. J.*, i (1946), 117–19.

23: Ryle, *op. cit.* (ref. 13), 30.
24. Ryle, *op. cit.* (ref. 1), 12.
25. J. A. Ryle, 'Social Medicine its Meaning and its Scope', *B. M. J.*, ii (1943), 633–6; *idem*, *op. cit.* (ref. 1), 28–47.
26. Philip Abrams, *The Origins of British Sociology 1834–1914*, (Chicago: Chicago University Press, 1968); Philip Boardman, *The Worlds of Patrick Geddes. Biologist, Town Planner, Re-educator, Peace-Warrior* (London: Routledge & Kegan Paul, 1978).
27. J. A. Ryle, 'Socio-Medical Surveys', *Lancet*, i (1946), 64–6, 64.
28. *Ibid.*, 65–6.
29. J. A. Ryle, *op. cit.* (ref. 1), vii I have not yet discovered any evidence that Ryle was widely erudite in the social sciences or in the history of their development. However Ryle's conception of social science had many parallels with British and American progressive evolutionary sociologists who linked social science with humanist ethics.

At the turn of the twentieth century some of the founders of sociology in Britain and the United States, such as L. T. Hobhouse, Albion Small and the early Chicago sociologists believed that social evolution was based on 'mutual aid'. In their view the sociologist was both a social philosopher and a social scientist who permanently confronted the dialectical tension between evolution and progress. They believed that purposive social evolution could be achieved through rational, scientific political decision-making. Progressive evolutionism attempted to develop a synthetic, naturalistic account of man and society which incorporated idealism, moralism and religious thought into a scientific framework. This chimed with Ryle's conception of holistic social inquiry into the historical evolutionary rhythms of human development which fuelled his perception of the new social physician as a natural historian of man in his ecological habitat, with a mission to use knowledge to educate and improve. Ryle believed that social medicine built upon social science would turn medicine into scientific humanism. For discussion of Hobhouse see Stefan Collini, *Liberalism and Sociology. L. T. Hobhouse and Political Argument in England 1880–1914* (Cambridge: Cambridge University Press, 1979). On Chicago sociology see Robert C. Bannister, *Sociology and Scientism. The American Quest for Objectivity 1880–1940* (Chapel Hill: University of North Carolina Press, 1987); Lester R. Kurtz, *Evaluating Chicago Sociology* (Chicago: Chicago University Press, 1984); J. David Lewis and Richard L. Smith, *American Sociology and Pragmatism.* Mead, *Chicago Sociology and Symbolic Interaction* (Chicago: Chicago University Press, 1978); Julius Weinberg, *Edward Alsworth Ross and the Sociology of Progressivism* (Madison: University of Wisconsin Press, 1972); Dennis Smith, *The Chicago School. A Liberal Critique of Capitalism* (London: Macmillan, 1988).

30. Ryle, *op. cit.* (ref. 25), 634–5.
31. J. A. Ryle, 'The Science of Health', *B.M.J* ii (1942), 745–8.
32. *Ibid.*, 745.
33. For discussion of the political-epistemology of the book see, Mikulás Teich, 'Reflecting on the Golden Jubilee of Bernal's *Social Function of Science*', *History of Science*, xxviii (1990), 411–18. For Bernal himself see Maurice Goldsmith, *Sage. A Life of J. D. Bernal* (London: Hutchinson, 1980). For discussion of Bernal's circle of socialist scientists see Werskey, *op. cit.* (ref. 10).
34. J. D. Bernal, *The Social Function of Science* (London: Routledge, 1940; first edition, 1939), 353–6.
35. In some 'Notes for students' talk' which Ryle gave on 16 February – no other date – 'at home', he refers to the importance of both Bernal's book and Huxley's book *The Uniqueness of Man*: 'There has been a rather rude awakening of recent years to the fact that we have allowed our scientists to run away with us and our intellectual interests, at the expense of our human interests. Private ownership in knowledge can, like private ownership of wealth, lead to great injustices. (refer to Bernal's 'Social Function of Science') Now we are beginning to look ahead and see how we might do better. (refer to Julian Huxley and 'scientific humanism' – *Uniqueness of Man*).
36. J. A. Ryle, 'The Meaning of the Normal', *Lancet*, i (1947), 1–5; Ryle, *op. cit.* (ref. 1) 66–83.
37. *Ibid.*
38. *Ibid.*, 2.
39. *Ibid.*, 3.
40. J. A. Ryle, 'Diathesis, or Variation and Disease in Man', reproduced in J. A. Ryle, *The Natural History of Disease* (1st edition, 1936; second edition 1946; reprinted London: The Keynes Press, 1988), 375–83.
41. J. A. Ryle, 'Constitution as a Factor in Morbidity', *Clinical Journal*, lx (1931), 73–81.
42. Ryle, *op. cit.* (ref. 36), 3.
43. Ryle, *op. cit.* (ref. 40), 11.
44. For Galton see D. W. Forrest, *Francis Galton: The Life and Work of a Genius* (London: Paul Elek, 1974); for Galton and eugenics see Daniel Kevles, *In the Name of Eugenics. Genetics and the Uses of Human Heredity* (New York: Knopf, 1985); Geoffrey R. Searle, *Eugenics and Politics in Britain 1900–1914* (Leyden: Noordhoff, 1976); C. Webster (ed.), *Biology, Medicine and Society 1840–1940*

(Cambridge: Cambridge University Press, 1981); Donald MacKenzie, *Statistics in Britain, 1865–1930* (Edinburgh: Edinburgh University Press, 1981). For discussion of eugenics and preventive medicine see Greta Jones, *Social Darwinism and English Thought: the Interaction between Biological and Social Theory* (Brighton: Harvester Press, 1980); *idem., Social Hygiene in Britain* (London: Croom Helm, 1986); Dorothy Porter, '"Enemies of the Race": Biologism, Environmentalism and the Public Health in Edwardian England', *Victorian Studies*, xxiv (1991), 159–78.

45. For a recent discussion of Huxley's life and work see Milo Keynes and G. Ainsworth Harrison (eds), *Evolutionary Studies. A Centenary Celebration of the Life of Julian Huxley* (London: Macmillan, 1989). On Huxley's eugenics see David Hubback, 'Julian Huxley and Eugenics', in *ibid.*, 194–206. See also Huxley's autobiographical *memoirs*, J. S. Huxley, *Memories*, 2 vols (London: Allen & Unwin, 1970 and 1973).
46. Julian Huxley, *The Uniqueness of Man* (London: Chatto and Windus, 1941), 34–83.
47. J. A. Ryle, 'Medicine and Eugenics', *Eugenics Review*, xxx (xi new series) (1938–9), 9–19.
48. Ryle, *op. cit.* (ref. 31), 747.
49. See J. Huxley, *Essays of a Biologist* (London: Chatto & Windus, 1923), 67–101.
50. Ryle's synthesis of Darwinism and eugenics is typical of the twentieth-century 'evolutionary synthesis' brilliantly examined by Peter Bowler, *Evolution, the History of an Idea* (Berkeley: University of California Press, 1984), 288–316.
51. J. A. Ryle to Miriam Ryle, 14 October, 1917.
52. *Ibid.*
53. See Miriam Ryle, *John A. Ryle* (Unpublished typescript biography in the possession of Anthony Ryle), 164–5:
'John was on the Medical Planning Commission of the National Health Service, from early in 1942. His large practice in London with many consultations in the poorer districts and his years of out-patients at Guy's had made him familiar with and sympathetic towards the great difficulties of general practitioners but also conscious of their short comings, particularly in the poorer areas. He had watched young and enthusiastic doctors being gradually defeated by the impossibility of doing first class work. Dirt and poverty and ignorance were ever present among the patients and fatigue and the hopelessness of doing good work weeded out most of the good doctors. Those who stayed made the best arrangements they could to

enable them to survive.... The Committee of the Royal College of Physicians studying proposals for the National Health Service were on the whole critical of John's ideas, particularly of his wish to abolish the great difference in the proposed remuneration and prestige of the general practitioner and the consultant. One infuriated member's remark "so now that you've climbed to the top of the ladder, you want to kick it down" amused him but it was a pointer that emphasized where much of the obstinate hostility lay.'

54. See also J. A. Ryle, 'A Fundamental Principle', *B. M. J.*, ii (1945), 936; *idem.*, 'A Fundamental Principle', *B. M. J.*, i (1946), 105.
55. J. A. Ryle to 'X' 22 March, 1942. The debate with Horder surfaced later in published form: see J. A. Ryle, 'Shall We Nationalize Medicine?', *B. M. J.*, i (1945), 456.
56. Ryle, *op. cit.* (ref. 25), 635.
57. J. A. Ryle to Miriam Ryle, 21 October, 1942. The emphasis highlighted in the quotes is Ryle's.
58. Ryle, *op. cit.* (ref. 31), 747.
59. Ryle, *op. cit.* (ref. 47).
60. J. A. Ryle to his father-in-Law, 21 December, 1941.
61. J. A. Ryle, *op. cit.* (ref. 31), 633.
62. *Ibid.*, 636.
63. J. A. Ryle, *Fears May Be Liars* (London: Allen & Unwin, 1941), 44–54; Huxley, *op. cit.* (ref. 46), 222–76.
64. *Ibid.*, Ryle, 27–43.
65. Huxley, *op. cit.* (ref. 46), 224.
66. J. A. Ryle, 'Today and To-morrow', *B. M. J.*, ii (1940), 657–9, 659.
67. Ryle, *op. cit.* (ref. 1).
68. Ryle, *op. cit.* (ref. 25), 635.
69. Although he was disappointed with regard to the provision for health centres, Ryle was very supportive of the pioneering health centre at Peckham developed before the War. See J. A. Ryle, 'Health Centres', *B.M.J* i (1948), 1003. For discussion of Peckham see J. Lewis and B. Brookes, 'A Reassessment of the Work of the Peckham Health Centre, 1926–51', *Milbank Memorial Quarterly, Health and Society*, lxi (1983), 307–50; Innes H. Pearse and Lucy H. Crocker, *The Peckham Experiment. A Study in the Living Structure of Society* (London: Allen & Unwin, 1943).
70. Ryle, *op. cit.* (ref. 25), 635.
71. *Ibid.*
72. *Ibid.*, 636.
73. *Ibid.*
74. Harrington, *op. cit.* (ref. 6).

75. See also, Robert M. Young, *Mind, Brain and Adaptation in the Nineteenth Century* (Oxford: Clarendon Press, 1970); E. Clarke and S. Jacyna, *Nineteenth Century Origins of Neuroscientific Concepts* (Berkeley: University of California Press, 1987).
76. Harrington, *op. cit.* (ref. 6).
77. See also F. Wyatt and H. L. Teuber, 'German Psychology Under the Nazi System: 1933–40', *Psychological Review*, li (1944), 229–47; Paul Weindling, *Health, Race and Politics Between National Unification and Nazism, 1870–1945* (Cambridge: Cambridge University Press, 1989).
78. Werskey, *op. cit.* (ref. 10), 179–84.
79. See also Robert M. Young, 'Science *is* Social Relations', *Radical Science Journal*, v (1977), 65–129.
80. Werskey, *op. cit.* (ref. 10), 52–9, 92–100.
81. See J. B. S. Haldane, 'The Scientific Work of J. S. Haldane (1860–1936)', *Nature*, 187 (1960), 103.
82. Ronald Clark, *J. B. S. The Life and Work of J. B. S. Haldane* (London: Hodder & Stoughton, 1968).
83. Bowler, *op. cit.* (ref. 50), 291–6. Bowler is of course following Huxley's categorization. See J. S. Huxley (ed.), *Evolution: The Modern Synthesis* (London: Allen & Unwin, 1963).
84. Gary Werskey, 'Haldane and Huxley: the First Appraisals', *Journal of the History of Biology*, (1971), 171–83; Krishna R. Dronamraju, *The Life and Work of J. B. S. Haldane, With Special Reference to India* (Aberdeen: Aberdeen University Press, 1985), 39–111.
85. See Pauline M. H. Mazumdar, *Eugenics, Human Genetics and Human Failings. The Eugenics Society, its Sources and its Critics in Britain* (London: Routledge, 1992). See also J. B. S. Haldane, *Heredity and Politics* (New York: Norton, 1938); *idem*, *Human Biology and Politics* (London: British Science Guild, 1935); F. A. E. Crew, J. B. S. Haldane, L. T. Hogben and J. S. Huxley *et al*, 'Social Biology and Population Improvement', *Nature*, (1939), 521-2.
86. *Ibid.*, Mazumdar, 149ff. Werskey, *op. cit.* (ref. 10), 60–7. See also Lancelot Hogben, *Science for the Citizen: A Self-Educator Based on the Social Background of Scientific Discovery* (London: Allen & Unwin, 1938).
87. Werskey, *op. cit.* (ref. 10), 103.
88. *Ibid.*, 60–7.
89. *Ibid.*, 110–15.
90. *Ibid.*, 111.
91. W. K. Hancock, *Smuts. the Sanguine Years 1870–1919* (Cambridge: Cambridge University Press, 1962); F. S. Crafford, *Jan Smuts. A Biography* (London: Allen & Unwin, 1946).

92. Werskey, *op. cit.* (ref. 10), 113.
93. *Ibid.*, 176–211.
94. Huxley, *op. cit.* (ref. 46), 277–90.
95. Bernal, *op. cit.* (ref. 34); Werskey, *op. cit.* (ref. 10), 185–99.
96. J. A. Ryle, 'Man and the Machine', *B.M.J* ii (1949), 176; *idem, op. cit.* (ref. 12).
97. J. C. Smuts, *Holism and Evolution* (Westport, Conn.: Greenwood Press, 1973, 1st edition, 1926).
98. *Ibid.*, 179.
99. *Ibid.*, 180.
100. *Ibid.*, 184.
101. *Ibid.*, 190.
102. *Ibid.*, 220.
103. *Ibid.*
104. *Ibid.*
105. *Ibid.*, 221.
106. Ryle, *op. cit.* (ref. 36).
107. When he was the principal of the London School of Economics William Beveridge appointed Hogben to fill a new chair in social biology. Beveridge believed that Hogben was uniquely qualified to enhance the movement toward greater interdisciplinary co-operation between the natural and the social sciences. See Werskey, *op. cit.* (ref. 10), 110.
108. Jürgen Habermas, *Toward a Rational Society* (London: Heinemann, 1972, 1st edition 1968); Herbert Marcuse, *One Dimensional Man: Studies in the Ideology of Advanced Societies* (London: Routledge, 1991, 1st edition 1964).
109. David Armstrong, *Political Anatomy of the Body* (Cambridge: Cambridge University Press, 1983).
110. Armstrong is drawing upon the analysis of knowledge and power offered by Michel Foucault in *Discipline and Punish, The Birth of the Prison* (London, Tavistock, 1977), 198–208.
111. Armstrong, *op. cit.* (ref. 109), 1–6.
112. *Ibid.*, 42–92.
113. N. Jewson, 'The Disappearance of the Sick Man from Medical Cosmology 1770–1870', *Sociology*, x (1976), 225–44.
114. Armstrong, *op. cit.* (ref. 109), 10–13; 101–17.
115. *Ibid.*, 73–84.
116. R. Strauss, 'The Nature and Status of Medical Sociology', *American Sociological Review*, xxii (1957), 200–04.
117. Raymond Illsley, 'Promotion to Observer Status', *Social Science and Medicine*, ix (1975), 63–7. (Originally prepared as the Opening Address delivered to the 4th International Conference on Social

Science and Medicine, Elsinore, August, 1974); see also Derek G. Gill, 'Medical Sociology: What's in a Name?', *International Social Science Journal*, xix (1977), 369–85.

118. See for example Brian Turner, *Medical Power and Social Knowledge* (London: Sage, 1987).
119. For discussion see C. Booth, 'Smoking and the Gold Headed Cane', in *Balancing Act*: *Essays to Honour Stephen Lock* (London: Keynes Press, 1991), 49–55; A. M. Brandt, 'The Cigarette, Risk and American Culture', *Daedalus*, cxix (1990), 155–76.
120. See M. Foucault, *The Order of Things* (London: Tavistock, 1974); *idem*, *Madness and Civilization* (London: Tavistock, 1965); *idem*, *The Birth of the Clinic* (London: Tavistock, 1973); I. Illich, *The Limits to Medicine* (Harmondsworth: Penguin Books, 1978).
121. J. Lewis, *What Price Community Medicine?* (Brighton: Wheatsheaf, 1986), 35–56, 100–20.
122. *Ibid.*
123. John Pemberton, *Will Pickles of Wensleydale. The Life of a Country Doctor* (Newton Abbot: Country Book Club, 1970).

# 11

# Doing History, Making Revolution: the Aspirations of Henry E. Sigerist and George Rosen

*Elizabeth Fee and Edward T. Morman*

This paper discusses the lives and contributions of two physician-historians who believed that the history of medicine could change the world by altering the ways in which doctors thought and practised. Both maintained that medical history could transform physicians' attitudes by demonstrating that medicine was, above all, a social endeavour; that health and illness were primarily determined by political and economic forces; and that the physician's responsibility necessarily extended beyond care of the individual patient to embrace the kinds of social reforms that could mean improved health for all. The medical history these men advocated was not a celebratory history for self-congratulation; it was a critical history for social transformation.

Henry Sigerist was the more active in the medical politics of his day as an advocate of Soviet medicine and a spokesman for national health insurance and 'socialized medicine'; George Rosen was a leading voice in the social medicine movement and in public health. Both men were energetic, enormously prolific, and well known in their respective professional circles of medicine and public health. Both men spent time in Europe as well as the United States – the Paris-born Sigerist studied in Zurich and held the medical history chair in Leipzig before coming to America in 1932; and Rosen, a native New Yorker, earned his MD degree in Berlin. Sigerist found his social and political optimism sorely tried by his own experiences in the United States in the late 1940s when the adulation he had originally received as an articulate and impassioned advocate of medical and social reform turned into sour suspicion and official rejection of his 'subversive' views. Discouraged, he left America and went to Switzerland where he hoped to complete his masterwork, a projected eight-volume history of medicine; he died with the project unfinished and the political world wrapped up in the intense Cold War paranoia of the 1950s. George Rosen had also been disappointed by the failure of social medicine and the more radical versions of medical reform envisioned in the 1930s and 1940s. Rosen, however, lived through the 1970s, remained productive as a scholar, and died at a moment when there still seemed reason to be hopeful about the possibility of social and medical transformation in the United States.

Sigerist and Rosen shared many of the same ideas. Both saw themselves as rewriting the history of medicine and public health in order to contribute to the creation of a new, socially-oriented system of health care. First, they wanted to demonstrate that health and disease were social phenomena, not simply biological processes. Every illness, they said, was as much a social fact as a biological one; to understand only the biological basis of disease was to grasp a single, limited aspect of reality. Second, they argued that medicine as a social endeavour did not consist simply of the curative treatment of diseased individuals – physicians had larger social and political responsibilities to the public health and, as social actors, should be expected to contribute to the historical progress of civilization. Their view of the physician's role was at the same time radical and also heroic, even grandiose. Third, they wanted to use medical history as a tool to reconceptualize the nature of medicine, to help reorganize the system of medical care, and – in Sigerist's case – to contribute to building social revolution on the Soviet model.

This paper will examine the ways in which each attempted to use medical history as a form of social criticism, discuss their personal and political relationship, and evaluate the extent to which each was able to achieve his goals. We begin with a brief sketch of the diverse family backgrounds, early careers, and political views of the two men.

### Henry Sigerist's Background and Early Career

Henry Sigerist was a European scholar of wide erudition and an enthusiastic approach to all aspects of culture. He was born to a wealthy Swiss family living in Paris, ever his favourite city, in 1891. One of Sigerist's grandfathers had been a wine dealer, the other a goldsmith who had opened a small metal-plating factory. His father was a successful businessman, the founder and director of a shoe company, Chaussures Raoul, and owner of over one hundred stores in France and abroad. When his father died while Sigerist was still a boy, his mother moved herself and the two children back to Switzerland. The family was well provided for; the children had everything they wanted or needed, the best private education available, and opportunities to travel. Sigerist described himself at that age:

> I was ten years old, to be sure, but I was and felt myself a Parisian. I was used to being called monsieur, and when I went out I wore a bowler hat and kid gloves and had a cane with a silver handle.[1]

The rich young man loved books and learning. As he grew older, he was able to study what interested him and to prepare for the future possibility of an academic position without having to face the immediate necessity of earning a living.[2] At the age of 25 he would marry Emmy Escher, the daughter of a prominent Swiss family, and then spend the next eight years as an independent scholar. His studies began at the University of Zurich in 1910 when he began to work in oriental philology; he then continued to study Sanskrit, Hebrew, Arabic, and Chinese at the University of London. He resisted his teachers' pressure to choose a field of specialization, instead returning to Zurich to study science and medicine. He completed his clinical studies in Munich and, while on a trip to Venice, had the sudden realization that by choosing the field of the history of medicine, he could essentially avoid specialization and combine his varied interests in languages, the humanities, history, science and medicine.

Back in Zurich, Sigerist was called into active duty in the Swiss army and was forced to divide his time between military service and university studies. Later, he remembered that he had first become aware of working-class perspectives during his two years of army service: 'So far I had lived the life of the middle class', he said, 'These anonymous soldiers became my teachers. They opened my eyes about many problems that I had not seen before and made me realize how little I knew about the world in which I was living ... it often struck me how much more convincing their interpretations were than those I heard in the officers' mess.'[3]

After completing his MD degree, Sigerist wrote to Karl Sudhoff in Leipzig to express his desire to study the history of medicine. Sudhoff, the most prominent medical historian of the era, encouraged the young man's interest and offered advice; in 1919, the two met for the first time and Sigerist became, even if informally, Sudhoff's student. Sigerist was immediately attracted to the study of the eighteenth century but, on Sudhoff's recommendation, turned instead to the philological study of early medieval texts. Living at home in Zurich, he worked as an independent scholar, kept up an active correspondence with Sudhoff, and began writing articles for medical and medical-historical journals and published the first of his many books on medical history.[4] In 1921, he became Privatdozent in the history of medicine at the University of Zurich and was licensed to offer lecture courses and seminars at the University.[5]

In 1925, Sigerist's dedication to his chosen field was amply recognized when he was named Sudhoff's successor as head of the Institute for the History of Medicine at Leipzig. Here he expanded the existing lecture series and added regular seminars on a variety of historical and contemporary topics. A brilliant and popular teacher, he made medical history appealing to other members of the faculty and practising physicians, as well as to large numbers of eager students. Sigerist also threw numerous parties, sponsored social and intellectual gatherings, and was generous in using his own resources to assist more impoverished scholars.[6] He initiated and nurtured a highly productive programme of research and publishing, and encouraged members of the Institute to explore a wide variety of research topics from philological commentaries, to investigations of ancient drugs and herbaria, to cultural studies and the history of ideas.[7]

During the Leipzig period, Sigerist displayed clear left-wing sympathies and was hostile to the rising power of the Nazis. Erwin Ackerknecht, a member of the Institute and a leader of the Trotskyist youth movement in Germany, recalled in the 1970s that Sigerist had initially been a Christian socialist. Ackerknecht complained wryly that he had 'sold Marxism to him (Sigerist) and later could not get him back from it'.[8] As political and economic tensions grew in Germany, and as the Institute's budget was being cut back, Sigerist became increasingly worried about the future: 'I knew my name was on all the black lists and that I could not remain in Germany if Hitler came to power. In the summer of 1926, in Weimar, I had participated at the meeting of republican university professors who had decided to support, and not to sabotage, the German Republic. I had helped to publish the *Neue Blätter für den Sozialismus* (New Socialist Journal); and in the summer semester of 1932 I myself had thrown out two fat Nazis who appeared in full uniform in my lecture room, contrary to the rector's rule that party shirts could not be worn in the lecture halls. This was a clear case of provocation. I knew what was ahead of me and that I could expect no mercy from the Nazis.'[9]

By 1931, the political climate in Germany was increasingly gloomy and when, during Sigerist's successful lecture tour in

America, William Henry Welch proffered an invitation to become his successor as professor of the history of medicine and director of the Institute of the History of Medicine at Johns Hopkins, Sigerist was happy to accept the appointment. At that time, he insisted that America was the country of the future – a country with an optimistic and rational outlook, while Europe was becoming more and more reactionary and mystical.

Sigerist completely charmed his American audiences. He was perceived as a brilliant medieval scholar and as a humane physician with a wide-ranging knowledge of the history of medicine and a clear sense of its contemporary relevance. Americans also saw him as a European scholar in the old tradition, a man who spoke many languages fluently, cited his texts in the original, displayed an encyclopaedic knowledge, lectured with energy, erudition, and passion, and spoke with enthusiasm and authority on a multiplicity of subjects. While Sigerist was obviously sophisticated and cosmopolitan, he always seemed open and thoroughly interested in everybody and everything. Not the least element in Sigerist's charm was the fact that he seemed delighted with America and things American.

## George Rosen: Background and Early Career

George Rosen's background is a study in contrasts. Born in Brooklyn in 1910, Rosen's early life was typical of first generation American Jews of Eastern European background. His parents spoke Yiddish at home; George only learned English and was given an English first name when he entered the New York City public schools. His father, a presser in a laundry, was an ardent trade unionist who took the boy to union functions. To motivate his own children, Rosen later claimed that a grade school teacher had told him that he 'would never amount to anything'. His family moved several times during his childhood and youth; he commuted to high school from East Harlem and to college from the Bronx.[10]

At Stuyvesant High School, a selective public school for boys interested in science and engineering, Rosen affiliated with the left, but did not seem especially interested in politics. His closest friends knew him to devour books on any subject and a required course in drafting left him with a lifetime hobby of drawing and painting. After graduating from Stuyvesant in 1926, he proceeded to the College of the City of New York – for bright young men (largely Jews) of the city's working class, simultaneously a gateway to the petit bourgeois life and a centre of radical politics.[11] At college, outside of a few friendships, Rosen devoted himself to schoolwork, his job at a post office in Brooklyn, the college swimming team, and his voracious reading.[12]

With a relative on the attending staff of Brooklyn's Beth-El Hospital serving as a model for upward mobility, Rosen followed the pre-medical programme at City College. Upon graduation, however, he and his two closest friends found themselves excluded from medical school because of the anti-Semitic admissions policies then prevailing in American medical education.[13] All three decided to enroll at the University of Berlin, joining what was, in effect, the final migration of Americans to Europe in search of a high quality medical education.[14]

Late in the summer of 1930, the three City College boys booked passage on the Hamburg-American Line. None was aware of the developing political situation in Germany, but they soon became familiar with Nazism – as a parliamentary force in the Reichstag and as a social movement on the streets of Berlin. Rosen's experience in Germany was necessarily political; a Jew exposed to an atmosphere of growing anti-Semitism could not avoid politics. In Berlin, he began to take an interest in Marxism both as a political philosophy and as historical methodology. He developed a general familiarity with German scholarship in sociology, philosophy, and literature. He was also favourably impressed with the workings of the German national health insurance system in the late years of the Weimar Republic.[15]

Jewish-American medical students in Berlin had the chance to enjoy the cultural amenities of a European capital but they could see that conditions for German Jews were steadily getting worse. Rosen clearly understood this as he became involved with a fellow medical student, Beate Caspari, the daughter of a successful Berlin physician who was also an observant Jew. Rosen proposed marriage after only a few weeks – his haste motivated by a desire to lend her and her family some of the protection he had as an American citizen.

In his father-in-law Rosen had a potential model of a compassionate, politically alert physician who maintained a Jewish identity within a very comfortable household, while participating in the broader secular culture of his city and nation. Though himself an atheist,[16] indifferent to Zionism, and an aspiring cosmopolite, Rosen always acknowledged his Jewish roots.[17] When he moved into the Caspari home after his marriage, Rosen would have found the kosher food customs familiar, although the presence of a servant and the atmosphere of genteel culture were a far cry from his parents' proletarian apartment in the Bronx. He had no trouble accustoming himself to the relative luxury of his in-laws' household, although pride prevented him from allowing the older Dr Caspari to pay for first-class passage when he and Beate returned to America.

Not long after meeting Dr Caspari, Rosen encountered Henry Sigerist – another cultured, humane, gentleman-physician. Sigerist was a gentile, and thus perhaps less suitable as a role-model; on the other hand, as the leading scholar in his field, he appealed to the intellectually curious and ambitious younger man. By his third year in medical school, Rosen's interest in history was sufficiently developed that he asked the medical historian Paul Diepgen to supervise his medical thesis. Diepgen agreed, and in turn urged Rosen to contact Sigerist (by then already settled in Baltimore) for advice on choosing a topic in American medicine that could be studied using the library resources of Berlin.[18]

Sigerist quickly responded to Rosen's inquiry, proposing that the younger man investigate the European reception of Beaumont's discoveries in gastric physiology. Rosen proceeded to write a well-received thesis on this subject,[19] and thereby established himself as Sigerist's informal student. During his final months in Berlin, Rosen wrote asking Sigerist to suggest further topics for historical research and requesting a letter of reference for an internship.[20]

After his return to New York, Rosen continued to practise a form of *lernfreiheit;* Sigerist would suggest topics and readings, and Rosen would send what he wrote to Sigerist for review and criticism.[21] In essence, Sigerist re-established the kind of relationship he had earlier had with Sudhoff; this time, he was the mentor and Rosen the student by correspondence. Sigerist agreed to publish Rosen's work in the *Bulletin* and invited him to visit the Institute in Baltimore.[22] The two men met for the first time in January, 1936, following one of Sigerist's lectures in New York.

Rosen was an energetic and talented disciple. Sigerist saw that the younger man was bright and hard-working; he continued to encourage him, provide advice on his work, and recommend further topics for research – including miners' diseases, the subject of Rosen's first major book.[23] To Sigerist, Rosen was obviously a devoted admirer, someone who could be taught, and who would pursue virtually whatever research directions he suggested. In his turn, Sigerist was willing to publish almost anything Rosen sent, including some very brief and almost trivial items.[24] Rosen was indeed hard-working and generally deferential, but he could also be demanding, and he regularly asked Sigerist and the Institute staff to mail him books from the Institute library.[25]

Early in their relationship, while he was still in Germany, Rosen had let Sigerist know that he planned to continue serious work in medical history.[26] Several years later, while struggling to establish a private practice,[27] he explicitly asked Sigerist to recommend him for an academic position. Although Sigerist could not help him directly, he assured Rosen that if a place were open at the Johns Hopkins Institute, he would have liked to have him there.[28] What Sigerist could do, however, was to help provide Rosen with scholarly means to supplement his income. Sigerist thus recommended Rosen to the publisher Alfred A. Knopf as a translator, and to the Ciba-Geigy drug firm as an editor.[29] Knopf eventually published four books translated by Rosen,[30] and Rosen and his wife drew a significant income from Ciba, editing *Ciba Symposia* from 1939 to 1951.

Uncertain of ever finding a formal position in medical history, Rosen enrolled as a Ph.D. candidate in sociology at Columbia University in September, 1939 and began to study with Robert Merton, Robert Lynd, Robert MacIver, and Bernhard Stern. At the same time, he continued avidly to work on medical history; he would soon have three books published within as many years.[31] Even as Rosen developed an independent reputation in the field of medical history, Sigerist remained for him a larger-than-life figure. In their correspondence, it is clear that at some level, Rosen always perceived himself as the struggling son of immigrants, and saw Sigerist as the natural European gentleman and renowned scholar who had the power not only to help him but to bestow distinction.

## Medical Care and Politics

In America, Sigerist's left-wing and anti-fascist politics were at first accepted, even welcomed by his medical and popular audiences. Sigerist's early years in America were years of depression and economic crisis in the capitalist west and of what he saw as an emerging struggle between socialism and fascism in Europe. Although Sigerist was enthusiastic about America and Americans, he believed that the economic and political system of capitalism had broken down and that, despite the production of great wealth for a few, it had proved incapable of meeting the majority of people's basic needs for food, shelter, employment, and health care.

If America was in crisis, European civilization seemed to Sigerist to be in its death throes. Observing the situation in Europe in the summer of 1933, after his first year in America, Sigerist wrote: 'There is no doubt that democracy doesn't work any longer. The choice is between communism and fascism.' In Paris, he met many old friends who had lost their jobs or been driven out of Germany.[32]

He began reading about fascism and trying to understand its development and the reasons for its appeal. Sigerist quickly decided that fascism was totally irrational. He described Hitler's *Mein Kampf* as 'the most stupid book of a political dilettante I've ever read' and drew the conclusion that the essence of fascism was mysticism, and that the idea that Germans were a superior race with a great mission to fulfil in the world was a national psychic compensation for the 'feeling of inferiority' derived from losing the Great War.[33]

While in Europe that summer, Sigerist met his friend, Adolf Meyer, the Hopkins psychiatrist, who had just returned from a visit to the Soviet Union. Meyer was enthusiastic about what he had seen and filled Sigerist with the desire to visit the country and see the revolution in medical care for himself.[34] The more Sigerist read and heard, the more he was convinced that the whole edifice of fascism was mystical nonsense, while socialism, by contrast, was rational and scientific. 'The real antagonism', he concluded, 'is between rationalism and mysticism.'[35]

The grand philosophical and political theme of a necessary choice between different world systems animated Sigerist as an intellectual and as a historian. By 1933, he was preparing a volume of his observations of American medicine, to appear first in German as *Amerika und die Medizin* and subsequently in English as *American Medicine.*[36] As soon as his American volume was finished, he decided, he would begin to write a book on Soviet medicine. His two books, at least for the realm of health and medicine, would together pose the great question of the age: capitalism or communism? Posing the issue in this way gave Sigerist a heady sense of being part of history in the making: 'It is thrilling to be a historian today when all over the world history is being made ... If I were younger I would probably want to play an active part in the development. Now my field of action is in literature and teaching and I hope that by just being detached and critical I can influence the development at least in the limited field of medicine.'[37] Sigerist may have believed himself 'detached and critical' but it is clear that by the summer of 1933, he had already made the political choices that would determine most of his subsequent career.

Sigerist resolved to learn Russian, spend his summers in the Soviet Union, and prepare his book about medicine under communism.[38] This, along with teaching medical students at Johns Hopkins, was to be his contribution to the coming revolution. In his diaries, he mused about the political limits and possibilities of his role as an intellectual. After teaching an introductory course in the history of medicine for medical students, for example, he remarked: 'I told the students about the future of medicine, about the great social tasks waiting for them. They seemed quite impressed and applauded very much. Well, this is one way of preparing the path for the social revolution.'[39]

As Sigerist absorbed Russian grammars, Soviet newspapers, and Marxist texts on economics, he gradually abandoned his study of medieval texts. In his own mind, he didn't abandon so much as postpone his philological studies – the immediate attractions of making history (or at least helping to influence others' perceptions of the great issues of the day) were too compelling. Throughout the mid-1930s, his attention was divided between his enthusiasm for what he perceived as the revolutionary successes of the Soviet Union, his worries about the growing influence of fascism in Europe, and his encouragement for the medical care reform movements associated with the New Deal in the United States.

America was embroiled in controversies over the organization and financing of medical care. The final report of the Committee on the Costs of Medical Care in 1932 had recommended the reorganization of medical care around group practice and had raised the question of covering costs either by insurance or taxation.[40] This, and the subsequent national debates over unemployment insurance, old age pensions, public health infrastructure and other social and health reforms had placed the issues of medical care organization on the national political agenda. Sigerist, with his desire to be politically active, became heavily involved in the debates over national health insurance – he spoke to countless groups, gave radio addresses, and appeared everywhere as a representative of the progressive wing of the medical profession. Dorothy and Roy Porter have commented that Sigerist reduced the problems of social medicine to national health insurance, but this accusation seems to us unfair.[41] Sigerist was fairly realistic (if not overly optimistic) about the possibilities of medical and social reform in the United States; he understood that national health insurance was a 'conservative' measure but felt that it was the best that could be hoped for at the time.

One of Sigerist's projects intended to contribute to medical care reform was a series of articles, written for the short-lived left-liberal New York daily, *PM*, about group health plans around the United States.[42] The newspaper articles were written in a lively and popular style and leave no doubt of Sigerist's views about different aspects of medical care organization. Describing one health insurance plan, for example, he says: 'The plan has been blessed by all the bigwigs of organized medicine because it guarantees the free choice of physicians, in other words, permits the patient to consult incompetent doctors if he so desires.'[43]

Championing the issue of health insurance or 'socialized medicine' certainly gave Sigerist a reputation as a 'medical bolshevik', especially after 1939 when the reform impulses of the New Deal era seemed to have played themselves out. But whatever his theoretical views, which always tended toward the utopian, Sigerist was ready to dedicate himself to the political battles of his day. He worked on national health insurance committees as assiduously as he appeared at rallies for republican Spain and made anti-fascist speeches about European politics.[44]

Sigerist and many of his contemporaries perceived science and medicine as a positive and liberating force; science was constrained under capitalism, perverted under fascism, and would only be fully developed under socialism.[45] They believed that science and medical knowledge were themselves value-free but that the uses of science were determined by the structures of social and economic power. Capitalism thus thwarted the socially beneficial role of science by forcing it to serve the ends of private profit and military production rather than human needs. Science and technology – the forces of production – were the main motor of history; the contradiction between the development of these productive forces and outdated social relations would eventually lead to a new mode of production under socialism.

Different positions on the politics and epistemology of science may in part account for the surprising range of opinion that subsequent commentators have expressed about Sigerist's politics: he has been variously described as a liberal, a radical reformer, a Fabian, a socialist, a Marxist, a communist, and a 'twentieth-century philosopher'.[46]

Sigerist's speeches on medical care, reported enthusiastically in the popular press, and his two books on the Soviet Union would bring him trouble. In 1943, just two months after he had become a United States citizen, he was called before a Special Hearing of the Civil Service Commission, accused of being actively engaged in 'Communist Front Organizations' and of being 'very much interested and in sympathy with the Communist Form of Government'.[47] Sigerist explained that he had studied public health in Russia and had travelled there several times, and added, probably truthfully, that he had never been a member of the Communist Party.[48]

Sigerist's answers were deemed unsatisfactory. Several months later, he was told that his eligibility for government service had been cancelled because 'you do not measure up to the general standards of suitability and fitness maintained for government employees'.[49]

This was the beginning of the end of Sigerist's career in America. As he became aware of the increasing hostility of many medical colleagues and of the resistance of the university administration, now embarrassed by his political reputation and activities, he realized that his welcome in America had turned sour. He stayed in the United States for three more years but, as the political climate became steadily more unfriendly, he made plans to retire to Switzerland where he hoped to complete his masterwork, a comprehensive history of medicine in eight volumes.

Was Sigerist a Marxist? He was certainly influenced by Marxism and maintained his enthusiasm about the Soviet Union at least until late in his life. His first volume on the Soviet Union contains a lengthy discussion of dialectical materialism and the class struggle, written as though Sigerist were simultaneously trying to convince himself and his readers of the truth.[50] The text is somewhat self-consciously strained and lacks Sigerist's usually easy style. Intellectually accepting Marxist analyses, Sigerist was nonetheless by temperament an idealist, an inveterate personal and social optimist. Yet he was also capable of believing in 'iron laws of history' when they seemed to support his passionate desire for social progress. As he fervently informed one former student, 'History is developing with iron logic almost like a mathematical equation. The polarization of society is going on inexorably.'[51]

In his American period, Sigerist belonged to the penumbra of the Communist Party, a serious fellow-traveller, although he was probably too independent to join that organization. In his final years, when he was working on Indian medicine, he became very interested in Buddhism and vacillated between his older left-wing and adamantly anti-mystical views and a new curiosity about things spiritual. In the end, Sigerist is perhaps fully consistent only as an enthusiast – an intellectual who desired a grand vision of the future, who wanted to believe in a better world, and tried, in the ways he knew how, to help bring it into being.

In contrast to Sigerist, Rosen was not an activist by temperament, nor was he particularly attracted by Russian communism or the Communist Party of the United States. At different times in his life he might have characterized himself as a left-liberal or a social democrat; but there is no evidence that he was ever victimized for his political beliefs.[52] Whereas Sigerist was specifically ruled unsuitable for government service during the Second World War, Rosen joined the Army and was assigned to the medical intelligence service. For about two years between 1943 and

1945, he worked at the Surgeon-General's Office in Washington, frequently taking the opportunity to visit Sigerist in nearby Baltimore and becoming increasingly integrated into Sigerist's circle of protégés and students.

There is no doubt that Rosen was a Marxist, in the sense of regarding Marxism as the analytical tool most useful for understanding the social world. For a period in the 1930s and 1940s, even after he became immersed in American functionalist sociology, this is explicit in his writings;[53] later in his life, he was more eclectic, but it is evident that certain Marxian concepts continued to inform his approach to problems ranging from urban health to mental illness.

With his working class background, Rosen's path to Marxism was very different from Sigerist's. On the one hand, Marxism was an intellectual extension of his uneducated father's labour activism. On the other, Rosen's interest in Marxism was associated with his broad reading in German philosophy and sociology and with a set of intellectual interests quite divorced from any direct commitment to political activity. He found Marxism useful as a theoretical approach to history – one that could potentially help set the intellectual content of medicine and public health within a broader social framework.

Rosen took Marxism seriously enough in the early 1940s that he wrote two essays – his only extant work not concerned with public health or history of medicine – articulating his understanding of Marx's view of history. In these pieces, he argued that Marx had rejected simplistic economic determinism, and that the core of Marxism was a much richer and more sophisticated view of the relations between material production and the broader culture. He submitted these pieces to *Science and Society* – a scholarly journal friendly to Marxism whose editorial staff at that time included people associated with the Communist Party, USA – but they were rejected and remain unpublished.[54]

Despite some political differences with Sigerist himself, Rosen shared with Sigerist and his group of disciples a deep interest in social medicine. He planned a book that would trace its history; by thus appropriating the role of historian of social medicine, he hoped to be able to specify its intellectual lineage and thereby define its content. In 1947, as a preliminary exercise, he published an essay on the history of social medicine.[55] Although his continuing research in this area yielded some important detailed empirical studies, he never completed a projected book-length treatment of the subject. Long after Sigerist had returned to Europe, he continued to encourage Rosen to publish a book, or collection of essays, on the history of social medicine and to continue working in this area. Rosen, by now embedded in the world of public health, chose instead to use much of the material he had collected in his classic text, *A History of Public Health*.[56]

Rosen, as the intellectual, upwardly mobile son of a trade unionist, tried to remain faithful to his roots by translating political activity into political theorizing. His early attraction to Sigerist as a politically-informed intellectual lasted thoughout his career as Rosen continued to write to Sigerist as both mentor and friend; it is clear from their lengthy correspondence that Rosen both desired and needed Sigerist's continuing praise and approval. Rosen also wanted what seemed to come naturally to Sigerist – to be financially comfortable, to be more socially at ease, to be a recognized scholar, to influence others, and to be appreciated and acclaimed for his accomplishments. Rosen was more insecure and less outgoing than Sigerist, and, as a political person, he chose a less activist path. He restricted himself to scholarship and writing, while often urging others to become politically active.

## Disease and Health as Social Phenomena

In moving from Germany to the United States, Sigerist had gradually made a transition from a cultural, even romantic, view of disease to a more materialist view. As Temkin notes, Sigerist, in his Leipzig period, tended to be both a romantic and a relativist.[57] In some of his more sweeping historical pronouncements, he argued that all cultural manifestations of a period, including that period's most characteristic diseases, were expressions of its cultural 'style'.[58] This somewhat vague, if provocative, approach worked best with forms of medical thought, where one could trace the parallels between medical ideas and philosophical, political, theological, and artistic preoccupations. William Harvey's work on the circulation of the blood, for example, could be related to the baroque artists' fascination with movement.[59] Some of Sigerist's later essays in *Civilization and Disease* take up the theme of the relationship between disease, medicine, and other aspects of culture – although not, perhaps, with the degree of philosophical abandon he expressed in the context of the German youth movement during the happier years of the Weimar Republic.[60]

Once Sigerist had arrived in the United States, the idea that disease was created by social and economic conditions began to assume a central importance in his writing. In the midst of the Depression, he increasingly emphasized the idea that poverty and malnutrition were major causes of disease. As he observed the organization of workers, applauded evidence of workers' resistance,[61] and read Marxist economic texts, Sigerist began to pay special attention to occupational health. In 1936, he outlined a programme for the study of occupational medicine. Rather than value civilizations according to their artistic achievements, while forgetting the 'blood and tears of thousands of human beings' who had laboured to build them, he proposed to judge each civilization by the living and working conditions of the masses.[62] He persuaded Rosen to write a history of miners' diseases; it was Rosen, rather than Sigerist, who would take up the serious study of occupational medicine.

Sigerist's more materialist view of disease suffused the text of *Socialized Medicine in the Soviet Union*, and no doubt fitted well with his, and his Soviet hosts', view of the future of health under socialism. Sigerist stressed the need to protect the health of industrial workers and also outlined broad new categories of 'social diseases' caused by poor economic conditions.[63] He argued that venereal diseases were linked to prostitution and ultimately caused by the lack of economic opportunities for women.[64] Alcoholism and crime were social diseases resulting from poverty and unemployment; the 'treatment' for crime was full employment.[65]

At some of his more enthusiastic moments, Sigerist was willing to diagnose any social behaviour of which he disapproved as pathology. 'War', he said, 'is a social disease, like poverty or crime'.[66] Similarly, 'excessive individualism' was pathological. Individuals who insisted on their freedom at the expense of the social good were like cancer cells: 'As soon as a cell-group begins to lead an independent life without regard to the rest of the cells, a malignant tumour develops which will destroy the whole organism. This applies to society as well'.[67] The socially-minded physician would therefore be concerned with the total range of individual behaviour and social organization and could give medical counsel on such matters as war, crime, and excessive individualism.

Sigerist was clearly searching for a set of explanations of disease that fitted with his developing social and political philosophy. He succinctly presented his general view of the relation between social conditions and disease in 'The History of Medical History': 'When we study the history of disease we will soon find that its incidence is determined primarily by the economic and social conditions of a society.... The mode of production and the working conditions are largely responsible for whether a man's life will be healthy or not.... In other words: we must be thoroughly familiar with economic and social history before we can approach the history of disease.'[68] This view provided an obvious justification for a new kind of history of medicine; no longer the story of the 'great doctors', it was to be the history of civilization itself.[69] A generally Marxist approach (a Marxism more notable for the general ebullience of Sigerist's cultural and philosophical musings than for any strict adherence to orthodoxy), linked the material world of work, living conditions, and the experience of illness to the physicians' world of medical theory and social practice.[70]

Sigerist's analysis of disease as a social phenomenon interested Rosen; and Sigerist certainly gave the younger man much impetus in this direction by proposing that he work on the history of occupational health. Rosen was pleased to take on this project because it provided obvious examples of the social causation of disease. The correspondence between the two men shows that Rosen independently came to be concerned with the physician's ability to recognize the social etiology of organic disease. Rosen's view, best expressed in his theoretical 'Aperçu',[71] and based on his understanding of Marxist notions of class relations and the nature of history, was that a new, social, history of medicine must be dialectical and founded on an investigation of the economic structure of society. With Sigerist's encouragement, he applied this class perspective in a series of empirical studies including his book on miners' diseases and an early article on the health of seamen.[72]

Rejecting the ontological view of disease, Rosen argued that diseases were intelligible only within their social context.[73] He criticized an older historiography of medicine for viewing the patient as 'an accident in the history of the disease',[74] and insisted that patient, healer, and disease all be understood in their class context. This theme, first developed early in his career in connection with his work on social etiology, was informed by Marx's idea that history was made by human beings acting in accord with their own interests; it continually reappeared in Rosen's later writings.[75] Rosen's point of view is also evident in his late work on mental illness, in which he demonstrated that madness and irrationality are generally connected either to conflicts in social role, or to oppression or social calamity.[76]

Sigerist and Rosen both liked to quote Rudolf Virchow: 'Medicine is a social science, and politics is nothing else but medicine on a large scale.'[77] It followed that the physician treating patients must be able to perceive the social roots of their illnesses as well as the social conditions needed for recovery. Sigerist in particular wanted the physician to go further than simply an intellectual understanding of the social causation of disease and he urged medical students to become activists and work to bring about the social conditions necessary for health. Because physicians best understood the social relations of health and disease, they should take a leading role in social reform.[78] In his diaries, Sigerist frequently wrote about students' enthusiastic responses to his lectures and seminars and he understood his inspirational role for a younger generation as one of his more important political tasks and influences:

> The physician ... who is familiar with (working) conditions and knows the evil effects of such work on the people's health must assume leadership in the struggle for the improvement of conditions: His concern is not whether an enterprise is profitable or not. His place is with the workers, whose protector he is.[79]

Sigerist was somewhat ambivalent about the precise relationship of the 'new physician' to the working class; sometimes he was described as leader, sometimes as protector, sometimes as ally, and sometimes as expert adviser. Sigerist was certainly persuaded of the social and political value of medical experts to any popular movement; he also wanted to inspire his medical audiences to adopt a more activist and heroic image of their own historical possibilities. In general, he was quite uncritical (and unself-critical) about the role of intellectuals, physicians, and other professionals in left-wing or other popular movements. He did, however, caution members of his medical audiences that medical leadership would accomplish little unless the working class followed; the entire population would have to be 'permanently mobilized' in a people's war for health.[80]

Following Sigerist's lead, Rosen began collecting activist physicians for a kind of inspirational gallery of heroes that could be used to convince doctors of the long and honourable tradition of social critics within their profession. The first significant article he wrote, independent of a specific suggestion by Sigerist, was on Jacob Henle, the liberal revolutionary and theorist of contagionism.[81] Rosen hoped that the Henle article would be only the beginning of a major project on 'the physician as agitator'. He next intended to work on Georg Buchner,[82] but soon broadened his perspective to include four or even six such doctors.[83] Eventually, in his rambling, would-be seminal, 1947 essay on the history of social medicine,[84] Rosen took on a long series of physicians, from Rudolf Virchow to John Ryle, who might reasonably be claimed as social critics. As Dorothy and Roy Porter have noted, however, Rosen in this paper ignored all contradictions in their positions so as to construct what he hoped would be a seamless web of social commitment.[85]

Trying to demonstrate that the most astute physicians and the most successful healers were those who recognized the social etiology of disease,[86] Rosen constructed his pantheon of social medicine by appropriating all the famous and not-so-famous doctors he could find who had given the slightest attention to social factors in disease causation. He even enlisted William Osler to the cause of social medicine, citing Osler's recognition of the occupational origin of lung diseases among miners.[87] The purpose of Rosen's 60-page paper was to provide social medicine with a long and distinguished tradition and thus help strengthen the currents of social medical thought within contemporary medicine.[88]

Through the late 1930s and 1940s, while building his pantheon, Rosen tried to refine his approach to medicine as a social activity and the physician as social activist. In a 1944 essay he discussed both medical and non-medical advocates and opponents of factory legislation in New England; but he summarized his findings rather vaguely, indicating merely that he had presented some empirical evidence of 'the roles played by physicians and health problems in social criticism and social change'.[89] By this time, Rosen had pretty much determined that his own role was not to be as physician-agitator, but as historian. In 1941 Sigerist had invited him to deliver a paper on these issues at the Johns Hopkins Medical History Club.[90] In his talk, published as 'Disease and Social Criticism', Rosen attempted to construct an historical description of a self-consciously critical and reformist fraction of the medical profession, with the aim of convincing contemporaries that they should join the group.[91] To historians he assigned the role of pointing out the social relations of disease in order to convert open-minded physicians into social critics.[92]

One of Sigerist's most activist disciples, Milton Roemer, reacted sharply to some of the flaws in the argument. He wrote to Rosen, and subsequently published a paper in Sigerist's *Bulletin*, arguing that 'although it is actually in the interest of medicine and public health to promote social criticism', 'the class basis of the medical profession tends to drive the profession into the very opposite ideology'. [93] Rosen could not, however, afford to pay much attention to this critique – it undermined too much of the joint project he shared with Sigerist of persuading the medical profession to take a leading role in progressive causes.

Both Rosen and Sigerist lapsed into idealism whenever they contemplated the social role of the physician, hoping to use the social history of medicine as inspiration and as propaganda to prepare the way for a new era of medicine that would be social in outlook and preventive in orientation. The social history of medicine was to inspire physicians and turn them into social reformers, radicals, and revolutionaries; the new physicians would then help to create a truly social medicine of the future.

Sigerist often announced that the medicine of the future would be preventive in orientation; physicians would not only heal the sick but would work to keep people well. If, as he had often stated, the problems of disease were primarily caused by social and economic conditions, what were the implications of this insight for the future of medicine and for the task of the physician? Were physicians merely to treat the symptoms consequent upon social problems or were they to attempt to prevent disease at its source? In many of his writings, Sigerist followed his own positions to their logical consequence: since disease was created by social and economic conditions, preventive medicine would require social, economic, and political transformations. Here, Sigerist took inspiration from Rudolf Virchow and the German health movement of 1848, although he was critical of that movement for failing to involve the mass of the population in the struggle for health. Health reforms, he said, could not be carried out by physicians on behalf of the people; the population must be mobilized to fight a 'people's war' for health.

> The great, forceful, and promising German health movement with its far-reaching programme had broken down. Why? Chiefly because it was a movement of liberal middle-class physicians for the people but without the people....The war against disease and for health cannot be fought by physicians alone. It is a people's war in which the entire population must be mobilized permanently.[94]

Rosen took one step back from Sigerist's vision of the physician as revolutionary. He assigned himself, a non-practising physician, the role of historian, who would not be politically active, but who would convince his professional colleagues to be social critics and agitators.[95]

Ironically, it was Sigerist, who had a full-time professorship as a historian of medicine, who most enjoyed the role of reformer, agitator, and visionary – and who insisted on exercising it in the face of the disapproval of many professional colleagues. Rosen, who longed to make his living by working as a historian, was forced to accept paying jobs that obliged him to intervene in health politics and articulate positions on the future of health care.

When he learned of Sigerist's impending retirement early in

1947, Rosen had initially been hopeful of succeeding his mentor at Johns Hopkins; but by the time Sigerist left, Rosen knew that this was not likely. The most honest appraisal of his chances was provided by Erwin Ackerknecht, who had become Rosen's close friend while working at the Institute during the War. 'This holy institution', Ackerknecht warned Rosen about Hopkins, 'has not yet had a Jewish chair holder.'[96] Moreover, the administration and trustees of Hopkins had had enough of Sigerist's advocacy of socialized medicine and friendliness toward the Soviet Union. Rosen, who never joined any political organization, and whose concern for reforms in health care always remained a matter of scholarship rather than activism, was tarred with the same brush. But, regardless of his politics or other qualities, Rosen had once more come face-to-face with institutional anti-Semitism.[97]

With the Hopkins job closed to him and no other positions likely to open in the history of medicine, Rosen resolved to continue his historical scholarship on his own time, while earning his living in public health.[98] He had long since given up his private medical practice and was now rising within the bureaucracy of the New York City Department of Health. In 1949, he was appointed Director of Health Education, where he supervised public relations and developed exhibitions, radio broadcasts, and publications.[99] He left the city government in 1950 to found the department of Health Education and Preventive Services at the Health Insurance Plan of Greater New York (HIP).[100]

HIP, conceived as a medical care programme for families of moderate income enrolled through employee groups, had begun operations in 1947. While Rosen was working there, it consisted of about 30 semi-autonomous medical partnerships, compensated by capitation payments derived from enrollees' premiums, and co-ordinated through a central office. In some ways HIP resembled the health maintenance organizations (HMOs) that have developed in the US since the 1970s, but many of the planners and early administrators of HIP regarded it as a small-scale, privately organized model for a government-based national health system – in effect a pilot project for social medicine in the United States.[101] Not only was medical care at HIP based on the principles of prepayment and group practice, but medical care for the ill was only a part of its mission. Preventive medicine and health education were central to HIP's purpose and ideology, and Rosen, as Director of Health Education and Preventive Services, was responsible for developing an innovative and effective programme, faithful to the general principles espoused by Sigerist and other medical care reformers. Rosen took his administrative responsibilities seriously. His passion remained history and his goal a faculty position, but he realized that he had achieved real status within the world of public health – a position from which he could attempt to apply the theories and principles of social medicine that he had long advocated.[102]

Rosen became increasingly active in the American Public Health Association while working for the Department of Health and HIP. He was invited to join the Editorial Board of the *American Journal of Public Health* in 1948, and as a national figure, regularly contributed to the *AJPH* and participated at APHA meetings. He was appointed editor of the journal in 1957 and remained in that position until 1973. His paid editorial position at the *AJPH* allowed Rosen to leave HIP and take a full-time faculty position at the Columbia University School of Public Health, where he had taught part-time since 1951. In 1969, after having turned down offers from other universities farther from New York City, Rosen acceded to the chair of history of medicine at Yale – where he also accepted an appointment as professor of public health and epidemiology.

During the time that Rosen presided over the *AJPH*, he perceived that expanded federal programmes were undermining the responsibilities and importance of state and local health agencies, the traditional base of support of the APHA. As public health work in America became increasingly fragmented, he struggled against tendencies toward narrow specialization and tried to forge a broad vision of what public health could be.[103] As editor, Rosen happily published a steadily increasing number of papers by women; he regretted that, as more papers were coming from the universities, fewer were coming from health workers in the field. In an effort to broaden the scope of the journal, he initiated new features such as 'Public Health and the Law' and 'Public Health Then and Now' – the latter an attempt to cultivate a sense of professional solidarity among public health workers by providing them evidence of a common heritage.[104]

The editorials that Rosen prepared during his 16 years at the journal were consistently well-written expressions of his social and political commitment, his understanding of history,[105] and his vision of the future. In early editorials, he criticized those who would prefer to moralize about 'charity abuse' than provide medical care to indigent patients and he expressed cautious optimism about the decline in infectious diseases in the developing world.[106] Using historical examples such as Britain's adoption of national health insurance in 1911, he urged public health workers to play a political role and to collaborate with social scientists.[107] He wanted to expand public health concern to include traffic safety and to regain public health control over air pollution, housing inspection, and industrial hygiene.[108]

In the November, 1969 issue of the *AJPH*, Rosen returned to a central theme of any system of social medicine: the problem of universal health coverage. Reviewing a proposal from organized labour that would have extended the 1965 medical care for the aged programme to the entire American population, Rosen complained that a market-based medical care system might have been appropriate for Germany in the 1880s or Britain in 1911, but was not sufficient to address the needs of the United States in his day: 'The basic fact is that scientific knowledge and complex technology have created a situation where the economic, social and political mechanisms upon which we have depended for the distribution of health services are no longer adequate.'[109] Framed in more respectable language, this is exactly what Sigerist and his disciples had been saying some 35 years earlier.

Rejecting the market as incapable of guaranteeing adequate health care, Rosen argued that health insurance should be centrally and rationally organized in relationship to demographic factors, manpower planning, and equity. Just as he opposed purely individualistic notions of responsibility for health and disease, so too was he wary of voluntarism and decentralization.[110] Coming from an older socialist and public health tradition, Rosen emphasized the rational basis of global, strategic planning. In a sense, he had become a typical mid-century planner who believed that enlightened public leaders (most often liberal Democrats) could solve social problems using efficiently organized government bureaucracies. Ultimately, for Rosen, it was the state that must guarantee health through such measures as health education, housing reform, occupational medicine, food inspection, and the provision of medical care.

## Conclusion

Sigerist and Rosen left a significant legacy in the history of medicine. Sigerist's initial interest in using history to illuminate the problems of contemporary medicine had led him to propose and outline a new approach to the historiography of medicine. In Leipzig, his student Erwin Ackerknecht exemplified this programme in his dissertation on medicine and the German revolution of 1848.[111] In the United States, George Rosen eagerly accepted the task of helping to create the new social history of medicine.

Sigerist's historical work can be divided into archival and empirical studies (mainly on the Middle Ages and the early modern period), programmatic and synthetic works outlining the new social history of medicine, and writings on the organization of medical care in the United States and the Soviet Union. Many of his works, from the biographical sketches of *The Great Doctors* to the broad cultural essays of *Civilization and Disease*, were oriented to young physicians and served to present medicine in a new light and to situate it in a broad and often inspirational context.[112] Sigerist also ranged from short, playful essays on such matters as truffles and tea, to serious forays into the sociology and economics of medicine.[113]

Rosen went beyond Sigerist in developing a corpus of scholarly works – on occupational diseases, urban health, mental illness, and public health – whose foundation was an appreciation of the social character of disease and medicine.[114] During the 1930s, Rosen attempted to formulate a theory of the historiography of medicine based on his understanding of Marx, Mannheim, and other authors he had come to appreciate while a student in Germany. At the same time, he started work on a series of empirical studies on the role of the physician, the social etiology of disease, and the economic basis of medical practice. By the mid-1940s Rosen had envisaged the culmination of these projects as a treatise on the history of social medicine.

Disappointed in his aspirations of finding a position in medical history, Rosen determined to make a career in academic public health just as the post-war social medicine movement was evaporating. He then applied his findings in social medicine toward public health, ultimately producing his idiosyncratic but authoritative *A History of Public Health* in 1958.[115]

The product of what might be called Rosen's 'late period', the last 20 years of his life, shows no break with his earlier work. If he was less enthusiastic about applying Marxism to medical history, his work still implicitly demonstrated the lessons he had learned as a young man, not only from his extracurricular readings in Germany, but also from his graduate training in sociology at Columbia. He continued writing on the history of occupational health;[116] while his work on social medicine and public health led to *Preventive Medicine in the United States* [117] and his magisterial essay on health in the Victorian city.[118] The project that began with *Fees and Fee Bills* [119] in the early 1940s was concluded with the posthumous *The Structure of American Medical Practice*.[120]

Even Rosen's project on the history of irrationality and mental illness, manifested as a series of essays that began appearing in 1959,[121] represents no break with the motivations or methods of the earnest medical student or intern of the 1930s. In this corpus Rosen tried to understand the function of irrational behaviour in society and to identify the social and political origins of madness and irrationality. Not surprisingly, as in his work on social medicine and public health, Rosen frequently turned to Rudolf Virchow to illustrate his points about the social basis of madness.[122]

Henry Sigerist and his protégé George Rosen were successful in creating the social history of medicine in the United States. Sigerist built the professional structure of the history of medicine, including the American Association of the History of Medicine, the Johns Hopkins Institute of the History of Medicine, and the *Bulletin of the History of Medicine;* he helped Rosen launch the *Journal of the History of Medicine and Allied Sciences.* Rosen, extending the work of Sigerist, left a body of work for the new crop of social historians, many of them products of the 1960s who were coming of age when he died in 1977.[123] The work of Sigerist and Rosen articulated the possibility of a 'left' history of medicine and opened a space for broader, more critical, and more inclusive social approaches to historical scholarship. Together, their work helped redefine the history of medicine in the United States.

On the other hand, if the purpose of medical history was to influence the medical profession, to become a 'living force in contemporary medicine' and to prepare the way for a new socially-oriented medicine, that larger aim has failed – or perhaps, is yet unfulfilled. A significant group of physicians who were inspired by Sigerist's views did try to implement his programme in medical care, social medicine, and public health. George Rosen, Milton Roemer, Leslie Falk, Milton Terris, George Silver, Cecil Sheps, and many others, working within public health and medicine, tried to live the vision that Sigerist projected.[124] As seen from 1993, the best efforts of these physician agitators have failed – even what Sigerist termed the 'conservative reform' of national health insurance is perennially being proposed and perennially rejected. While the social causes of disease are ever more evident, they are usually addressed, if at all, by individually-oriented, high technology medicine. In recent years, the tendency to blame individuals for causing disease through 'unhealthy behaviours' has become an American obsession.

Henry Sigerist, whose picture was on the cover of *Time* magazine in 1939, is now little known outside the community of medical historians and the left wing of public health, where Rosen too, is best remembered. Both Sigerist and Rosen, we may conclude, were successful as historians but were far too optimistic about what they thought the history of medicine could accomplish.

## Notes

1. Nora Sigerist Beeson, (ed.), *Henry E. Sigerist: Autobiographical Writings* (Montreal: McGill University Press, 1966), 37.
2. This and other details come from the rich account of Sigerist's early career in Marcel H. Bickel, 'Sigerist's Family Background and Early Years in Paris and Zurich, 1891–1925', in *Making Medical History: The Life and Work of Henry E. Sigerist,* Elizabeth Fee and Theodore M. Brown (eds), (Baltimore: Johns Hopkins University Press, in preparation).
3. N. Sigerist Beeson *op. cit.* (ref. 1), 59–60.
4. H. E. Sigerist, 'Studien und Texte zur frühmittelalterlichen Rezeptliteratur', *Studien zur Geschichtc der Medizin herausgegeben von der Puschmann-Stiftung an der Universität Leipzig* (Barth, Leipzig: Heft 13, Verlag Johann Ambrosius, 1923).
5. Bickel, *op. cit.* (ref. 2).
6. Owsei Temkin, personal communication. See also Owsei Temkin, 'The Double Face of Janus', in *The Double Face of Janus and Other Essays* (Baltimore: Johns Hopkins University Press, 1977), 3–37.
7. For a detailed account of the activities of the Leipzig Institute, see Ingrid Kästner, 'Henry Ernest Sigerist: The Leipzig Period, 1925–1932', in *op. cit.* (ref. 2).
8. H. H. Walser and H. M. Koelbing, 'Introduction: An Interview with Erwin H. Ackerknecht', in Ackerknecht, *Medicine and Ethnology: Selected Essays* (Bern: Verlag Hans Huber, 1971), 10; Ackerknecht, 'Recollections of a Former Leipzig Student', *Journal of the History of Medicine and Allied Sciences,* xiii (1958), 147–50.
9. Sigerist Beeson, *op. cit.* (ref. 1) 81.
10. Information on Rosen's early life in this and the following paragraphs is abstracted from a series of interviews by Edward Morman and from Saul Benison's essay 'Dr George Rosen: An Appreciation', in *Healing and History: Essays for George Rosen,* Charles Rosenberg (ed.) (New York: Science History, 1979), 242–51. Benison has told us that everything he wrote of Rosen's childhood was derived from conversations he had had with Rosen. Other interviews were held with Dr Beate Caspari Rosen (Rosen's widow, interviewed 9 and 12 June, 1991), Dr Thomas Patrick (medical school classmate of Rosen's, interviewed 21 June, 1991), Dr Louis Schneider (classmate of Rosen in high school, college and medical school, interviewed 27 June,

1991), Arnold Koslow (Rosen's former-son-in-law, interviewed 22 August, 1991), and Susan Rosen-Olejarz (Rosen's daughter, interviewed 8 September, 1991).

11. There are many discussions of the intellectual atmosphere and student life at City College in the first half of this century. One that might particularly help illuminate George Rosen's experience is David Hollinger, *Morris Raphael Cohen and the Scientific Ideal* (Cambridge, Mass.: MIT Press, 1975).
12. Rosen's habits in high school and college were reported by Dr Louis Schneider. Susan Rosen-Olejarz confirms that her father's youthful enthusiasm for reading almost anything never abated.
13. Dr Schneider estimates that less than five per cent of the approximately 400 pre-medical students who graduated from City College in 1926 were admitted to medical school in the United States.
14. Apparently several dozen young American men were studying medicine in Berlin when Rosen arrived. From what is now known of these expatriates, all but one (an African American) were Jews who had been excluded from American medical schools.
15. Erich Meyerhoff, a German Jewish emigré who got to know Rosen in the 1950s, has remarked that Rosen 'knew everything there was to know about German sociology' (interview with Edward Morman, 17 June,1991). Arnold Koslow has alluded to Rosen's familiarity with German philosophy, and Saul Benison claims that 'knowing German poetry and literature can provide an insight into George Rosen'. Beate Caspari-Rosen noted Rosen's impressions of the German health care system, and Rosen discusses this himself in 'Medicine under Hitler', *Bulletin of the New York Academy of Medicine,* xxv (1949), 125–9.
16. Rosen complained about having a clergyman deliver an invocation at the banquet of the 1975 meeting of the American Association of the History of Medicine. 'Not only am I a non-believer, but I object strenuously to the pouring out of "Christian love" at a time when any such mention is almost obscene. The same would apply to Rabbis, Mullahs or any other type of cleric.' Rosen to Lester King, 12 May, 1975. Yale University Library, George Rosen Papers (hereinafter GRP), Addition of 28 August, 1978, Box I. Beate Caspari-Rosen also reports that George did not want a religious wedding, and took out all his anger at being obliged to do so by crushing the traditional glass with great fury.
17. According to Arnold Koslow, Rosen, who was literate in Hebrew, enjoyed presiding over the ritual Passover dinner, with its prayers, blessings and readings.

18. This introduction may have been a friendly and complimentary gesture from Diepgen to Sigerist; Sigerist had been deeply disappointed when Diepgen was awarded the Berlin chair which Sigerist himself had hoped to attain.
19. *Die Aufnahme der Endeckung William Beaumont's durch die europäische Medizin* (Berlin: Ebering, 1935); Rosen later translated the thesis and published it as *The Reception of William Beaumont's Discovery in Europe* (New York: Schuman's, 1942).
20. The entire correspondence between Sigerist and Rosen, from Rosen's initial letter through Sigerist's departure from Baltimore in 1947, is preserved in the records of the Institute of the History of Medicine at the Alan Mason Chesney Archives of the Johns Hopkins Medical Institutions. The 11 letters between them from 16 November, 1933 through 29 October, 1934 concern Rosen's medical thesis; Sigerist declares the thesis 'excellent' in his letter of 29 October, 1934.
21. Sigerist's position as holder of the only history of medicine chair in the United States made him the natural person for Rosen to turn to for guidance, and his editorship of the *Bulletin of the History of Medicine* made him the natural person to whom Rosen would send his own writing. Owsei Temkin acknowledged that Rosen's relationship with Sigerist resembled his own when he was enrolled as Sigerist's student at Leipzig (personal interview, 22 July, 1991).
22. Rosen's first piece in the *Bulletin* was 'John Elliotson – Physician and Hypnotist', published in the 'Notes and Comments' section of the July, 1936 issue.
23. George Rosen, *The History of Miners' Diseases: A Medical and Social Interpretation* (New York: Schuman's, 1943). Sigerist proposed that Rosen investigate miners' diseases just around the time that he was preparing his own lecture on the history of occupational disease (Sigerist to Rosen, 13 October, 1936).
24. See, for example, 'A Note on the Reception of the Stethoscope in England', *Bulletin of the History of Medicine,* vii (1939), 93–4; or 'Left-Wing Puritanism and Science', *Bulletin of the History of Medicine,* xv (1944), 375–80.
25. There are many examples of Rosen's appetite for hard work. As an intern, and while working on one topic already approved by Sigerist, he requested another, since 'I have time to work at two problems simultaneously'. Rosen to Sigerist, 6 October, 1936. For Rosen's continuing requests for books from the Institute Library, see, for example, Rosen to Sigerist (2 February, 1937, 17 March, 1937, 25 May, 1938, 6 January, 1939), Rosen to Hope Trebing (27 September, 1937), and Rosen to Genevieve Miller (23 February, 1947).

26. Rosen to Sigerist, 2 December, 1934.
27. Rosen did not remain in practice long, taking part-time and ultimately full-time salaried positions with the New York City Department of Health. People who were very fond of Rosen acknowledged that he did not have a temperament suitable for medical practice (interview with Susan Rosen-Olejarz, 8 September, 1991; see also Benison, *Dr George Rosen: An Appreciation,* 244).
28. Rosen to Sigerist, 3 December, 1937; Sigerist to Rosen, 17 December, 1937.
29. Rosen to Sigerist, 28 December, 1937; Sigerist to Rosen, 24 March, 1938.
30. Fritz Kahn, *Our Sex Life: A Guide and Counselor for Everyone* (1939); Arthur Rosenberg, *Democracy and Socialism* (1939); Fritz Kahn, *Man in Structure and Function* (1943); and Philip Frankl, *Einstein, His Life and Times* (1947).
31. *The Reception of William Beaumont's Discovery* (1942); *The History of Miners' Diseases* (1943); and *The Specialization of Medicine with Particular Reference to Ophthalmology* (New York: Froben, 1944).
32. Walter Pagel, for example, had lost his job and was working at the Pasteur Institute without salary. Henry E. Sigerist, Diary, 13 June, 1933.
33. H. E. Sigerist, Diary, 19 July, 1933. Yale University Library, H. E. Sigerist Papers, Addition (June, 1987), Biographical Data and Memorabilia, Group 788, Box 1.
34. Sigerist recorded in his diary: 'Adolf Meyer and Mrs. Meyer came to see us. They are in St Moritz. He is just back from Russia and most enthusiastic about what he saw particularly the psychiatric service ... I was extremely interested in all he said. There is no doubt that Russia is a unique opportunity. There are new ideas, new trends in all fields and while we talk they act there. In the medicine of the fascist countries I didn't find any new ideas. They are just following the beaten tracks, while Russia is opening up new horizons. I must go there, see and study a world in *statu nascendi.*' 22 July, 1933.
35. H. E. Sigerist, Diary, 6 August, 1933.
36. H. E. Sigerist, *American Medicine* (New York: W.W. Norton, 1934).
37. H. E. Sigerist, Diary, 20 July, 1933.
38. In 1937, after his first two summer trips to Russia, Sigerist published *Socialized Medicine in the Soviet Union* (New York: W. W. Norton, 1937).
39. H. E. Sigerist, Diary, 28 November, 1933.
40. Committee on the Costs of Medical Care, *Medical Care for the American People: The Final Report of the Committee on the Costs of Medical Care* (Chicago: University of Chicago Press, 1932).
41. Dorothy Porter and Roy Porter, 'What Was Social Medicine? An Historiographical Essay', *Journal of Historical Sociology*, i (1989), 90–106.

42. 'Dr Sigerist Surveys the Health Plan at the Endicott-Johnson Shoe Factory: Staff of 100, Three Medical Centers Care for 50,000 Workers and Their Families', *PM,* 15 July, 1940, 25; 'Dr Sigerist Compares and Analyzes Three Upstate Group Health Plans: Visits Industrial Plants in Binghamton ... Reports Results of Survey in Detail', *PM,* 17 July, 1940, 27; 'Dr Sigerist Finds Utica Health Plan Costly to Members for What It Gives: He Views Similar Plans as Fee Insurance Rather Than Health Insurance', *PM,* 19 July, 1940, 27; '"Ideal Rural Hospital" Discovered at Cooperstown, N.Y., by Dr Sigerist: He Says Local Health Plan Similar to That of Bassett Hospital Is Workable for Others', *PM,* 22 July, 1940, 27; 'Dr Sigerist Finds Greenbelt Health Plan Excellent But Project Group Too Small for Complete Treatment', *PM,* 22 July, 1940, 27; 'Dr Sigerist Examines Health Plan Set Up by CIO Detroit Auto Workers', *PM,* 26 July, 1940, 27. Sigerist planned to compile these articles into a book, to be entitled *Medical Service Plans in the United States,* but like many of his other ambitious schemes, this project was never completed.
43. 'Dr Sigerist Compares and Analyzes Three Upstate Group Health Plans: Visits Industrial Plants in Binghamton ... Reports Results of Survey in Detail', *PM,* 17 July, 1940, 27.
44. Sigerist's support for the Spanish republic and general anti-fascist politics brought him to the penumbra of the Communist Party, USA. He organized or participated in the Soviet-American Friendship League, the Physicians Forum, the Soviet-American Medical Association, and the Committees for National Health Insurance.
45. P. J. Kuznick, *Beyond the Laboratory: Scientists as Political Activists in 1930s America* (Chicago: University of Chicago Press, 1987); G. Werskey, *The Visible College: The Collective Biography of British Scientific Socialists of the 1930s* (New York: Holt, Rinehart & Winston, 1978).
46. See, for example, R. Frankenberg, 'Functionalism and After? Theory and Developments in Social Science Applied to the Health Field', *International Journal of Health Services,* iv (1974), 411–27; M. Terris, 'The Contributions of Henry E. Sigerist to Health Service Organization', *Milbank Memorial Fund Quarterly,* liii (1975), 489–530; F. G. Vescia, 'Henry E. Sigerist: The Years in America', *Medizinhistorisches Journal,* xiv (1979), 218–32; G. Rosen, 'Toward a Historical Sociology of Medicine: The Endeavor of Henry E. Sigerist', *Bulletin of the History of Medicine,* xxxii (1958), 500–16.
47. Fourth United States Civil Service Region Investigations Division, 'Report of Partial Hearing and Special Hearing', 15 November, 1943. Yale University Library, H. E. Sigerist Papers, Professional

Activities, Group 788, Series II, Box 31.

48. *Ibid.*, 2. The accusations against Sigerist included the fact that he had given speeches to 'subversive' audiences, had written articles for the *New Masses* and *Soviet Russia Today*, and had been quoted in *The Daily Worker* and *The Sunday Worker*. He had been a sponsor of the American League for Peace and Democracy and the American Committee for Democracy and Intellectual Freedom. To these, and other similar accusations, Sigerist gave measured and intelligent responses, concluding with the summary of his position: 'I never was connected with the Communist Party and ... am not a member and I feel absolutely independent. As far as medicine is concerned I feel that everybody should have the best medical care that the country can provide' (*ibid.*, 4).
49. United States Civil Service Commission to Henry E. Sigerist, 3 June, 1944. Yale University Library, H. E. Sigerist Papers, Professional Activities, Group 788, Series II, Box 31.
50. *Op. cit.* (ref. 38).
51. H. E. Sigerist to Leslie A. Falk, 12 June, 1948, 1. H. E. Sigerist Papers, Yale University Library, General Correspondence, 1947–57, Group 788, Series 1, Box 11.
52. In the summer of 1992 we asked the FBI, under the Freedom of Information Act, to send us photocopies of material the agency may have collected on Rosen; but as of December, 1992 the only response has been a form letter suggesting that many more months may still pass before the request is fulfilled.
53. 'According to that theory which appears most promising for the historical investigation of occupational medicine the productive forces at any given time are the basis of the social structure of that time.' Rosen, 'On the Historical Investigation of Occupational Diseases: An Aperçu'. *Bulletin of the History of Medicine,* v (1937), 943.
54. George Rosen, 'Some Pre-Suppositions of Marxian Socialism' and 'An Analysis of Certain Sections of Marx's *Kritik der Hegelschen Rechtsphilosophie*' (GRP, addition of 15 June, 1979, Box 1). *Science and Society* rejected these essays 'because of dire lack of space.' Bernhard Stern to Rosen, 23 July, 1942 (GRP, Addition of October 26, 1978). In the files adjacent to where he left these typescripts are several contemporary left-wing newspaper articles and pamphlets, dating to the 1930s, with annotations in Rosen's hand.
55. George Rosen, 'What is Social Medicine? A Genetic Analysis of the Concept', *Bulletin of the History of Medicine,* xxi (1947), 674–733.
56. George Rosen, *A History of Public Health* (New York: MD Publications, 1958) incorporated many of the findings of his articles

on social medicine, and is probably a substitute for the planned but unwritten book. See Edward T. Morman, 'George Rosen, Public Health and History', in Rosen, *A History of Public Health,* reprint edition (Baltimore: Johns Hopkins University Press, 1993).

57. Owsei Temkin, 'H. E. Sigerist and Aspects of Medical Historiography', *Bulletin of the History of Medicine,* 32 (1958), 485–99; see also Owsei Temkin, 'The Double Face of Janus', in *The Double Face of Janus and Other Essays* (Baltimore: Johns Hopkins University Press, 1977), 3–37.
58. H.E. Sigerist, 'Kultur und Krankheit', *Kyklos,* 1 (1928), 147–56.
59. H.E. Sigerist, 'William Harvey's Stellung in der europäischen Geistesgeschichte', *Archiv für Kulturgeschichte,* xix (1928), 158–68.
60 . H. E. Sigerist. *Civilization and Disease* (Chicago and London: University of Chicago Press, 1943).
61 . Sigerist noted various strikes and other evidence of popular 'revolutionary' activity in his diary, as in the following note: 'The strike in San Francisco is spreading. There are strikes going on in 38 states, the first symptoms of a revolutionary movement. The workers are fighting for what Roosevelt promised them, higher wages, shorter working hours, recognition of the unions. The employers are sabotaging Roosevelt's programme and the workers revolt. This is quite natural.' H. E. Sigerist, Diary, 17 July, 1934.
62. H. E. Sigerist, 'Historical Background of Industrial and Occupational Diseases', B*ulletin of the New York Academy of Medicine,* xii (1936), 597–609.
63. *Op. cit.* (ref. 38).
64. *Ibid.*, 228.
65. The physician, who understood that disease was itself both social and biological, could thus readily extend the concept of health from the biological individual to the social individual. Sigerist thus thought it perfectly reasonable that physicians should treat criminals with the aim of curing the social disease of their criminality and restoring them to healthy social behaviour. 'It may seem farfetched to extend the concept of health into the social field. And yet there can be no doubt that an individual who is maladjusted socially does not possess the balance that constitutes health ... the criminal ... is sick and in need of a physician.... The goal of medicine is social and medicine is actually a social science.' H. E. Sigerist, *Medicine and Human Welfare* (New Haven: Yale University Press, 1941; reprinted, New York: Arno Press, 1970), 100–01.
66. *Ibid.,* 135.
67. *Op. cit.* (ref. 38), 20.

68. H. E. Sigerist, 'The History of Medical History', in *Milestones in Medicine* (New York Academy of Medicine, New York: D. Appleton-Century Company, 1938), 163–84.
69. Sigerist's *Great Doctors,* while a series of biographical studies of famous physicians, is by no means a dry study of scientific ideas but seeks to place the physicians in their social, cultural, and even class context. H. E. Sigerist, *The Great Doctors: A Biographical History of Medicine* (New York: W.W. Norton, 1933).
70. As noted elsewhere, Sigerist's approach to the infectious diseases, occupational diseases, and nutritional diseases is fairly consistent and informed by this generally Marxist orientation. When dealing with the chronic diseases, however, he lost his critical edge and often referred to heart diseases as though they were the natural, biological consequence of maturity and old age. See, for example, H. E. Sigerist, 'Remarks on Social Medicine in Medical Education', in *Henry E. Sigerist on the Sociology of Medicine,* Milton I. Roemer (ed.), (New York: MD Publications, 1960), 361. See also Elizabeth Fee, 'Henry E. Sigerist: From the Social Production of Disease to Medical Management and Scientific Socialism', *The Milbank Quarterly,* lxvii Suppl. 1 (1989), 127–50.
71. G. Rosen, 'On the Historical Investigation of Occupational Diseases: An Aperçu', *Bulletin of the History of Medicine,* v (1937), 943.
72. G. Rosen, 'Occupational Diseases of English Seamen during the Seventeenth and Eighteenth Centuries', *Bulletin of the History of Medicine,* vii (1939), 751–8.
73. G. Rosen, 'A Theory of Medical Historiography', *Bulletin of the History of Medicine,* viii (1940), 655–65.
74. G. Rosen, 'Disease and Social Criticism: A Contribution to a Theory of Medical History', *Bulletin of the History of Medicine,* x (1941), 5–15.
75. In 1957, he discussed and rejected a variety of ways in which biological phenomena might be seen as crucial in human history; and in 1975 he urged a publisher not to publish a book manuscript which claimed that human history was reducible to parasitism operating on several levels of organization. G. Rosen, 'The Biological Element in Human History', *Medical History,* i (1957), 150–9; Rosen to Geoffrey House, 16 January 1975. GRP, Addition of 28 August, 1978, Box V.
76. Rosen did acknowledge that certain forms of mental illness were directly caused by nutritional deficiency, hormonal imbalance or microscopic pathogens (see Rosen, 'Patterns of Discovery and Control of Mental Illness', *American Journal of Public Health,* l (1960), 855–66 (reprinted in *Madness in Society* [Chicago: University

of Chicago Press, 1968], 247–62); but this no more committed him to an ontological view than did his recognition that infection by the bacillus was a necessary condition for a case of tuberculosis. As a materialist Rosen believed that both somatic and mental disease were caused by social conditions as mediated by material conditions.

77. *Op. cit.* (ref. 65) 93.
78. 'The social causes of illness are just as important as the physical ones. Etiological therapy means more than killing a few bugs. The medical officer of health and the practitioners of a distressed area are the natural advocates of the people.... They are not only scientists but also responsible citizens, and if they did not raise their voice, who else should?' *Ibid.*, 134.
79. *Ibid.*, 133.
80. *Ibid.*, 96.
81. 'Social Aspects of Jacob Henle's Medical Thought', *Bulletin of the History of Medicine,* v (1937), 509–37. Mervyn Susser has suggested that Rosen felt a particular affinity for Henle because of his politics and his Jewish background. See Susser, 'The Work of George Rosen: Observations on a Very Small Sample', *International Journal of Health Services,* x (1980), 323–7.
82. Rosen to Sigerist, 17 March, 1937.
83. Rosen to Sigerist, 4 October, 1937. The Rosen papers at Yale also contain extensive notes on this project, which never came to fruition.
84. See note 55.
85. Dorothy Porter and Roy Porter, 'What Was Social Medicine? An Historiographical Essay', *Journal of Historical Sociology,* i (1989), 90–106.
86. See, for example, the discussion of Lind and Blane in 'Occupational Diseases of English Seamen during the Seventeenth and Eighteenth Centuries', *Bulletin of the History of Medicine,* vii (1939), 751–8.
87. G. Rosen, 'Osler on Miner's Phthisis', *Journal of the History of Medicine and Allied Sciences,* iv (1949), 259–66.
88. 'If the major objectives in teaching the history of medicine to students are to orient them in the here and now, and to show them how we got here, then the social approach is the method of choice.' G. Rosen, 'An Orientation Course in the History of Medicine', *Journal of Medical Education,* xxxi (1956), 683.
89. G. Rosen, 'The Medical Aspects of the Controversy over Factory Conditions in New England, 1840–50', *Bulletin of the History of Medicine,* xv (1944), 483–97.
90. Sigerist to Rosen, 19 March, 1941.
91. G. Rosen, 'Disease and Social Criticism: A Contribution to a Theory of Medical History', *Bulletin of the History of Medicine,* x (1941), 5–15.

92. 'The story of disease must be written, or rewritten, to include both the medical and social aspects of the problem. From the standpoint of action in our own society, a recognition of the social relations of disease leads to a realization of the necessity for a co-ordination of medical, social and economic effort to cope with the problem of disease.' *Ibid.*, 15.
93. Roemer to Rosen, 17 July, 1941. GRP, Addition of 26 October, 1978. In Roemer's published reply he claimed that organized factions from the left which have tried to influence medicine have sometimes succeeded. Roemer effectively took a Leninist position and advocated being a political activist within medicine, a position that made Rosen – who preferred scholarship to activism – very uncomfortable. Milton I. Roemer, 'Medicine and Social Criticism: A Comment on George Rosen's Article', *Bulletin of the History of Medicine,* xi (1942), 228–34.
94. H. E. Sigerist, *Medicine and Human Welfare* (New Haven: Yale University Press, 1941), 96.
95. G. Rosen, 'Disease and Social Criticism: A Contribution to a Theory of Medical History', *Bulletin of the History of Medicine,* x (1941), 15.
96. Ackerknecht to Rosen, 7 March, 1947, 17 March, 1947. GRP, Addition of 4 June, 1979, Box II. Ackerknecht, who was not Jewish but had been a political refugee from Nazi Germany, admired Rosen's continuing self-identification as a Jew. See Ackerknecht's obituary, 'G. Rosen as I Knew Him', *Journal of the History of Medicine and Allied Sciences,* xxxiii (1978), 254–5.
97. Sigerist's position finally went to Richard H. Shryock, a native-born American Protestant of acceptable liberal academic political views who came from the history faculty at the University of Pennsylvania. Not a physician, Shryock had become a leading historian of medicine by approaching it from American history, rather than health care. He was, in fact, a good choice for the Hopkins job; and Rosen maintained friendly relations with him until Shryock's death in 1972 (personal communication from Beate Caspari-Rosen).
98. 'As you probably realize, I have given up any thought of being able to teach medical history and am concentrating on public health but continuing to carry on my historical studies privately as I have done until now.' Rosen to Sigerist, 14 November, 1948. Sigerist Papers, General Correspondence, 1947–57 (Yale University Library, Group 788, Series I, Box 21).
99. Rosen to Jean A. Curran, 31 March, 1950 (GRP, Addition of January, 1978, Box 2).
100. Rosen's responsibilities at HIP are described in G. Baehr's letter offering him the position. See Baehr to Rosen, 12 July, 1950 (GRP,

Addition of 4 June, 1979, Box 2).

101. John Z. Bowers claims that both Rosen and George Baehr (first president of HIP) 'thought of HIP as a model for a national system of high-quality low-cost care.' See Bowers, 'Remarks at George Rosen Memorial Service, 14 October, 1977, Yale University', *Journal of the History of Medicine and Allied Sciences,* xxxiii (1978), 256. When Rosen took his position at HIP, E. Ashworth Underwood wrote from London to congratulate him, and likened HIP to the new British National Health Service. Underwood to Rosen, 3 November, 1951. GRP, Addition of October, 26, 1978.

102. A good source on the early history of HIP is Louis L. Feldman, 'Organization of a Medical Group Practice Prepayment Program in New York City' (New York: Health Insurance Plan of Greater New York, 1953), mimeographed. See also *Health and Medical Care in New York City: A Report by the Committee for the Special Research Project in the Health Insurance Plan of Greater New York* (Cambridge, Mass.: published for the Commonwealth Fund by Harvard University Press, 1957). For Rosen's view of health education, see 'The Health Educator's Bookshelf ', *American Journal of Public Health,* xxxix (1949), 433–42. While working at both the municipal health department and at HIP, Rosen took time out from writing history to publish articles on immediate issues in health education and medical care. He was concerned, for example, about the psychological effects of community-based multiphasic screening in the absence of adequate patient education. See his 'Letter to the Editor (Multiphasic Screening)', *American Journal of Public Health,* xli (1951), 94–5; 'Clear Thinking and Multiple Screening' (editorial), *American Journal of Public Health,* xlii (1952), 304–05; 'Health Education and Preventive Medicine – " New Horizons in Medical Care"', *American Journal of Public Health,* xlii (1952), 687–93; and 'A Conceptual Framework and a Code for the Analysis and Evaluation of Preventive Care', in C. G. Sheps and E. H. Taylor, *Needed Research in Health and Medical Care, A Bio-Social Approach* (Chapel Hill: University of North Carolina Press, 1954), 199–211.

103. 'Science, Values and Public Issues' (editorial), *American Journal of Public Health,* lv (1965), 1508–09.

104. Rosen's contributions as editor of the *AJPH* have been assessed by Alfred Yankauer, his successor, and by Milton Terris, a former president of the APHA. See Yankauer, 'The American Journal of Public Health 1957–73', in *Healing and History: Essays for George Rosen* (New York: Science History Publications, 1979), 229–41; and Terris, 'George Rosen and the American Public Health Tradition', *American Journal of*

*Public Health,* lxix (1979), 173–6. In *The Sanitarians: A History of American Public Health* (Urbana: University of Illinois Press, 1990), John Duffy also describes the fragmentation of public health authority in late twentieth century America. See especially 294–309.

105. See particularly his March, 1958 (editorial), 'Clio and Hygiea', *American Journal of Public Health,* xlviii (1958), 369–70.
106. 'Measuring Ability to Pay for Health and Social Services', *American Journal of Public Health,* xlviii. (1958), 83–5; 'The Retreat of Mass Diseases', *American Journal of Public Health,* xlviii (1958), 232–4; 'The Health of Nations', *American Journal of Public Health,* xlviii (1958), 495–6.
107. 'Lloyd George's Ambulance Wagon', *American Journal of Public Health,* xlvii (1958), 922–3; 'The Politics of Public Health', *American Journal of Public Health,* xlix (1959), 364–5.
108. 'Environmental Health Services – Yesterday, Today, Tomorrow', *American Journal of Public Health,* liii (1963), 1453–4.
109. 'National Health Insurance – Yes! But is it Enough?', *American Journal of Public Health,* lix (1969), 1977–8.
110. G. Rosen, 'The First Neighborhood Health Center Movement – Its Rise and Fall', *American Journal of Public Health,* lxi (1971), 1620–37.
111. Erwin H. Ackerknecht, 'Beiträg zur Geschichte der Medizinalreform von 1848', *Sudhoffs Archiv,* xxv (1932), 61–109 and 113–83.
112. In his preface to *The Great Doctors,* for example, Sigerist says he has written the book for the 'practicing physician' and he dedicates it to the 'unknown doctor'. Henry E. Sigerist, *The Great Doctors: A Biographical History of Medicine* (New York: W.W. Norton, 1933; reprint edition, New York: Dover, 1971), 19.
113. See the two collections of Sigerist's articles: F. Marti-Ibañez, (ed.), *H. E. Sigerist on the History of Medicine* (New York: MD Publications, 1960), and Milton I. Roemer, (ed.), *H. E. Sigerist on the Sociology of Medicine* (New York: MD Publications, 1960); for a complete bibliography of Sigerist's work, see Genevieve Miller, *A Bibliography of the Writings of H. E. Sigerist* (Montreal: McGill University Press, 1966).
114. See the bibliography of Rosen's writings in *Healing and History: Essays for George Rosen* (New York: Science History, 1979), 252–62.
115. G. Rosen, *A History of Public Health* (New York: MD Publications, 1958; reprint edition with new introductory material by Elizabeth Fee and Edward T. Morman, Baltimore: Johns Hopkins University Press, 1993).
116. See, for example, his final article, 'Urbanization, Occupation and Disease in the United States 1870–1920: The Case of New York City', in E. G. Forbes, (ed.), *Human Implications of Scientific Advance* (Edinburgh: Edinburgh University Press, 1978), 224–50. Reprinted in *Journal of the*

*History of Medicine and Allied Sciences,* xliii (1988), 391–425.

117. G. Rosen, *Preventive Medicine in the United States, 1900–1975: Trends and Interpretations* (New York: Science History, 1975). Revised edition published as Bonnie Bullough and G. Rosen, *Preventive Medicine in the United States, 1900–1990: Trends and Interpretations* (Canton, Mass.: Science History, 1992).
118. G. Rosen, 'Disease, Debility and Death', in: *The Victorian City: Images and Reality,* H. J. Dyos and Michael Wolff (eds), (London: Routledge & Kegan Paul, 1973), ii 625–67.
119. G. Rosen, *Fees & Fee Bills: Some Economic Aspects of Medical Practice in 19th-Century America* (Baltimore: Johns Hopkins Press, 1946).
120. G. Rosen, *The Structure of American Medical Practice, 1875–1941,* C. E. Rosenberg (ed.), (Philadelphia: University of Pennsylvania Press, 1983).
121. Several of the most important of these were collected in *Madness in Society: Chapters in the Historical Sociology of Mental Illness* (London: Routledge & Kegan Paul; Chicago: University of Chicago Press, 1968). For a critique of Rosen as a psychiatric historian, see Edward T. Morman, 'George Rosen and the History of Mental Illness', in Roy Porter and Mark S. Micale (eds), *Discovering the History of Psychiatry* (New York: Oxford University Press, 1993).
122. See, for example, G. Rosen, 'Social Stress and Mental Disease from the 18th Century to the Present: Some Origins of Social Psychiatry', *Milbank Memorial Fund Quarterly,* xxxvii (1959), 14.
123. The influence of Sigerist, Rosen, and other social historians born before the First World War, such as Erwin Ackerknecht and Richard Shryock, was also felt by the generation of American medical historians who came of age after the Second World War. See for example, Thomas Bonner, *Medicine in Chicago: A Chapter in the Social and Scientific Development of a City* (Madison, Wisc.: American History Research Center, 1957; revised edition Urbana: University of Illinois Press, 1991).
124. A number of these men have written about Sigerist's contributions to social medicine and his influence on medical care organization. See Leslie A. Falk, 'Medical Sociology: The Contributions of Dr Henry E. Sigerist', *Journal of the History of Medicine and Allied Sciences,* xiii (1958), 214–88; Milton I. Roemer, 'Henry Ernest Sigerist; Internationalist of Social Medicine', *Journal of the History of Medicine and Allied Sciences,* xiii (1958), 229–43; Milton I. Roemer, 'Medical Care Programs in Other Countries: Henry Sigerist and International Medicine', *American Journal of Public Health,* xlviii (1958), 425–7; Milton Terris, 'The Contributions of Henry E. Sigerist to Health Service Organization', *Milbank Memorial Fund Quarterly,* liii (1975), 489–530; George Silver, 'Social Medicine and Social Policy', *Yale Journal of Biology and Medicine,* (1984), 851–64.

# *ARCHIVES INTERNATIONALES D'HISTOIRE DES SCIENCES*

No. 128, 1992


ARTICLES: SYMPOSIUM 'HISTORIOGRAPHIE ET HISTOIRE DES MATHÉMATIQUES' (18e Congrès international d'histoire des sciences, Hambourg-Munich, 1-9 août 1989). **Introduction** (S.S. Demidov, M. Folkerts); Ch. J. Scriba – **Historiographie der Mathematik als Wissenschaft, Kunst – und Macht?**; S. Brentjes – **Historiographie der Mathematik im islamischen Mittelalter**; I. Schneider – **Hintergrund und Formen der Mathematikgeschichte des 18. Jahrhunderts**; L.M.R. Saraiva – **Garção Stockler and the First History of Mathematics in Portugal**; A.R. Garciadiego – **Should We Trust Primary Sources? Bertrand Russell: A Case Study**; S.S. Demidov – **Historiographie des mathématiques en Russie et en URSS avant 1941**; L. Nový – **Die Entwicklung der Geschichte der Mathematik in den böhmischen Ländern**; M.T. Borgato – **On the History of Mathematics in Italy Before Political Unification**; U. Bottazzini – **On the Historiography of Mathematics in Italy, 1860-1940. An Overview.**

IN MEMORIAM / INFORMATIONS / QUESTIONS, RÉPONSES ET RÉPLIQUES / BIBLIOGRAPHIE CRITIQUE / LIVRES REÇUS

---


Executive committee: G. Bernardini, V. Cappelletti (Director), M.D. Grmek, G. Montalenti†, J.D. North, G.E. Viola (Secretary). Editor: R. Halleux (Université de Liège, 15, avenue des Tilleuls, B-4000 Liège). Assistant editor: A. Postigliola (Italia). Editorial committee: P. Costabel†, R. Fox (England), S.R. Mikulinskii†, J. Murdoch (U.S.A.), J. Samsó (España), C.J. Scriba (Deutschland), J. Vernet-Ginés (España), A.-A.P. Yushkevich (Rossia). Editorial office: Servizio Attività Culturali, Istituto della Enciclopedia Italiana, piazza della Enciclopedia Italiana (già piazza Paganica), 4, I-00186 Roma. Académie internationale d'histoire des sciences: 12, rue Colbert, F-75002 Paris. Orders and subscriptions: Istituto della Enciclopedia Italiana, Settore gestione clienti, piazza della Enciclopedia Italiana (già piazza Paganica), 4, I-00186 Roma.

**Archives internationales d'histoire des sciences** is published twice each year. Subscriptions: $ 85 for one year.

*ISTITUTO DELLA ENCICLOPEDIA ITALIANA*

*FONDATA DA GIOVANNI TRECCANI*